COMMON PROBLEMS IN

PEDIATRIC SURGERY

COMMON PROBLEMS IN SURGERY SERIES

David C. Brewster/**Common Problems in Vascular Surgery**
Josef E. Fischer/**Common Problems in Gastrointestinal Surgery**
Jay L. Grosfeld/**Common Problems in Pediatric Surgery**
James M. Hurst/**Common Problems in Trauma**
Jonathan A. vanHeerden/**Common Problems in Endocrine Surgery**
Harold J. Wanebo/**Common Problems in Cancer Surgery**

COMMON PROBLEMS IN

PEDIATRIC SURGERY

JAY L. GROSFELD, M.D.
Professor and Chairman
Department of Surgery
Indiana University Medical Center
Surgeon-in-Chief
J.W. Riley Hospital for Children
Indianapolis, Indiana

Mosby Year Book

St. Louis Baltimore Boston Chicago London Philadelphia Sydney Toronto

Mosby Year Book

Dedicated to Publishing Excellence

Sponsoring Editor: Nancy E. Chorpenning
Associate Managing Editor, Manuscript Services: Deborah Thorp
Production Project Coordinator: Carol A. Reynolds
Proofroom Manager: Barbara Kelly

Mosby–Year Book, Inc.
11830 Westline Industrial Drive
St. Louis, MO 63146

1 2 3 4 5 6 7 8 9 0 CL MB 95 94 93 92 91

Library of Congress Cataloging-in-Publication Data

Common problems in pediatric surgery / [edited by] Jay L. Grosfeld.
p. cm.
Includes bibliographical references and index.
ISBN 0-8151-3949-7
1. Children—Surgery. I. Grosfeld, Jay L., 1935- .
[DNLM: 1. Surgery, Operative—in infancy & childhood. WO 925 C734]
RD93.5.C4C65 1991 91-13650
617.9′8—dc20 CIP
DNLM/DLC
for Library of Congress

This book is dedicated to my wife Margie and our five children, Lisa, Denise, Janice, Jeff, and Mark, whose love, understanding, unselfish loyalty, and faithful longstanding support over the many years of my training and practice of surgery has been deeply appreciated.

CONTRIBUTORS

R. PETER ALTMAN, M.D.
Professor of Surgery and Pediatrics, College of Physicians and Surgeons, Columbia University; Director, Pediatric Surgery, Babies Hospital Columbia-Presbyterian Medical Center, New York, New York

KATHRYN D. ANDERSON, M.D.
Professor of Surgery and Pediatrics, George Washington University; Senior Attending Surgeon, Children's National Medical Center, Washington, D.C.

KEITH W. ASHCRAFT, M.D.
Clinical Professor of Pediatric Surgery, University of Missouri at Kansas City; Chief of Urology, Children's Mercy Hospital, Kansas City, Missouri

RICHARD G. AZIZKHAN, M.D.
Associate Professor of Surgery and Pediatrics, Chief of Pediatric Surgery, University of North Carolina School of Medicine, Chapel Hill, North Carolina

MARGARET J. BLYTHE, M.D.
Assistant Clinical Professor, Department of Pediatrics, Indiana University Medical Center, Indianapolis, Indiana

SCOTT J. BOLEY, M.D.
Professor of Surgery and Pediatrics, Chief of Pediatric Surgical Services, Albert Einstein College of Medicine, Montefiore Medical Center, New York, New York

CHRISTOPHER P. BRANDT, M.D.
Senior Instructor of Surgery, Case Western Reserve University School of Medicine, Cleveland, Ohio

DONALD R. COONEY, M.D.
Professor of Surgery and Pediatrics, State University of New York and Buffalo; Head, Department of Pediatric Surgery, Children's Hospital of Buffalo, Buffalo, New York

ARNOLD G. CORAN, M.D.
Professor of Surgery, University of Michigan Medical School; Surgeon-in-Chief, C.S. Mott Children's Hospital, Ann Arbor, Michigan

DAVID E. M. DRUCKER, M.D.
Chief Resident in Pediatric Surgery, Children's Hospital of Michigan, Detroit, Michigan

STEPHEN P. DUNN, M.D.
Assistant Professor of Surgery, Department of Surgery, Temple University School of Medicine, Philadelphia, Pennsylvania

MARTIN R. EICHELBERGER, M.D.
Professor of Surgery, Division of Pediatric Surgery, George Washington University, Children's National Medical Center, Washington, D.C.

NEIL R. FEINS, M.D.
Clinical Professor of Pediatric Surgery, Boston University, Chief of Pediatric Surgery, Kennedy Medical Center, Boston, Massachusetts

ROBERT M. FILLER, M.D.
Surgeon-in-Chief, The Hospital for Sick Children, Toronto, Canada

HOWARD C. FILSTON, M.D.
Professor of Pediatric Surgery and Pediatrics, Chief of Pediatric Surgery Service, University of Tennessee, Knoxville, Tennessee

ERIC W. FONKALSRUD, M.D.
Professor and Chief of Pediatric Surgery, UCLA School of Medicine, Los Angeles, California

GEORGE GANESAN, M.D.
Instructor, Pediatric Urology, Children's Hospital and Medical Center, Seattle, Washington

MICHAEL W.L. GAUDERER, M.D.
Associate Professor of Pediatric Surgery and Pediatrics, Case Western Reserve University School of Medicine; Chief, Division of Pediatric Surgery, Rainbow Babies and Children's Hospital, Cleveland, Ohio

JAY L. GROSFELD, M.D.
Professor and Chairman, Department of Surgery, Indiana University Medical Center; Surgeon-in-Chief, J.W. Riley Hospital for Children, Indianapolis, Indiana

J. ALEX HALLER, JR., M.D.
Professor of Pediatric Surgery, Children's Surgeon-in-Charge, The Johns Hopkins University School of Medicine, Baltimore, Maryland

BURTON H. HARRIS, M.D.
Professor of Surgery, Tufts University School of Medicine; Chief of Pediatric Surgery and Pediatric Trauma, New England Medical Center; Director, Kiwanis Pediatric Trauma Institute, Boston, Massachusetts

THOMAS M. HOLDER, M.D.
Clinical Professor of Surgery, University of Missouri at Kansas City; Chief, Thoracic and Cardiovascular Surgery, Children's Mercy Hospital, Kansas City, Missouri

DALE G. JOHNSON, M.D.
Professor of Surgery and Pediatrics, University of Utah Medical Center; Surgeon-in-Chief, Primary Children's Medical Center, Salt Lake City, Utah

FREDERICK M. KARRER, M.D.
Assistant Professor, Department of Surgery, University of Colorado School of Medicine, Denver, Colorado

KEN KIMURA, M.D.
Associate Professor of Surgery, University of Iowa Hospitals and Clinics, Iowa City, Iowa

SYLVAIN KLEINHAUS, M.D.
Associate Professor of Surgery and Pediatrics, Montefiore Medical Center, New York, New York

JOHN R. LILLY, M.D.
Professor and Chief, Pediatric Surgery, University of Colorado School of Medicine, Denver, Colorado

PETER B. MANNING, M.D.
Chief Resident in Surgery, Children's Mercy Hospital, University of Missouri at Kansas City School of Medicine, Kansas City, Missouri

LESTER W. MARTIN, M.D.
Professor of Surgery and Pediatrics, College of Medicine, University of Cincinnati, Cincinnati, Ohio

MICHAEL E. MITCHELL, M.D.
Professor and Chief, Pediatric Urology, Children's Hospital and Medical Center, Seattle, Washington

JAMES A. O'NEILL, JR., M.D.
C. E. Koop Professor of Pediatric Surgery, University of Pennsylvania School of Medicine; Surgeon-in-Chief, Children's Hospital of Philadelphia, Philadelphia, Pennsylvania

H. BIEMANN OTHERSEN, JR., M.D.
Professor of Surgery and Pediatrics; Chief of Pediatric Surgery, Medical College of South Carolina; Medical Director, Children's Hospital, Charleston, South Carolina

ARVIN I. PHILIPPART, M.D.
Professor of Surgery, Wayne State University School of Medicine; Chairman of Surgical Services, Children's Hospital of Michigan, Detroit, Michigan

JOHN G. RAFFENSPERGER, M.D.
Professor of Surgery, Northwestern Hospital; Surgeon-in-Chief, Childrens Memorial Hospital, Chicago, Illinois

FREDERICK J. RESCORLA, M.D.
Assistant Professor of Surgery (Pediatric), Indiana University Medical Center, Indianapolis, Indiana

HERNAN M. REYES, M.D.
Professor of Surgery and Pediatrics, University of Illinois at Chicago; Chairman, Department of Surgery and Division of Pediatrics, Cook County Hospital, Chicago, Illinois

MARC I. ROWE, M.D.
Professor of Surgery, University of Pittsburgh School of Medicine; Chief of Surgery Services, Children's Hospital of Pittsburgh, Pittsburgh, Pennsylvania

L. R. SCHERER III, M.D.
Assistant Professor, Division of Pediatric Surgery, The Johns Hopkins University School of Medicine, Baltimore, Maryland

MARSHALL Z. SCHWARTZ, M.D.
Professor of Surgery and Pediatrics, Chief, Division of Pediatric Surgery, University of California at Davis, Davis, California

AMY SHAPIRO, M.D.
Assistant Professor of Pediatrics, Hematology/Oncology Division, Indiana University School of Medicine, Indianapolis, Indiana

DONALD B. SHAUL, M.D.
Fellow in Pediatric Surgery, Children's Hospital of Los Angeles, Los Angeles, California

DENNIS W. SHERMETA, M.D.
Cactus Pediatric Surgeons, Ltd., Phoenix, Arizona

ROBERT T. SOPER, M.D.
Professor of Surgery, Director, Pediatric Surgery, University of Iowa Hospitals and Clinics, Iowa City, Iowa

CHARLES H. STOLAR, M.D.
Associate Professor of Surgery, Columbia University; Associate Attending Surgeon, The Babies Hospital, Columbia-Presbyterian Medical Center, New York, New York

STEVEN STYLIANOS, M.D.
Instructor in Surgery, Tufts University School of Medicine; Trauma Fellow, Kiwanis Pediatric Trauma Institute, Philadelphia, Pennsylvania

EDWARD P. TAGGE, M.D.
Instructor in Pediatric Surgery, University of Pittsburgh School of Medicine; Children's Hospital of Pittsburgh, Pittsburgh, Pennsylvania

ROBERT L. TELANDER, M.D.
Professor of Surgery, University of North Dakota School of Medicine; Chief of Surgery, Fargo Clinic, Fargo, North Dakota

DENNIS W. VANE, M.D.
Associate Professor of Surgery, Section of Pediatric Surgery, Indiana University School of Medicine, Indianapolis, Indiana

DAVID E. WESSON, M.D.
Associate Professor of Surgery, University of Toronto; Staff Surgeon and Director, Trauma Program, The Hospital for Sick Children, Toronto, Canada

KAREN W. WEST, M.D.
Assistant Professor of Surgery, Department of Surgery, Indiana University School of Medicine, Indianapolis, Indiana

MORTON M. WOOLEY, M.D.
Surgeon-in-Chief and Head, Department of Surgery, Children's Hospital of Los Angeles, Los Angeles, California

PREFACE

The purpose of *Common Problems in Pediatric Surgery* is to make available an affordable, concise, current, and easy-to-read reference concerning common pediatric surgical problems. The chapters are relatively short and to the point, and are organized to give the reader an orderly access to various related topic areas or conditions.

Each of the chapters is written by an author with contemporary expertise, and represents the authors' current techniques for evaluation and management of commonly encountered pediatric surgical problems. Topics are introduced by specific clinical case presentations, which are carefully discussed by expert consultants. Both mundane and complex subjects are included, such as inguinoscrotal conditions and umbilical hernia, the acute abdomen in infants and children, gastroesophageal disorders, hepatobiliary and pancreatic conditions, trauma, and common congenital and acquired disorders of the head and neck, as well as important patient care topics that are encountered on a day-to-day basis, such as vascular access, nutrition support, coagulation defects, and airway problems.

The text is by no means all-inclusive, and while there are obviously many other subjects of pediatric surgical importance, we considered them beyond the scope of this treatise. The book was primarily written for general surgical and pediatric surgical residents, practicing surgeons who care for infants and children, pediatricians, and family physicians. The text should also prove useful to students in surgery and pediatrics and to nurses who care for infants and children.

I am grateful to my colleagues in pediatric surgery who have contributed chapters to this book: to Sandy Davis, my administrative assistant, for collating the chapters and participating in the organizational process, and to Nancy Chorpenning, Executive Editor at Mosby–Year Book, Inc., and her staff for support and encouragement.

Jay L. Grosfeld, M.D.

CONTENTS

Preface *xi*

PART I: Inguinal and Umbilical Hernia; Testes *1*

1 / Inguinal Hernia in the Premature Neonate *3*
Jay L. Grosfeld

2 / Incarcerated Hernia in an Infant *9*
Frederick J. Rescorla

3 / Repair of Inguinal Hernia in Children With Ventriculoperitoneal Shunts *17*
Donald R. Cooney

4 / Recurrent Inguinal Hernia in Children *29*
Sylvain Kleinhaus and Scott J. Boley

5 / Umbilical Hernia in Infants and Children *36*
Christopher P. Brandt and Michael W.L. Gauderer

6 / Management of Unilateral Cryptorchid Testicle *51*
Eric W. Fonkalsrud

7 / Bilaterally Undescended Testes *55*
Michael E. Mitchell and George Ganesan

8 / Testicular Torsion *60*
Robert T. Soper

PART II: Acute Abdominal Conditions *69*

9 / Acute Appendicitis *71*
Robert M. Filler

10 / Intussusception *77*
Karen W. West

11 / Malrotation with Midgut Volvulus *84*
Frederick J. Rescorla and Jay L. Grosfeld

12 / Pelvic Inflammatory Disease *92*
Margaret J. Blythe

13 / Torsion of the Ovary *100*
Neil R. Feins

14 / Hydrometrocolpos *104*
John G. Raffensperger

15 / Abdominal Pain in the Immunosuppressed Patient *108*
Marc I. Rowe and Edward P. Tagge

16 / Inflammatory Bowel Disease *113*
Robert L. Telander

17 / Hirschsprung's Disease With Superimposed Enterocolitis *119*
Lester W. Martin

18 / Meckel's Diverticulum *127*
Dennis W. Vane

19 / Necrotizing Enterocolitis *132*
James A. O'Neill, Jr.

PART III Gastroesophageal Disorders *139*

20 / Esophageal Atresia With Tracheoesophageal Fistula *141*
Thomas M. Holder and Peter B. Manning

21 / Type A Esophageal Atresia *148*
Morton M. Woolley

22 / Esophageal Replacement Procedures *154*
Kathryn D. Anderson

23 / Achalasia of the Esophagus *162*
Richard G. Azizkhan

24 / Gastroesophageal Reflux *169*
Dale G. Johnson

25 / Caustic Stricture of the Esophagus *175*
Hernan M. Reyes

26 / Hypertrophic Pyloric Stenosis *184*
Marshall Z. Schwartz and Donald B. Shaul

27 / Acute Peptic Ulcer in Infants and Children *190*
Stephen P. Dunn

PART IV: Hepatobiliary and Pancreatic Disorders *195*

28 / Biliary Atresia *197*
F. M. Karrer and John R. Lilly

29 / Choledochal Cyst *206*
Ken Kimura

30 / Cholelithiasis in Children 214
David E.M. Drucker and Arvin I. Philippart

31 / Pancreatic Pseudocysts 222
H. Biemann Othersen, Jr.

PART V: Pediatric Trauma 229

32 / Resuscitation of the Injured Child 231
Burton H. Harris and Steven Stylianos

33 / Blunt Abdominal Trauma 236
L.R. Scherer III and J. Alex Haller, Jr.

34 / Thoracic Trauma in Children 244
Martin R. Eichelberger

35 / Pancreatic and Duodenal Trauma 249
David E. Wesson

PART VI: Head and Neck Lesions 255

36 / Congenital Cysts and Sinuses of the Neck 257
Charles H. Stolar

37 / Cystic Hygroma 260
Dennis W. Shermeta

38 / Management of Cervical Lymphadenopathy 264
R. Peter Altman

39 / Vascular Access 267
Howard C. Filston

40 / Parenteral Nutrition 276
Arnold G. Coran

41 / Airway Management 290
Keith W. Ashcraft

42 / Bleeding and Clotting Disorders 295
Amy Shapiro

Index 301

PART ONE

Inguinal and Umbilical Hernia; Testes

1

Inguinal Hernia in the Premature Neonate

Jay L. Grosfeld, M.D.

A 1.5-kg premature infant boy was born at 33 weeks' gestation. He developed severe respiratory distress syndrome requiring intubation and ventilator support for 3 weeks. He was subsequently weaned from the ventilator but had some evidence of bronchopulmonary dysplasia. Episodes of apnea and bradycardia required continuous monitoring. The infant had a large inguinal hernia that initially was easily reducible. With time, however, the hernia became more difficult to reduce.

The development of modern neonatal intensive care unit (NICU) facilities has resulted in the survival of many seriously ill premature infants. Many premature infants present with a clinically symptomatic inguinal hernia during their initial hospitalization in the NICU.[1-3] The incidence of inguinal hernia in preterm infants is 9% to 11%, which is considerably higher than in full-term babies (3.5% to 5.0%).[4] Hernia in the immediate perinatal period is more common in boys than girls, and frequently presents on the right side (60%). The incidence of bilateral inguinal hernias in the premature infant has been reported to range from 44% to 55%.[1] This is compared to an 8% to 10% incidence of bilateral presentation in older infants and children.

Cryptorchidism occurs more frequently in the preterm (30%) than in the full-term infant (2.0% to 3.0%).[4] A congenital indirect inguinal hernia is almost always present in these cases (>90%). The undescended testis, complicated by a symptomatic inguinal hernia, makes the cryptorchid gonad more vulnerable to vascular compromise and atrophy, especially if incarceration of the hernia occurs.[3, 4]

The major complication of an inguinal hernia is incarceration of bowel, with the resultant risk of intestinal ischemia and infarction. The risk of incarceration in the premature infant is quite high (31%)[3-5] (Fig 1–1). This high

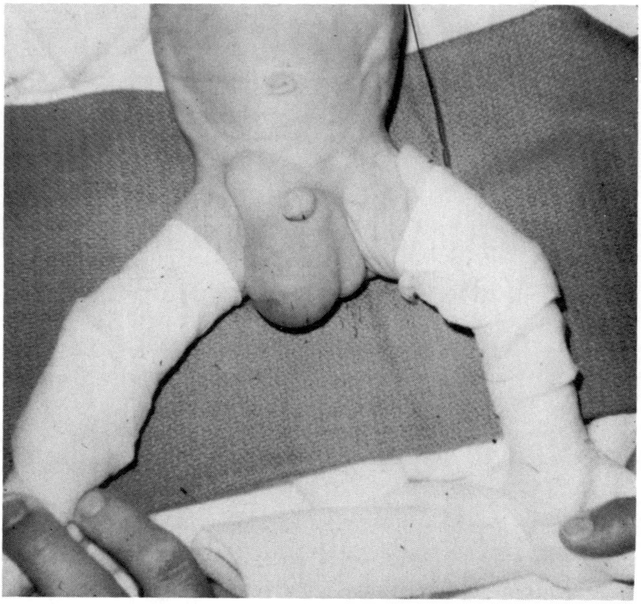

FIG 1–1.
Large right inguinal hernia in a 3 lb infant with congenital heart disease who required ventilator support after delivery. The hernia was incarcerated. After reduction on a few occasions, the hernia was repaired prior to hospital discharge. (From Grosfeld JL: Groin hernia in infants and children, in Nyhus LM, Condon RE (eds): *Hernia*. Philadelphia, JB Lippincott, 1989, pp 81–96. Used with permission.)

incidence of incarceration may persist for the first year of life, and is two to five times the 6% to 18% rate of incarceration reported in older children.[4] In addition to the increased risk of gonadal infarction from an inguinal hernia, bowel obstruction is reported in 9% of cases and strangulated bowel in 3% to 7% of reported cases[3] (Fig 1–2).

Because babies in the NICU are often severely ill with other problems, including hyaline membrane disease, sepsis, necrotizing enterocolitis, and other causes of respiratory distress requiring ventilator support, symptomatic clinical hernia may complicate their course. Fortunately, unlike adults, infants with incarcerated hernias can undergo safe reduction of the hernia in more than 70% of cases.[2, 3] Close observation and prompt reduction of the hernia in the NICU will often allow the infant to recover from its underlying illness without being subjected to the stress of an emergency operative procedure. The complication rate following emergency surgical care of an incarcerated hernia in infancy and childhood is greater than 22%.[3] This compares to a postoperative complication rate of 1.7% after elective repair. Because of the high rate of incarceration and

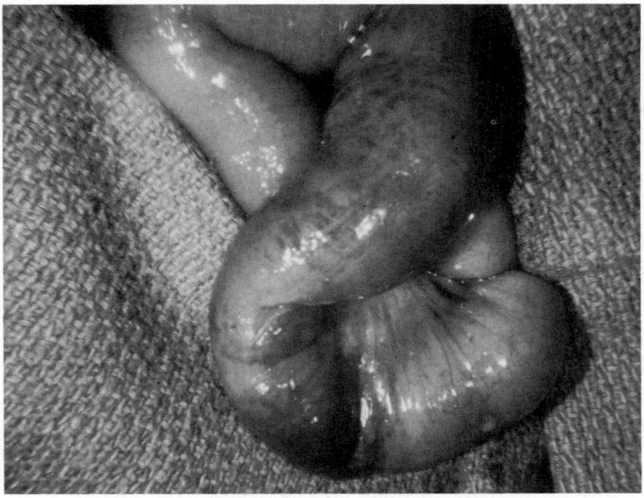

FIG 1–2.
Intraoperative view of a loop of small bowel incarcerated in an inguinal hernia in a premature infant in the NICU recovering from respiratory distress. Although the trapped bowel was initially discolored, it eventually appeared normal and resection was not necessary.

other complications (e.g., obstruction and gonadal infarction) in this age group, inguinal hernia in infants is repaired electively prior to discharge from the hospital.

In those instances in which reduction is unsuccessful, an emergency procedure may be necessary. The operative procedure is similar to that described for older infants and children.[5] A transverse incision is made in the lowest inguinal crease. The superficial fascia is incised, exposing the external inguinal ring. The external oblique fascia is incised in the long axis of its fibers, perpendicular to the external inguinal ring. The cremasteric muscle is opened and the anteromedially located indirect hernia sac is identified and carefully separated from the vas deferens and spermatic vessels. High ligation of the sac is accomplished at the level of the internal inguinal ring with suture ligatures of 4–0 silk. If the internal inguinal ring is excessively large, the transversalis fascia inferior to the cord structures is made snug with an additional 4–0 silk suture to reduce the risk of hernia recurrence. Wound closure is affected with interrupted 4–0 Vicryl sutures on the external oblique and Scarpa's fasciae, and a subcuticular 4–0 Vicryl suture is used to oppose the skin edges. A collodion seal dressing is applied to protect the wound from urine.

A number of factors must be considered in evaluating the preterm infant's overall care, particularly in the perioperative period. Respiratory control is poorly developed in the premature infant. Immature respiratory control mechanisms can predispose the neonate to potentially life-threatening respiratory complications. The compliant rib cage in the neonate may tend to collapse, reducing air inflow during respiration and creating a negative pleural pressure. The rib cage in the premature infant is more circular than the elliptical configuration present in adults; this anatomic characteristic may result in inadequate contraction of the diaphragm.[6] In addition, there are other unfavorable factors that affect newborn respiration, including a relative deficiency of type I fatigue-resistant muscular fibers in the diaphragm. The adult diaphragm has 55% type I fibers, the full-term infant diaphragm 25%, and the premature infant diaphragm only 10%.[6] The premature infant's intercostal muscles show a similar developmental pattern, predisposing the infant to fatigue of the main respiratory muscles. The combination of a high work of breathing, increased oxygen consumption, decreased functional residual capacity, and decreased resistance to muscle fatigue noted in the premature infant may result in abnormal breathing patterns, including periodic breathing or apneic episodes.[6] The incidence of apneic episodes may be increased in the malnourished premature infant with a reduced energy reserve.

Neonates with respiratory distress syndrome are also subject to a decrease in lung compliance and atelectasis. Longstanding use of ventilator support in the premature infant may be associated with oxygen toxicity and barotrauma resulting from positive pressure ventilation. These factors have been implicated in the development of bronchopulmonary dysplasia (BPD). The neonate with BPD can have severe lower airway obstruction resulting in air trapping, carbon dioxide retention, atelectasis, and bronchopneumonia, and may require supplemental inspired oxygen when stressed.[6] The infant who requires an anesthetic must therefore be carefully monitored with a pulse oximeter to monitor oxygen saturation, evaluated for end-tidal volume to judge the adequacy of respiratory exchange, and have available a nerve stimulator to evaluate the effects of a neuromuscular blockade.

In the operating room setting, other factors must also be considered. The premature infant has a depressed carbon dioxide response curve and will not show a rapid response to hypercapnea. Brief exposure to hypoxia may lead to hyperventilation followed by hypoventilation, resulting in periodic breathing and apnea.[6] The Hering-Breuer reflex (inflation of the lung resulting in apnea) is more prominent in the premature infant. Periodic breathing is noted in 50% of pre-term infants but occurs less often in infants older than 36 weeks gestation. The pre-term infant also has a large ratio of deadspace to tidal volume (V_D/V_T) because of an uneven distribution of ventilation and capillary perfusion. The fact that babies with BPD and air trapping are more susceptible to pneumothorax indicates that nitrous oxide should be avoided or, if necessary, must be carefully administered. Because of the premature infant's increased rate of insensible losses and fluid requirements (e.g., 140 to 150 cc/kg/day), adequate hydration and avoidance of hypothermia are other important intraoperative considerations.

Postoperatively, premature infants are more prone to postanesthetic complications. Steward reported an 18% incidence of apnea in preterm infants under 38 weeks gestation during the first 12 hours after operative procedures.[7] Liu et al., in a prospective study, reported that a history of apnea and a postconceptual age of 44 weeks or less was associated with prolonged postoperative apnea.[8] Kurth and associates described a 37% incidence of postanesthetic apnea in infants who were premature and had a postconceptual age that varied from 32 to 55 weeks.[9] They recommended monitoring for 36 hours postoperatively for infants who had been premature and were less than 44 postconceptual weeks of age, and for 24 hours for those older than 44 weeks. They suggested that monitoring be continued to a postconceptual age of 60 weeks.

Welborn et al. noted a 63.6% rate of periodic breathing, but not apnea, in healthy premature infants who were less than 44 postconceptual weeks of age.[10] Postoperative narcotics and residual anesthesia may also play a role in the development of apneic episodes in the premature infant with immature metabolic degradation pathways.

These observations suggest that premature infants with inguinal hernias must be carefully monitored for at least 24 hours following their operative repair within the hospital environment. For infants in the NICU, hernia repair should be performed just prior to discharge from the hospital, to avoid the significant 31% risk of incarceration at home. If the hernia was not observed prior to NICU discharge, and is noted for the first time at home, the infant should reenter the hospital setting via a morning admission program through the ambulatory surgery area.[3, 4] Hospital admission would then take place postoperatively for a 24-hour observation period, with the infant being carefully monitored for episodes of apnea, bradycardia, and periodic breathing. Rescorla and Grosfeld reported that 4 of 100 (4%) premature infants of less than 2 months postconceptual age at operation required overnight ventilator support after their hernia repair, including 2 infants with periods of apnea and bradycardia, 1 with BPD associated with transient hypoxia, and 1 with digoxin toxicity and an arrythmia.[3] This suggests that in addition to the premature infant, those NICU patients with BPD should also be treated in an inpatient setting because of reactive airway disease and the risk of bronchospasm resulting in hypoxia.

These observations have led some children's surgeons to recommend either local or spinal anesthesia for hernia repair in the neonate, particularly if a skilled pediatric anesthesiologist is not available. In more than 200 neonates given a general anesthetic for inguinal hernia repair, we have not experienced a death. The availability of a very strong group of skilled pediatric anesthesiologists at our hospital plays a role in these results, and has led us to continue to prefer the use of carefully monitored general anesthesia in these cases. If appropriate precautions are followed, elective hernia repair can be done safely in infants hospitalized in the NICU before their discharge from the hospital, or through a carefully monitored morning admission program for infants whose hernia is first observed following NICU discharge.[2–4] This will avoid the risk of bowel incarceration and potential strangulation, which is much higher in this age group. If the guidelines noted above are followed, inguinal hernia repair is associated with a very low morbidity and no mortality.

REFERENCES

1. Harper RG, Garcia A, Sih C: Inguinal hernia a common problem of premature infants weighing 1000 grams or less at birth. *Pediatrics* 1975; 56:112.
2. Groff D, Nagaraj HS, Pietsch JB: Inguinal hernias in premature infants operated on before discharge from the neonatal intensive care unit. *Arch Surg* 1985; 120:962.
3. Rescorla FG, Grosfeld JL: Inguinal hernia repair in the perinatal period and early infancy. *J Pediatr Surg* 1984; 19:382.
4. Grosfeld JL: Current concepts in inguinal hernia in infants and children. *World J Surg* 1989; 13:506.
5. Grosfeld JL: Groin hernia in infants and children in, Nyhus LM, Condon RE (eds): *Hernia*. Philadelphia, JB Lippincott, 1989, pp 81–96.
6. Bikhazi GB, Davis PJ: Anesthesia of neonates and premature infants in, Motoyama EK, Davis PJ (eds): *Smith's Anesthesia for Infants and Children,* ed 5. St Louis, CV Mosby, 1990, pp 427–462.
7. Steward DJ: Preterm infants are more prone to complications following minor surgery than are term infants. *Anesthesiology* 1982; 56:304.
8. Liu LMP, Cote CJ, Goudsonzian NG, et al: Life-threatening apnea in infants recovering from anesthesia. *Anesthesiology* 1983; 59:506.
9. Kurth CD, Spitzer AR, Broeunle AM, et al: Postoperative apnea in preterm infants. *Anesthesiology* 1987; 66:483.
10. Welborn LG, Ramirez N, Oh TH, et al: Postanesthetic apnea and periodic breathing infants. *Anesthesiology* 1986; 65:658.

2

Incarcerated Inguinal Hernia in an Infant

Frederick J. Rescorla, M.D.

A 6-month-old boy is referred for evaluation of an irreducible left inguinoscrotal mass. The infant's mother had previously observed the mass when the infant cried or strained, and noted that the swelling resolved when the infant took a nap. On physical examination, the left scrotal mass was discolored, painful on palpation, and remained irreducible. An x-ray of the abdomen showed a dilated small-bowel loop and air in the groin.

An infant presenting with the signs and symptoms described above most likely has an incarcerated inguinal hernia, perhaps with strangulation of the intestinal contents. This represents a true pediatric surgical emergency requiring prompt intervention to prevent bowel loss. This chapter will review the embryology, diagnosis, management options, and complications of incarcerated inguinal hernias.

EMBRYOLOGY

The basic defect that allows development of an indirect inguinal hernia is persistent patency of the embryonic processus vaginalis. The processus vaginalis appears at the third fetal month as an outpouching of peritoneum at the internal ring.[1] As the testes descend through the internal inguinal ring during the seventh month of fetal life, the processus vaginalis accompanies it to the scrotum, with the distal portion of the processus forming the tunica vaginalis. The proximal processus is patent in over 80% of neonates at birth, with a decreasing patency rate throughout infancy and childhood.[2] Patency persists into adulthood in approximately 20% of individuals, and a hernia through this area remains the most common type of hernia in adults.[3] The clinical problems related to this patency can include herniation of abdominal contents through the internal ring into the inguinal canal or scrotum (depending on whether the patency extends to the level of the testes). If the processus vaginalis obliterates proximally, a hydrocele may develop as fluid fills the remaining portion. This is usually adjacent and continuous with the tunica vaginalis, but can occur anywhere along the path of descent of the processus. In cases in which only a small opening persists, allowing fluid but not intestinal contents into the scrotum, the child will have a communicating hydrocele.

CLINICAL PRESENTATION

A hernia generally appears as a bulge in the area of the lowest abdominal crease, with varying degrees of extension toward the respective hemiscrotum. As the history in the child described above demonstrates, the parents frequently notice the bulge when the child cries or strains. The hernia bulge often reduces spontaneously when the child relaxes, or may be manually reduced by gentle pressure. The major complication of an inguinal hernia is incarceration of abdominal contents, as noted in the present case. These contained structures can include small bowel, a Meckel's diverticulum (Littre's hernia), the appendix or colon, or an ovary, Fallopian tube or both. Incarceration may lead to strangulation, with intestinal ischemia and gonadal compromise either from incarceration and strangulation of an ovary in girls or from vascular compromise of the testes due to compression applied to its vessels by the distended bowel in boys. The latter occurrence is commonly observed in instances of incarceration with cryptorchid testes. The incidence of incarceration in several large series involving general pediatric populations has ranged from 6.4% to 20%, with the highest incidence observed in newborns and infants. In a review of 511 hernias in infants less than 1 year of age, Puri et al. noted a 31% rate of incarceration.[4] This is similar to the 31% rate of incarceration noted in a review of 100 infants less than 2 months of age treated at our institution.[5] Rowe, in a review of 351 incarcerated hernias, noted a 28% rate of incarceration during the first 2 months of life, which decreased to 14% by 1 to 2 years of age.[6]

As illustrated in the case described above, the presenting symptoms of an incarcerated inguinal hernia can include irritability, pain, abdominal distention, and vomiting. A tense tender mass is noted in the inguinal region, occasionally with extension into the scrotum. The mass will usually not transilluminate, thus distinguishing it from a hydrocele. In some instances a child may present with a relatively asymptomatic incarcerated inguinal hernia. In these cases the internal ring is of adequate size to allow normal intestinal function. In addition, girls are frequently seen with a palpable irreducible ovary (15%) presenting as an asymptomatic inguinal or labial mass. Plain films, although usually unnecessary, may demonstrate intraluminal intestinal gas (Fig 2–1). If the intestinal contents become compromised at the neck of the hernia, strangulation may develop. In these cases venous occlusion develops initially, followed by further distention and eventually arterial compromise. The abdominal distention then increases in association with bilious vomiting from a mechanical small-bowel obstruction. The mass becomes tender and firm with erythma and edema of the inguinal and scrotal skin. In a girl with an incarcerated ovary, torsion with strangulation may occur in the absence of intestinal symptoms.

Plain abdominal roentgenograms in patients with an incarcerated hernia may demonstrate bowel distention and air-fluid levels due to a mechanical bowel obstruction (Fig 2–2). The differential diagnosis includes torsion of the testes, acute hydrocele, and inguinal lymphadenopathy. In cases of torsion, the swollen testes is extremely tender, generally with extension into the inguinal canal. A hydrocele should transilluminate and is usually unassociated with gastrointestinal symptoms. In addition, there is commonly a distinct upper limit to the mass in cases of hydrocele and torsion. Inguinal lymphadenopathy usually develops in association with an active or resolving infectious process. On phys-

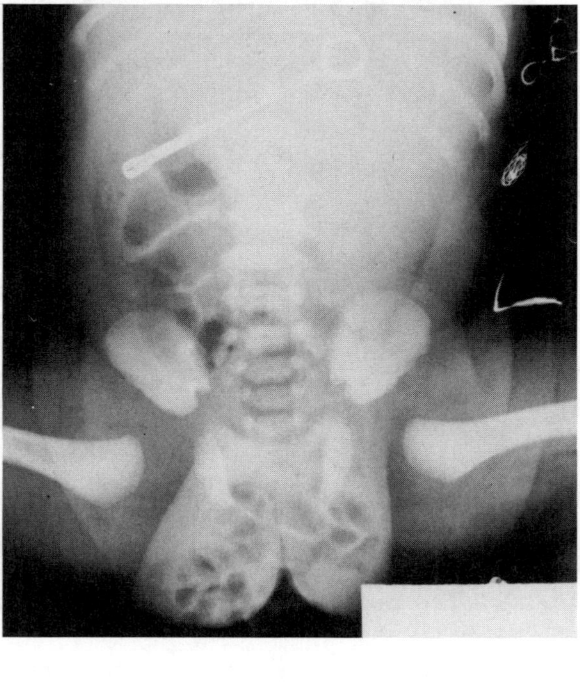

FIG 2–1.
Radiograph demonstrating intestinal contents within the scrotum of a newborn with bilateral inguinal hernias.

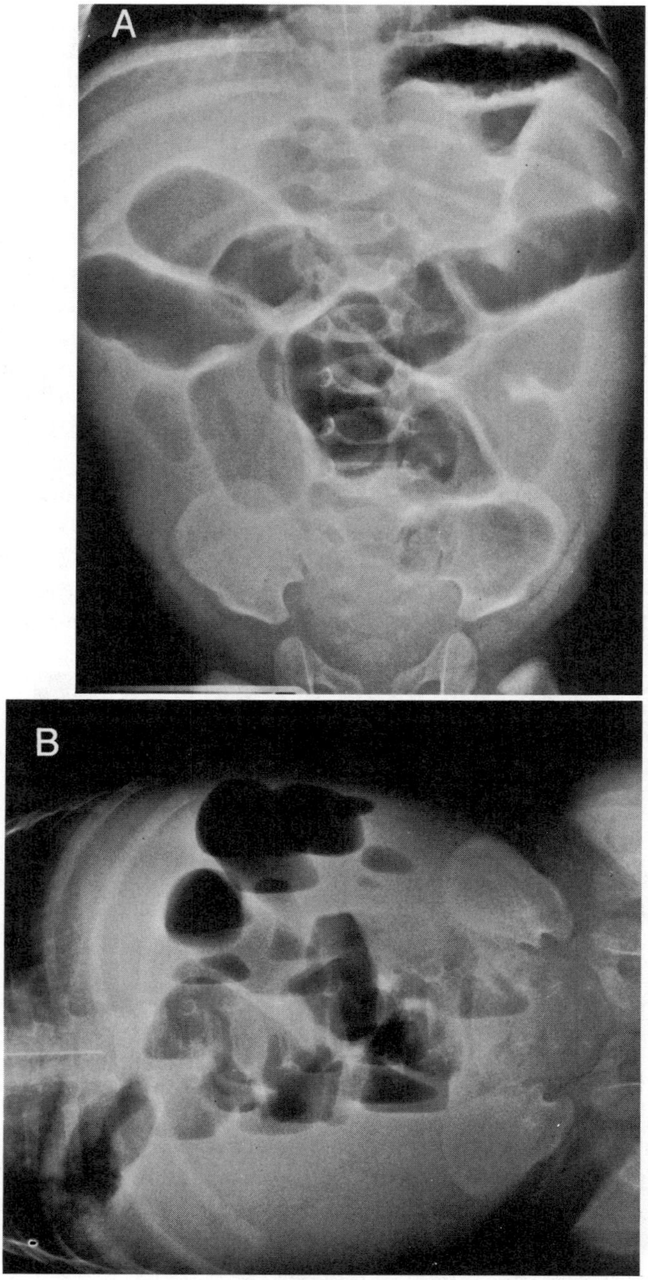

FIG 2–2.

Plain abdominal **(A)** and decubitus **(B)** radiographs demonstrating distended small bowel with air-fluid levels in a 6-month-old boy with an irreducible inguinal hernia. Operative reduction demonstrated discolored but viable small intestine within the hernia sac.

ical examination, the testes and inguinal structures should be normal to palpation and the abdomen soft and nontender. In girls it is occasionally difficult to differentiate incarcerated bowel from a strangulated ovary.

MANAGEMENT

Nonoperative

The history and physical examination of the child in the present case are consistent with an incarcerated inguinal hernia with evidence of impending strangulation. In most cases of incarcerated hernia in infants, nonoperative reduction should be attempted. As noted by Rowe and Marchildon in a survey of senior pediatric surgeons, all would attempt nonoperative reduction in stable patients without signs of peritoneal irritation.[7] Most would also do this even if the child had radiologic evidence of a bowel obstruction. The approach generally involves sedation, elevation, and gentle manual reduction.

Sedation is induced intramuscularly using meperidine hydrochloride (Demerol) (1 mg/kg) and secobarbital sodium (Seconal) (1 mg/kg) or morphine (0.1 to 0.2 mg/kg). We generally avoid morphine in younger infants (<3 months) because of the untoward effect of respiratory depression. Elevation may be effected with use of the Trendelenberg position, elevating the foot of the bed or suspending the child by the legs in the bed. It may also be achieved by holding the child in this position in the parent's arms. After the child is well relaxed and quiet (15 to 30 minutes), gentle pressure is applied initially downward and then with the fingers of the other hand over the area of the external ring (to prevent reduction superficial to the ring), and manual reduction is attempted. If the reduction is successful, the child is admitted to the hospital with operative repair of the hernia scheduled for the following day. This method has been effective in over 80% of incarcerations in infancy and childhood.[4, 6] If reduction is unsuccessful, the child is prepared for immediate operative reduction.

Operative Management

If attempts at hernia reduction are unsuccessful or if signs of peritoneal irritation are present, the child is taken to the operating suite for inguinal exploration. Occasionally the hernia reduces with induction of anesthesia. In these cases the child should undergo a standard exploration with high ligation of the sac at the level of the internal ring. Nonviable bowel is unlikely to reduce in this fashion, and we would not attempt to locate the bowel unless, upon opening the sac, cloudy fluid or a foul odor is noted. Under these circumstances (bloody fluid or a foul odor), the previously incarcerated bowel must be identified to assess its viability. This can most often be accomplished through the internal ring, but occasionally requires a counterincision and formal laparotomy. If the bowel does not reduce, the sac is opened distally and the bowel inspected. If the bowel is clearly viable it is reduced into the peritoneal cavity by enlarging the internal ring by retraction or actual incision. If the bowel is discolored or ischemic in appearance, it is temporarily covered with a warm, saline-soaked laparotomy pad (for at least 5 minutes) and is then re-evaluated. Viable bowel should be identified proximally and distally and delivered into the wound. The internal ring may need to be stretched or incised laterally to insure that the bowel is not compromised at the neck of the sac. The bowel is examined for signs of viability such as color, mesenteric and antimesenteric pulsations (with use of a Doppler flow probe), and peristalsis. If it is clearly viable it is reduced. If viability remains questionable or if the bowel is clearly necrotic, a resection with end-to-end anastomosis is performed. After reduction of the bowel into the peritoneal cavity, the hernia sac is suture ligated at the level of the internal ring. If the internal ring has been excessively dilated by the trapped viscera, or if it has been incised in order to reduce the incarcerated viscus, the ring should be narrowed by sutures across the floor of the canal inferior to the spermatic vessels and vas deferens, to prevent recurrence.

COMPLICATIONS

The incidence of intestinal complications requiring bowel resection is relatively low among the total group of children with incarcerated hernias. In Rowe and Clatworthy's series, 68 of 351 incarcerations were irreducible and required emergent operation. Of these, intestinal resection was required in five cases representing 1.4% of the total group of incarcerated hernias and 7% of the irreducible cases.[6] In a review of 165 incarcerated hernias, Farrow noted 77 irreducible cases.[8] Twenty-one had signs of strangulation of bowel, omentum, or an ovary. Three resections were required (one appendix, one small bowel, and one omentum), for an incidence of 1.8% among all of the incarcerations and 4% among the irreducible group.

The incidence of testicular infarction with incarceration varies between 2.2% and 14%. In Rowe and Clatworthy's report of 351 incarcerated hernias, 8 of 68 irreducible hernias were accompanied by vascular compromise of the testes. The incidence of testicular infarction was 2.2% among the 351 incarcerated hernias, but rose to 11.8% among the 68 irreducible cases. In an interesting review by Slowman and Mylius, 8 cases of testicular infarction occurred among 57 incarcerated hernias.[9] Of interest is that seven of the cases occurred in infants less than 3 months of age. Three cases with blue testes noted intraoperatively were found to have a normal testicular size on follow-up. A discolored testis is frequently observed at the time of exploration for an irreducible hernia, and we would generally leave such a testis in place at the time of hernia repair. In a long-term follow-up study of 87 boys with incarcerated hernias, Puri et al. noted only 2 (2.3%) with testicular atrophy.[4]

The incidence of recurrent inguinal hernias after repair of an incarcerated hernia is generally reported to be higher than the 0.3% to 1.0% recurrence rate observed with uncomplicated inguinal hernias. In a recent review at our institution, previous incarceration was a factor in 4 of 62 recurrent hernias.[10] In a review of 69 hernias, Clatworthy and Thompson noted a recurrence rate of 6%.[11] Farrow's review of 2,566 hernia repairs noted a recurrence rate of less than 0.5% following uncomplicated herniorraphy, but a 3% recurrence rate after repair of incarcerated hernias.[8]

CONCLUSION

In summary, an incarcerated inguinal hernia is a pediatric surgical emergency. Nonoperative reduction is usually successful in converting an emergent case into a semielective one. If nonoperative reduction fails, emergency operative intervention must be performed to prevent intestinal loss. In the current era, prompt attention to these details should result in minimal morbidity and no mortality associated with this condition.

REFERENCES

1. Shrock P: The processus vaginalis and gubernaculum. *Surg Clin North Am* 1971; 51:1263.
2. Snyder WH, Jr, Greaney EM, Jr: Inguinal hernia, in Mustard WT, Ravitch MM, Snyder WH, et al (eds): *Pediatric Surgery,* ed. 2. Chicago, Year Book Medical Publishers, 1969, p 692.
3. Morgan EH, Anson BJ: Anatomy of region of inguinal hernia. IV. The internal surface of the parietal layers. *Q Bull Northwestern Univ Med School* 1942; 16:20.
4. Puri P, Guiney EJ, O'Donnell B: Inguinal hernia in infants: The fate of the testis following incarceration. *J Pediatr Surg* 1984; 19:44–46.
5. Rescorla FJ, Grosfeld JL: Inguinal hernia repair in the perinatal period and early infancy: Clinical considerations. *J Pediatr Surg* 1984; 19:832–837.
6. Rowe MI, Clatworthy HW: Incarcerated and strangulated hernias in children. *Arch Surg* 1970; 101:136–139.
7. Rowe MI, Marchildon MD: Inguinal hernia and hydrocele in infants and children. *Surg Clin North Am* 1981; 61:1137–1145.
8. Farrow GA, Thompson S: Incarcerated inguinal hernia in infants and children: A five-year review at the Hospital for Sick Children, Toronto, 1955 to 1959 inclusive. *Can J Surg* 1963; 6:63–66.

9. Slowman JG, Mylius RE: Testicular infarction in infancy: Its association with irreducible inguinal hernia. *Med J Aust* 1958; 1:242–244.
10. Grosfeld JL, Minnick K, Shedd F, et al: Inguinal hernia in children: Factors affecting recurrence in 62 cases. *J Pediatr Surg* (in press).
11. Clatworthy HW, Thompson AG: Incarcerated and strangulated inguinal hernia in infants: A preventable risk. *JAMA* 1954; 154:123–126.

3

Repair of Inguinal Hernia in Children With Ventriculoperitoneal Shunts

Donald R. Cooney, M.D.

A 4-month-old boy with hydrocephalus was referred because of right inguinal swelling. A ventriculoperitoneal (VP) shunt procedure had been performed at age 3 months because of increasing head circumference. Scrotal swelling was not present prior to the shunt procedure. On physical examination the right scrotal area was enlarged and edematous, and a firm structure was palpated through the scrotal skin. An abdominal roentgenogram showed the shunt catheter in the scrotum.

Inguinal hernia is one of the most frequently diagnosed surgical conditions afflicting children. Fortunately, the physiologic and anatomic abnormalities related to the formation, circulation, and absorption of cerebrospinal fluid (CSF) are much less common. Decades ago, neurosurgeons utilized a variety of methods for shunting CSF into the peritoneal cavity. This practice fell into disfavor as a result of the high incidence of associated intra-abdominal complications and frequent "clogging" or obstruction of the peritoneal catheter. The adopted alternative was ventriculovenous (atrial) shunting. Unfortunately, this technique was found to be linked to a number of serious and potentially life-threatening complications, including septicemia, endocarditis, pulmonary embolization, pulmonary hypertension, and glomerulonephritis. Another disadvantage of these vascular catheters was related to the fact that they had to be periodically "revised" to compensate for the child's linear growth. With the advent of inert silastic peritoneal catheters in the mid 1950s, and improved variable pressure valves in the 1960s and 1970s, VP shunting became the preferred method of diverting CSF. Catheter obstruction, common prior to the use of silastic tubing, was encountered much less frequently. An extra length of catheter could be safely inserted into the peritoneal cavity to allow for growth. Most importantly, the complications associated with the venous shunting procedures were eliminated.[1]

The management of a child with a VP shunt who develops an inguinal hernia is a relatively uncommon clinical problem. During the last decade (1980 to 1990), 6,366 patients with inguinal hernias were treated at the Children's Hospital of Buffalo. Only 10 of these inguinal hernias occurred in VP shunt patients (Fig 3–1). Although this combination of clinical conditions is relatively rare, most surgeons caring for children will eventually be confronted with it. To provide for the most appropriate treatment, it is necessary to take the following precautions, which pertain to this particular clinical situation: (1) avoidance of shunt catheter damage or kinking during the herniorrhaphy; (2) adoption of measures aimed at decreasing the risk of shunt infection; (3) application of adjunctive surgical measures to strengthen the inguinal floor, aimed at decreasing the risk of recurrent hernia; and (4) a more impelling rationale for contralateral groin exploration.

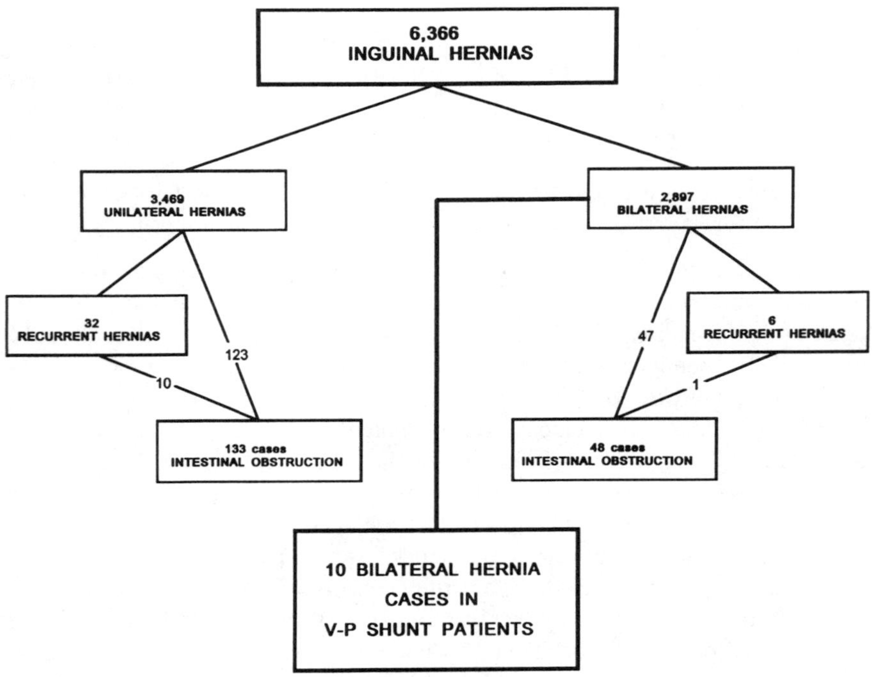

FIG 3–1.
A decade of experience with inguinal hernia at the Children's Hospital of Buffalo demonstrates that inguinal hernia in children with VP shunts was an infrequently encountered clinical problem. Bilateral inguinal hernias are common in these patients.

CLINICAL EXPERIENCE

The clinical experience with VP shunts and hernias at the James Whitcomb Riley and Buffalo Children's Hospitals is reviewed below in order to apply a clinical perspective to the problem.

During the years 1968 to 1972, 173 children underwent VP shunting procedures at the Riley Children's Hospital.[2] The mean age at the time of shunt insertion was 1½ months (range: 1 week to 7 years). Ventriculoperitoneal shunt operations performed for older children were usually revision procedures necessitated by malfunction of the shunt. Twenty-five of the 173 children (15%) undergoing VP shunting procedures developed an inguinal hernia. The mean interval from shunt insertion to the diagnosis of the hernia was 6.8 months. Twenty-one hernia patients were boys and 4 were girls. Twelve hernias occurred on the right, 9 on the left, and only 4 were bilateral. Incarceration occurred in five instances. There were no cases of strangulation. The VP shunt catheter was detected in the hernia sac by abdominal x-ray in four patients (Fig 3–2).

Four patients with bilateral hernias underwent high ligation of their indirect hernia sacs. Sixteen children with a clinically unilateral hernia had high ligation of the symptomatic side and a contralateral groin exploration. Thirteen of these 16 children were noted to have a patent processus vaginalis on the "silent" side

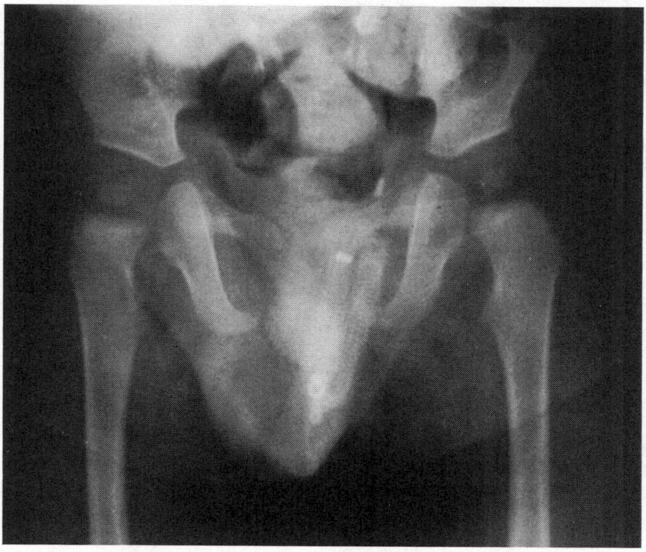

FIG 3–2.
Abdominal radiograph demonstrates the presence of a VP shunt catheter in an inguinal hernia sac.

(81%). In one instance, a disconnected catheter was located in a contralateral, clinically unrecognized hernia sac. Five further infants underwent urgent unilateral herniorrhaphy because of incarceration. Two of these infants later developed a symptomatic contralateral hernia requiring a remedial operation. In addition to the 4 patients who had clinically apparent bilateral hernias, 15 of the 21 patients with unilateral hernias had either a positive contralateral patent processus vaginalis, detected during exploration, or subsequently developed a contralateral hernia requiring treatment. In summarizing this series, it is important to recognize that 19 of the total of 25 children who had VP shunts (80%) had bilateral patent processes vaginalis.

Postoperative complications occurred in four instances. These included one superficial wound infection and three recurrent hernias. One recurrence was noted 4 months postoperatively in an infant with a wound infection, whose original operation was for an incarcerated hernia. In a second patient, recurrence was observed 3 months after the operation, at which time a prominent umbilical hernia was also noted. The third recurrence was diagnosed 5½ months postoperatively on the side of a contralateral, negative exploration. At re-exploration, large internal rings and pantaloon hernias were observed in the

TABLE 3–1.
Hernias Following CSF Shunting Procedures*

Medical Center	Years of Study	Shunt Procedures†	No. of Inguinal Hernias	Mean Interval Between VP Shunt and Hernia
Indiana University Medical Center—James Whitcomb Riley Children's Hospital	1968–1972	VP = 173	4 Bilateral 21 Unilateral	6.8
	1960–1968	VA = 242 Gallbladder = 29	3 0	— —
	1960–1972	Total = 444	28	—
University at Buffalo (SUNY)—Children's Hospital of Buffalo	1980–1990	Primary VP = 138 Revisions = 407 Total = 545	9 Bilateral 1 Unilateral 10	9.5 mo 24 mo —
Combined data for VP shunts	—	VP shunts only (revisions not included) = 311	13 Bilateral 22 Unilateral	7.3 mo

*Combined experience with inguinal hernias in ventriculoperitoneal shunt patients at the James
†VP = ventriculoperitoneal; VA = ventriculoatrial.

first two cases, and were treated by religation and transversalis fascia repairs. In the third case, a typical indirect sac was found and suture ligated at the normal-appearing internal ring.

During the 7 years prior to this study (1960 to 1968), 242 infants with hydrocephalus had ventriculovenous shunts into the jugular vein or atrium.[2] In contrast to the infants with VP shunts, only three (1.2%) of these patients developed a subsequent inguinal hernia. In addition, there were 29 infants with ventriculo-gallbladder shunts, none of whom developed an inguinal hernia (Table 3–1).

At the Children's Hospital of Buffalo, a total of 6,366 children with a diagnosis of inguinal hernia presented for treatment during the period 1980 to 1990. Of these, 3,469 had a unilateral inguinal hernia. Thirty two of these patients represented cases of recurrent hernia, 10 of which were complicated by the development of intestinal obstruction. An additional 123 unilateral hernia patients came to medical attention as the result of a developing bowel obstruction.

At the time of initial diagnosis, 2,897 of the patients had bilateral inguinal hernias. Forty seven of these children presented with intestinal obstruction. There were 6 cases (0.2%) of recurrent bilateral inguinal hernia, one of which

% Incidence of Hernia	Operations Performed	Patent Processus in VP Shunt Patients Who Were Explored	Developed Contralateral Hernia Later	Recurrent Hernias in VP Shunt Patients
15%	Bilat. herniorrhaphy = 4	4	—	0
	Herniorrhaphy and contralat. explor. = 16	13	—	2
	Unilat. herniorrhaphy = 5	?	2 (40%)	1
1.2%	Bilat. herniorrhaphy = 3	—	—	—
0%				
—				
7.2%	Bilat. herniorrhaphy = 9	9	—	0
—	Bilat. herniorrhaphy = 1	1	—	0
—				
11.3%	Bilat. herniorrhaphy = 13 Herniorrhaphy and contralat. explor. = 16 Unilat. herniorrhaphy = 5	27/30 (90%)	2/5 (40%)	3/35 (8.5%)

Whitcomb Riley and Buffalo Children's Hospitals.

also had associated intestinal obstruction. Only 10 of these inguinal hernia patients (0.15%) also had a VP shunt (Fig 3–1). Seven of these 10 children were boys and 3 were girls. In contrast to the Indiana series, it is significant to note that all of the Buffalo VP shunt patients had clinically apparent bilateral inguinal hernias. None of these shunted patients presented with any of the possible complications of inguinal hernia, such as incarceration, strangulation, or intestinal obstruction.

During this same period, 545 VP shunts were performed (Fig 3–3). One hundred thirty-eight of these operations were primary shunting procedures. The remaining 407 operations were remedial operations for patients whose shunts had malfunctioned, necessitating a shunt revision. Nine children (6 boys and 3 girls) (0.3%) developed hernias following a primary VP shunting procedure done to treat an interruption of CSF circulation. The mean age at diagnosis was 16 months (range: 3 to 26 months). The average age at the time of the initial shunting procedure was 5 months (range: 4 days to 24 months). The mean interval between the initial shunt operation and diagnosis of the hernia was 9 months (range: 1 month to 27 months). One additional shunt-dependent, 10-year-old boy developed bilateral hernias 2 years after his last shunt revision. All of the patients in this series underwent an operation to strengthen the inguinal floor (limited–modified Bassini operation), in addition to the standard

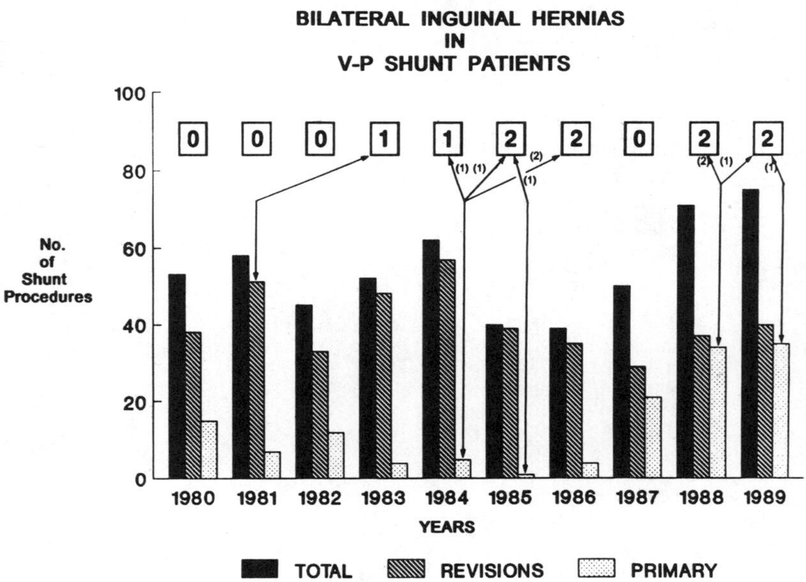

FIG 3–3.

Ten bilateral inguinal hernias developed in 545 VP shunt patients treated at the Children's Hospital of Buffalo from 1980 to 1989.

high ligation of the hernia sac. During the follow-up period, ranging from a few months to 6 years, no recurrent hernias or other complications were detected.

The combined experience from these two Children's Hospital series is shown in Table 3–1. Several conclusions may be derived from the data. The incidence of inguinal hernia for children in the "normal" population has been reported to range from 3.5% to 5.0%.[3] All small children with hernias and patients with hydrocephalus in the Buffalo metropolitan area are treated at the Children's Hospital. Through the use of population and diagnosis data collected by the State of New York, the actual incidence of inguinal hernia in children in the Buffalo area was confirmed to be 3%. The combined incidence (11.3%) of inguinal hernia in children with VP shunts is therefore three to five times greater than in the normal population. The Indiana experience documented the fact that these hernias are not directly related to the underlying abnormality in CSF circulation, since children undergoing ventriculovenous shunting had a low incidence (1.2%) of inguinal hernia. Clinically apparent bilateral hernias appear to be more common in VP shunt patients. These hernias usually develop following the initial shunting procedure and ordinarily become apparent within 6 to 12 months after the first VP shunt operation. A greater patency rate for the processus vaginalis on the "silent side" (90%), and an increased risk of hernia recurrence (85%), also appear to be characteristic clinical findings (Table 3–1).

DISCUSSION

Several identifiable, precipitating factors probably contribute to the development of inguinal hernias in VP shunt patients. The majority of ventriculoperitoneal shunts are inserted during the first few months of life, when the processus is patent in a large percentage of these infants. For a number of years, surgeons caring for children with inguinal hernias were hindered by conflicting sets of data related to the patency rate of the processus vaginalis.[3, 4, 5, 6] A landmark publication by Rowe and Clatworthy in 1969 essentially resolved the previous, longstanding controversy regarding patency rates, and established the present criteria for contralateral exploration.[4] By exploring the contralateral groin of all children undergoing inguinal herniorrhaphy, these authors observed that the processus vaginalis remained patent in a large percentage of children (70%) during the first few months of life. The patency rate declined to 35% to 40% by age 2 to 4 years and remained stable thereafter. Any skepticism based on an initial concern about these observers' objectivity in categorizing their operative findings was eliminated by a confirmatory clinical investigation by Jewett and Allen.[7] These authors demonstrated similar anatomic findings in an analysis of a large group of children undergoing herniography. The compatability of the Rowe-Clatworthy patency curve with the Jewett-Allen herniorrhaphy bar-graph data is striking (Fig 3–4). These two studies definitively established that the patency rate of the processus vaginalis was age dependent and declined to a plateau level by 2 to 4 years of age.

Another factor contributing to inguinal herniation in VP shunt patients is the continuous flow of CSF into the peritoneal cavity, which may increase intra-abdominal pressure. Increased intra-abdominal pressure has been cited as a factor contributing to increased patency rates of the contralateral processus vaginalis, and has also been implicated as causing the increased incidence of inguinal hernia observed in some groups of pediatric patients.[4] Supportive evidence for this theory may be obtained from reports of clinical experiences with peritoneal dialysis catheters in children. Stone et al. noted that 60 hernias (28 inguinal) developed in 93 children with end-stage renal disease being managed with continuous ambulatory peritoneal dialysis (CAPD).[8] In a similar series of CAPD patients, Tank and Hatch substantiated this observation by noting the occurence of 11 inguinal hernias in 9 children.[9] It is also significant to note that cases of "ascites" complicating VP shunting have been reported.[10] Cerebrospinal fluid accumulation (ascites) has been attributed either to an overproduction of fluid or to a decrease or threshold limit in the absorptive capacity of the peritoneum. Chronic catheter-induced peritoneal inflammation may interfere with

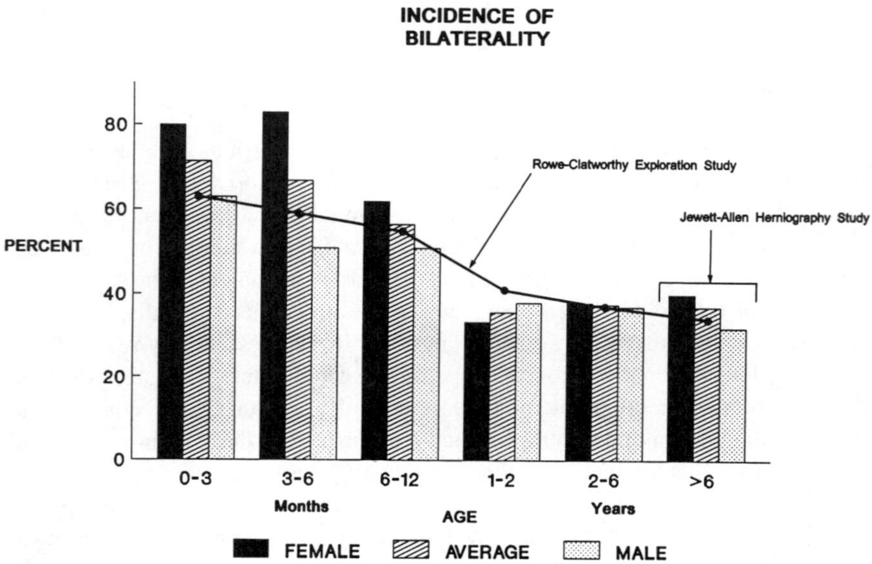

FIG 3–4.
The compatibility of the Rowe-Clatworthy exploration study and the Jewett-Allen herniography experience definitively established that patency rates were age dependent and plateaued by 2 to 4 years of age.

intra-abdominal lymphatic drainage. The resultant protein exudation can lead to a further increase in osmotic pressure and additional fluid accumulation. Many children with VP shunts have chronic states of low-grade peritoneal inflamation that may result in this type of subclinical "ascites" and increased intra-abdominal pressure.[11]

A very important management consideration is the avoidance of shunt infection acquired during the herniorrhaphy. Shunt infections are very serious and potentially fatal complications.[12] A 2% to 5% infection rate is currently associated with each shunt insertion. Mortality rates associated with shunt infections have ranged from 30% to 40%.[12] Moreover, prolonged morbidity and sequelae such as ventriculitis, partial shunt obstruction, chronic peritonitis, intermittent bacteremia, and psychomotor disability have been reported.[12] Surgeons managing these cases assume an added measure of responsibility for insuring that shunt infections do not occur. Since each pediatric center's experience is essentially limited to a few cases each year, recommendations regarding avoidance of this potential complication must be extrapolated from neurosurgical practice. The most common organisms causing shunt infections are *Staphylococcus epidermidis* and *S. aureus* (skin contaminants).[13] These two bacterial species account for approximately 85% of all shunt infections.[13] Approximately 10% to 20% of all infections are due to gram-negative bacteria.[12] Young infants, patients with immunologic deficiency, or children being treated with radiation, chemotherapy, or both are much more susceptible. These patients should also be considered at significant risk of developing a fatal shunt infection. Finally, dermatitis or abrasions at the incision site likewise increase the risk of postoperative infection.[12]

The efficacy of prophylactic antibiotics in providing protection against shunt infections has not been proven, and remains somewhat controversial.[14] Nevertheless, several nonrandomized longitudal studies indicate that the use of appropriate prophylactic antibiotics (administered before and at the time of operation, with topical antibiotic solutions applied to the shunt catheter) results in a threefold reduction in the infectious complication rate.[14] The choice of antibiotics should be guided in some measure by the local bacterial flora. Vancomycin or a cephalosporin may be the most appropriate choice for *S. epidermidis,* especially for infants in the newborn intensive care unit (NICU). Oxacillin or similar penicillinase-resistant agents may be the best choice if coagulase-positive *S. aureus* is a concern. Amminoglycosides should be considered in cases of incarceration, obstruction, or strangulation.

Shunt infections may present with the usual acute signs and symptoms of septicemia, meningitis, or peritonitis. On the other hand, it is just as common for children with these infections to come to medical attention with more insidious findings, such as low-grade fever, anorexia, failure to thrive, anemia, leukocytosis, shunt malfunction, and other subtle signs indicative of a chronic, in-

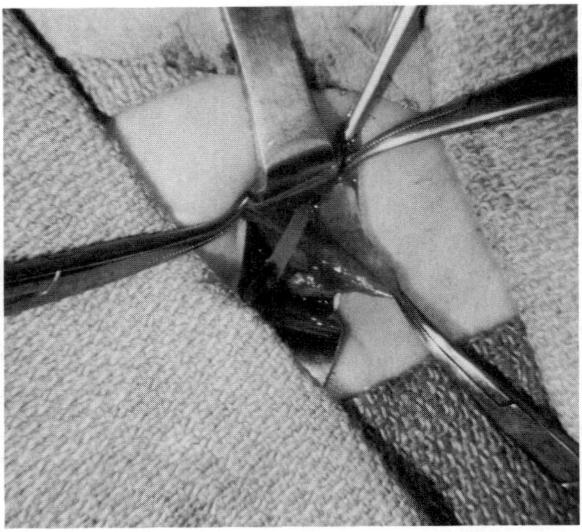

FIG 3–5.
An operative photograph demonstrates a shunt catheter exposed in the hernia sac during herniorrhaphy.

dolent, inflammatory process. Because of the seriousness of these infections and the frequent difficulty in establishing the diagnosis, the author has adopted the following principles: (1) An elective hernia operation should be undertaken only after skin pathology has resolved in the groin incision region. (2) Preoperative and intraoperative prophylactic parenteral antibiotics are administered to all patients. The antibiotics are chosen in accordance with the bacterial environment to which the patient has most recently been exposed. If the peritoneal catheter presents in the incision during conduct of the herniorrhaphy, it is bathed in a topical antibiotic solution (2 mg of cephapirin per cubic centimeter of irrigant) (Fig 3–5). (3) Additional attention is given to the skin prepping and draping of the incision. (4) If the catheter is exposed, a "break" in sterile technique occurs, or a long and difficult operation is necessary, cultures are obtained from the wound to be used as a therapeutic guide if infection ensues. (5) In cases of incarceration, obstruction, or strangulation, an aminoglycoside is added to the prophylactic antibiotic regimen to guard against infection by gastrointesinal organisms.

SUMMARY RECOMMENDATIONS FOR VENTRICULOPERITONEAL SHUNT PATIENTS

On the basis of the clinical data from two major children's hospitals and an extensive experience with shunting procedures, the following recommendations have been formulated to be applied to the management of children with VP shunts.

1. They should be examined frequently for the presence of inguinal hernia.
2. Expeditious operation immediately following diagnosis is mandatory to avoid the inherent risks from incarceration, obstruction, and strangulation, which are greatest during the first few months of life. The risk of life-threatening shunt infection is significantly increased if these complications ensue.
3. They should receive parenteral prophylactic antibiotics.
4. The surgeon should be alert to the possibility that catheters may be encountered in the hernia sac at the time of the operation. Care must be taken to avoid potential damage to the catheter or kinking and obstruction if an extra length of catheter must be returned to the peritoneal cavity. Preoperative abdominal x-rays may be helpful in identifying the location of the functional catheter or locating disconnected catheters that have been left in situ.
5. Contralateral exploration is advised in all cases of unilateral hernia because of the increased patency rate of contralateral processes vaginalis and development of hernias on the "silent side."
6. Recurrent hernias are more common in this group of patients. Additional surgical procedures aimed at strengthening the floor of the inguinal canal are recommended.
7. During the postoperative period, malaise, feeding problems, fever, or other nonspecific signs and symptoms suggest the possibility of an underlying shunt infection.

REFERENCES

1. Scott MR: *Concepts in Neurosurgery Hydrocephalus*. Baltimore, Williams & Wilkins, 1990.
2. Grosfeld JL, Cooney DR: Inguinal hernia after ventriculoperitoneal shunt for hydrocephalus. *J Pediatr Surg* 1974; 9:311–315.
3. Grosfeld JL: Current concepts in inguinal hernia in infants and children. *World J Surg* 1989; 13:506.
4. Rowe MI, Copelson LW, Clatworthy HW, Jr: The patent processus vaginalis and the inguinal hernia. *J Pediatr Surg* 1969; 4:102.
5. Rowe MI, Clatworthy HW, Jr: The other side of the pediatric inguinal hernia. *Surg Clin North Am* 1971; 51:1371–1376.
6. Grosfeld JL: Groin hernia in infants and children in, Nyhus LM, Condon RE (eds): *Hernia*. Philadelphia, JB Lippincott, 1989, pp 81–96.
7. Jewett TC, Jr, Kuhn JP, Allen JE: Herniography in children. *J Pediatr Surg* 1976; 11:451–454.

8. Stone MM, Fonkalsrud EW, Salusky IB, et al: Surgical management of peritoneal dialysis catheters in children: Five-year experience with 1,800 patient-month follow-up. *J Pediatr Surg* 1986; 21:1177–1181.
9. Tank ES, Hatch DA: Hernias complicating chronic ambulatory peritoneal dialysis in children. *J Pediatr Surg* 1986; 21:41–42.
10. Goodman GM, Gourley GR: Ascites complicating ventriculoperitoneal shunts. *J Pediatr Gastroenterol Nutr* 1988; 7:780–782.
11. Grosfeld JL, Cooney DR, Smith J, et al: Intra-abdominal complications following ventriculoperitoneal shunt procedures. *Pediatrics* 1974; 54:791–796.
12. Klein DM: Shunt infections, in Scott RM (ed): *Hydrocephalus*. Baltimore, Williams & Wilkins, 1990, pp 87–97.
13. Schoenbaum SC, Gardner P, Shillito J: Infections of cerebrospinal fluid shunts: Epidemiology, clinical manifestations, and therapy. *J Infect Dis* 1975; 131:543–552.
14. Klein DM: Comparison of antibiotic methods in the prophylaxis of operative shunt infections. *Concepts Pediatr Neurosurg* 1983; 4:131–141.

4

Recurrent Inguinal Hernia in Children

Sylvain Kleinhaus, M.D.
Scott J. Boley, M.D.

A 12-year-old girl with cystic fibrosis had a heavy cough and recurring episodes of respiratory infection. At age 2 years she underwent bilateral repair of an indirect inguinal hernia. Following a severe respiratory infection, the right inguinal hernia recurred, necessitating a second hernia operation at age 9 years. She now presents with a painful swelling in the upper portion of the right labia majora. The mass has bulged out on two recent occasions and was reduced with manual pressure.

Recurrent inguinal hernias in children are uncommon after elective herniorrhaphy. Various series have all reported an incidence of under 1% in these circumstances. Among conditions predisposing to recurrence are hereditary disorders of connective tissue (e.g., Marfan's syndrome) and conditions producing increased abdominal pressure, such as asthma, cystic fibrosis, or ventriculoperitoneal (VP) shunting and ascites. The emergency repair of an incarcerated hernia is the most common clinical situation leading to a recurrence. In incarcerated hernias the sac tends to be very friable, edematous, and tenuous, often being described as having the consistency of "wet tissue paper." In this situation identification of various tissue layers is more difficult, and small tears in the hernia sac occur more frequently and may be easily overlooked. In addition, with large incarcerated hernias, the internal ring is commonly enlarged, and even if the ring is tightened appropriately, the edema of the inflamed tissues may cause the closure to be inadequate when the edema recedes. This results in a residually dilated internal ring that may lead to a recurrence.

PREVENTION

Several technical points can be stressed in trying to eliminate or minimize recurrent inguinal hernias. First and foremost of these is an adequately high ligation of the sac. After the sac is ligated and transected, the stump should retract above the internal ring. If it does not and one cannot easily perform a higher ligation, the stump can be transplanted behind and lateral to the internal ring by placing a suture ligature through the stump and leaving both ends of the suture long. These two ends can then be passed through the internal ring and out through the internal oblique and transversus abdominis muscles so as to place the stump behind these two structures. An adequately high ligation can be assured by cleaning the peritoneal sac above the internal ring, twisting the sac so as to aid a higher ligation, and assuring that no tissues are included in the ligature on the sac that might fix the stump of the sac outside the internal ring. The last situation most frequently occurs today with the use of polyglycolic acid sutures, which tend to pick up any tissues adjacent to them when they are pulled through the sac. This complication can easily be avoided by inspection, and forceps can be used to assure that the ligature includes nothing but the hernia sac itself.

Another important facet of repairing an inguinal hernia in children is the snugging-up or tightening of the internal ring when a large hernia has dilated the ring. Such a dilated ring is easily identified when the high ligation is being performed. Tightening of the ring is facilitated by placing a hemostat on the medial angle of the internal ring prior to transecting the hernial sac. When this is done and the hemostat is elevated, the superior and inferior aspects of the ring are clearly delineated and can be closed appropriately with interrupted sutures. In the case described at the beginning of this chapter, of a recurrent inguinal hernia in a 12-year-old girl, the child's cystic fibrosis may have been a contributing factor. However, a properly performed operation in girls should be followed by an even lower incidence of recurrence than in boys, since one can completely close the internal ring. In girls, a sliding hernia is frequently encountered, most often involving the fallopian tube, but in some cases also involving the uterus and ovary. The absence of vasa deferentia and spermatic cords in the female makes it possible to completely reduce the peritoneal sac and to close the internal ring, so as to leave no opening for a recurrent hernia. A high ligation of the sac is not as crucial if one totally obliterates the internal ring, and the sliding nature of the hernia is therefore of no significance in its repair.

TREATMENT

Almost all recurrent inguinal hernias are diagnosed from months to years after the original repair; an exceptionally rare event is the immediate recurrence seen in the operating or recovery room. In these unusual circumstances it is preferable to retain the child or return it to the operating room and repair the hernia as soon as possible. The repair of these unusual recurrences is done with the same approach as in the original operation.

As in the original management of inguinal hernias in children, there is no urgency in operating on recurrences except when an incarceration is present. Both reoperation through the inguinal approach and preperitoneal repair of recurrent hernias have been used. In girls, in whom there is no risk to any important structure other than the ileoinguinal nerve, and in whom complete closure of the internal ring can be accomplished, most surgeons use the inguinal approach despite the residual scar tissue it leaves. As in the original operation for inguinal hernias in girls, emphasis is put on complete obliteration of the internal ring. This can be accomplished simply by closing the transversalis fascia, but is better done by utilizing a modified Bassini repair to reinforce the closure. The latter involves approximating the conjoint tendon to Poupart's ligament to reinforce the closure of the transversalis fascia.

In boys the risk of injury to the vas deferens or spermatic vessels in the presence of scar tissue is not negligible, and we have found the preperitoneal approach to be preferable. The preperitoneal approach permits one to repair the hernia without dissecting scar tissue, thereby minimizing the risk of injury to the cord structures. In addition, the preperitoneal approach allows the highest of all possible ligations to be done under direct vision, and any defect or laxity in the transversalis fascia and posterior wall of the inguinal canal can be identified and repaired. In the rare instance in which use of a prosthetic material becomes necessary after multiple recurrences, it can be placed without difficulty using the preperitoneal approach. In the illustrative case discussed at the beginning of the chapter, a preperitoneal approach would be ideal. The management of this second recurrence by the preperitoneal approach would permit operating through untouched tissues and would enable a high ligation, and closure of the internal ring would be facilitated by approaching it from the inner aspect of the abdominal wall. Initially, the surgeon may find the preperitoneal approach confusing, and identification of the internal ring and its contents may appear difficult. After two or three operations, however, the anatomy becomes familiar and one can quickly find the ring and separate the sac from the surrounding structures.

TECHNIQUE

Briefly, the technique for preperitoneal repair of a unilateral inguinal hernia is as follows:

A transverse skin incision is made one or two fingerbreadths above the pubic ramus. About one third of the incision is over the rectus muscle and two thirds are lateral to it (Fig 4–1). The incision is carried down to expose the external oblique aponeurosis, which is incised transversely along the entire length of the incision, exposing the lateral border of the rectus muscle. This is retracted medially and the internal oblique and transversus abdominis muscles and the transversalis fascia are then incised (Fig 4–2). The preperitoneal fat is then encountered and the peritoneum is pushed posteriorly and cephalad by blunt dissection, using cotton or gauze pledgets. The posterior aspect of the inguinal canal is exposed and the internal inguinal ring is identified. The indirect hernia sac can be seen entering the canal (Fig 4–3). The sac can usually be freed from the cord structures by gentle traction and dissection. If the sac cannot be withdrawn from the canal, it can be transected (Fig 4–4) under direct vision and repaired with purse-string or interrupted sutures. We prefer polyglycolic acid sutures for ligation of the sac. The posterior wall of the inguinal canal is then inspected for any direct inguinal hernia, and the femoral vessels and sheath are inspected for the presence of a femoral hernia. Any defect is repaired using nonabsorbable sutures, and the internal inguinal ring is appropriately tightened in boys and completely closed in girls. The sutures are placed on the medial aspect of the ring, laterally displacing the vas deferens and spermatic vessels. If the ring is very large, sutures may also be placed lat-

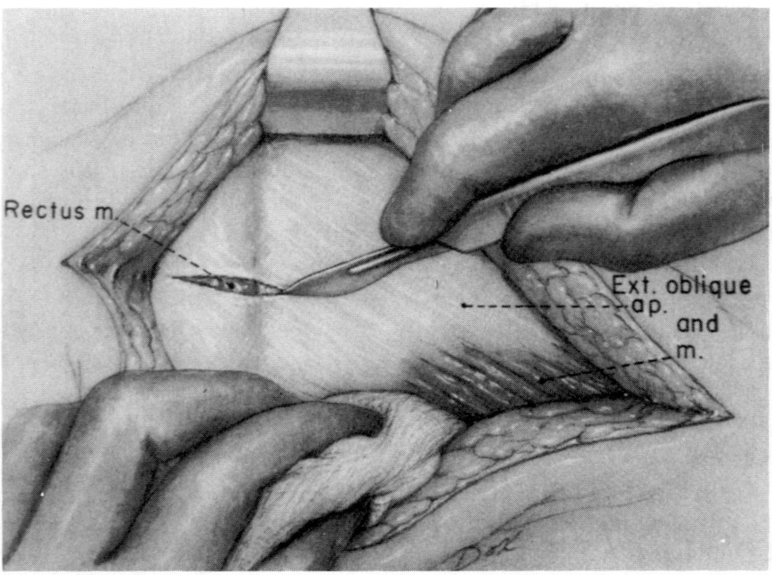

FIG 4–1.
The fascial incision begins over the middle of the rectus abdominis muscle and extends laterally onto the external oblique muscle. (From Nyhus LM, Bombeck CT: *GP* 1966; 33:115. Used by permission.)

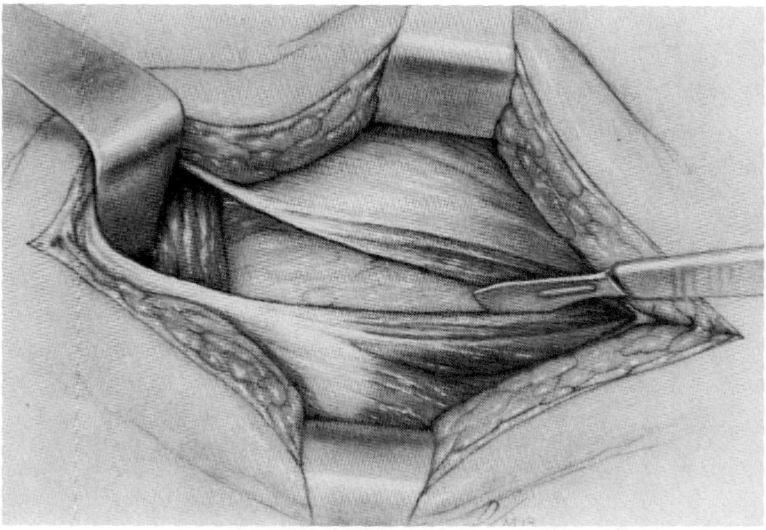

FIG 4–2.
The incision is carried through the internal oblique and transversus abdominis muscles and transversalis fascia, exposing the preperitoneal fat. (From Nyhus LM, Bombeck CT: *GP* 1966; 33:115. Used by permission.)

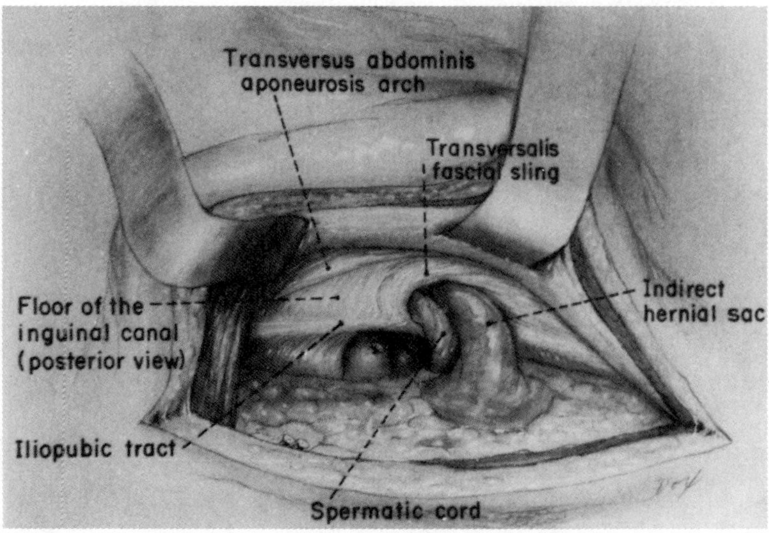

FIG 4–3.
The view is from above downward. All layers of the abdominal wall except the peritoneum and preperitoneal fat are elevated by retractors, revealing the floor of the inguinal canal from above and within. Note the sac of the indirect hernia protruding into the inguinal canal at the superolateral aspect of the internal ring. (From Nyhus LM, Bombeck CT: *GP* 1966; 33:115. Used by permission.)

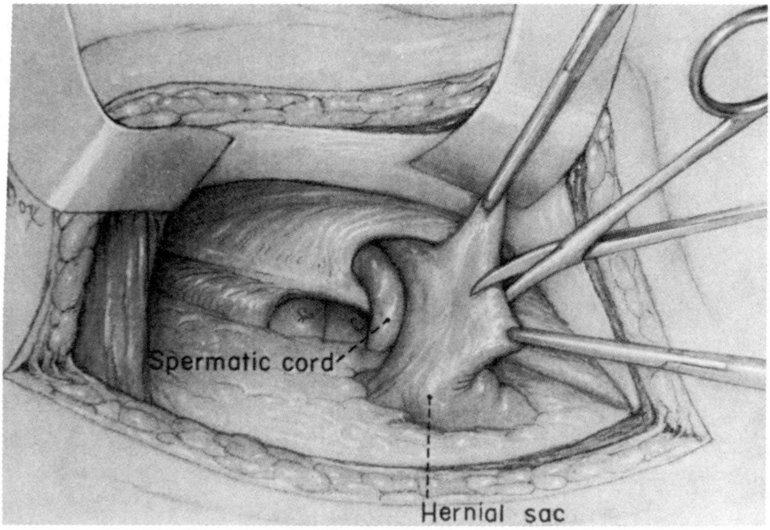

FIG 4–4.
The peritoneum is opened after the hernial sac is identified and separated from the spermatic cord. The hernia sac is ligated under direct vision. (From Nyhus LM, Bombeck CT: *GP* 1966; 33:115. Used by permission.)

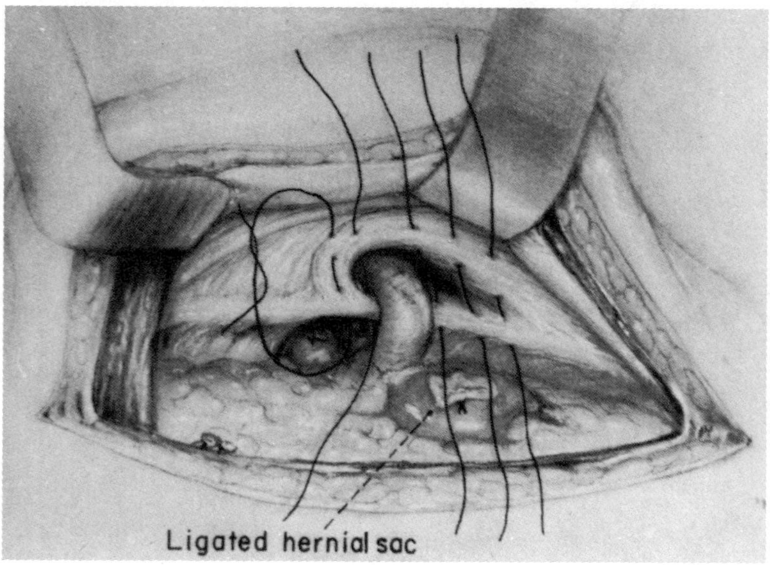

FIG 4–5.
The internal ring is tightened with interrupted nonabsorbable sutures. The sutures shown are placed both medially and laterally to cord structures. (From Nyhus LM, Bombeck CT: *GP* 1966; 33:115. Used by permission.)

eral to the vas deferens and spermatic vessels (Fig 4–5). The inferior epigastric vessels may be sacrificed to facilitate the repair, although this is rarely necessary. In the unusual case in which the structures of the posterior inguinal canal have been injured or scarred, precluding their use in the repair of the defect, the preperitoneal approach is also ideal for placement of a prosthetic patch through which the vas and vessels can pass.

Bilateral recurrences may be treated by the preperitoneal approach through a single incision extending from one linea semilunaris to another, not unlike a Pfannenstiehl incision. Although not recommended for primary repair of an inguinal hernia, the preperitoneal approach has many advantages in the repair of recurrent inguinal hernias and even of primary incarcerated hernias.

REFERENCES

1. Boley SJ, Kleinhaus S: A place for the Cheatle-Henry approach in pediatric surgery? *J Pediatr Surg* 1966; 1:394–397.
2. Nyhus LM, Bombeck CT: The anastomosis and physiologic repair of groin hernia. *GP* 1966; 33:114–121.
3. Shandling B, Thomson S: The Cheatle-Henry approach for inguinal herniotomy in infants and children. The Hospital for Sick Children, Toronto. *Can J Surg* 1963; 6:484–489.

5

Umbilical Hernia in Infants and Children

Christopher P. Brandt, M.D.
Michael W.L. Gauderer, M.D.

A 5-year-old girl presents with complaints of an umbilical swelling. Examination of the umbilicus shows a skin-covered mass protruding from the umbilical ring. The hernial sac contains bowel. The contents are reducible and a 2.5 cm fascial defect is palpable at the umbilical ring.

Umbilical hernia is a condition commonly seen in the pediatric population. While pediatric umbilical hernias may in many respects, be considered benign or incidental lesions, they are often the source of considerable anxiety and concern to parents and other relatives. In addition, disparity of opinion does exist about the natural history and proper treatment of this condition, and which hernias, if any, should undergo surgical repair.

Although umbilical hernias have a tendency for spontaneous closure, it is unlikely that a 2.5 cm fascial defect in a 5-year-old child will close without surgery. Repair can therefore be recommended.

EMBRYOLOGY

In the 5-week embryo, the yolk sac and body stalk enter the ventral surface of the embryo through a small circular area. The omphalomesenteric, or vitelline, duct develops as an outgrowth of the yolk sac, and the umbilical vessels develop from the mesenchyma of the body stalk. As the embryo grows, the omphalomesenteric duct and the body stalk are pressed together, elongate, and are covered by portions of the enlarging amnionic sac.[8] The resultant tubular structure represents the umbilical cord. During the fifth through tenth weeks, the intestines extrude into the umbilical cord, then return into the abdomen by the eleventh week. The omphalomesenteric duct normally closes by the seventh week and the right umbilical vein is obliterated by the sixth week.[14] The full-term cord consists mostly of connective tissue as well as the two arteries, one vein, vitelline duct remnant, and occasionally other small arteries (omphalomesenteric or urachal).

After birth, the cut umbilical cord dries up and heals to become the umbilical cicatrix. The umbilical orifice is a defect in the linea alba, which is formed from intraembryonic mesoderm. The fibrous remnants of the umbilical arteries are firmly attached to the inferior portion of the orifice, while the vein remnants are more loosely attached to the superior edge.[41] The ultimate closure of the umbilical ring is felt to be due to contraction of fibers arising from the obliterated arteries, as well as to fibrous proliferation of surrounding lateral connective-tissue plates.[5, 17] This closure may in part occur as a direct response to local mechanical stress and the tone of the rectus muscles.

An umbilical hernia occurs with incomplete closure or weakness at the umbilical ring, where protrusion of intra-abdominal contents may occur. In contrast to omphaloceles, this happens in an otherwise normally developed abdominal wall, and the protruding area is covered by skin.

ANATOMY

In dissections of the umbilical region, an umbilical canal has been described that passes obliquely through the abdominal wall, and through which runs the umbilical vein.[5] This canal is formed anteriorly by the linea alba, posteriorly by the transversalis (umbilical) fascia and peritoneum, and laterally by the medial edges of the rectus sheaths. It has been noted that the transversalis fascia is thickened and stronger inferior to the umbilical orifice and superior to the entrance of the umbilical vein into the canal, whereas the fascia directly posterior to the canal is thinner, creating an area of weakness. It has been proposed that a congenital or direct hernia occurs in this area, while herniation down through the umbilical canal leads to an indirect or acquired type of hernia.[5, 41] The direct hernia would be the type commonly seen in infants (Fig 5–1), while the acquired type would occur in later infancy, childhood, or adulthood. Spontaneous closure would be less likely to occur in this latter, less common type of hernia. Unfortunately, it is often impossible to distinguish the two types on clinical evaluation, although the indirect or more supraumbilical type of hernia may appear to be more ovoid, with a slightly higher and more sharply defined fascial defect. Occasionally, supraumbilical hernias coexist with umbilical hernias (Fig 5–2).

Small, midline bulges between the umbilicus and the xyphoid process are

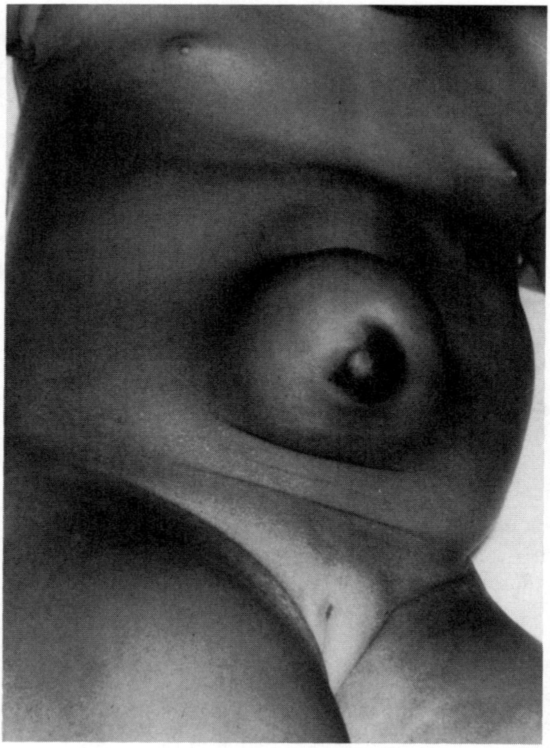

FIG 5–1.
Ten-month-old child with typical direct umbilical hernia. Note the pronounced diastasis recti. This defect (2 cm) closed spontaneously at age 5 years.

commonly known as "epigastric hernias." In this situation there is a protrusion of preperitoneal fat through a small fascial defect, without a hernia sac. Entrapment of fat may cause acute pain. These lesions do not close spontaneously.

A wide variety of other lesions may be located in the region of the umbilicus, including patent omphalomesenteric ducts, urachal cysts, skin-covered umbilical granulomas, and omphaloceles.[8] The physician involved in the treatment of umbilical hernias should be aware of the various congenital and acquired lesions that can occur in this area. The presence of an umbilical hernia should be distinguishable by careful physical examination.

INCIDENCE

The reported incidence of umbilical hernias varies with the population studied, and appears to be significantly higher in black children. In studies of blacks in

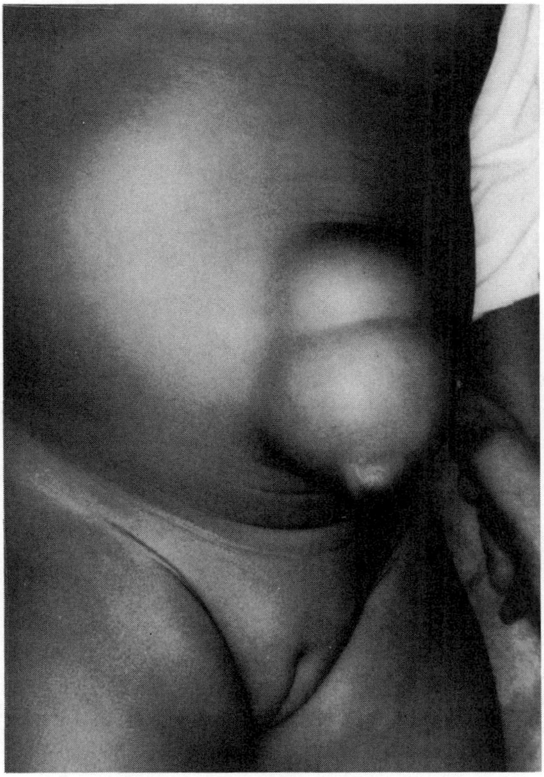

FIG 5–2.
A 1-year-old child with umbilical and supraumbilical defects. Surgical closure was eventually required.

the United States, the incidence in children from 0 to 1 year old ranged from 24.7% to 58.0%,[10, 11, 22] whereas in predominantly white populations an incidence of 1.9% to 18.5% has been found.[11, 41] In select African races, even higher incidences of 75% to 91% have been noted.[19, 21] A significant difference between males and females has not been seen in most studies, but umbilical hernias do appear to be more frequent in premature, low-birthweight infants.[11, 38] Vohr[38] found that 75% of infants with a birthweight of 500 to 1500 g had umbilical hernias, and that in this same group, all had closed by 1 year of age.

Although most umbilical hernias are isolated findings, they can be associated with other pathologic conditions, including Beckwith–Wiedemann syndrome, hypothyroidism, Hurler's syndrome, and trisomy 13, 18, and 21.[23] Concomitant inguinal hernias have been noted in about 15% of children with umbilical hernias.[25, 30] It also seems likely that any condition that increases intra-abdominal pressure may contribute to the formation of an umbilical hernia. This can include other pathologic processes (e.g., ascites secondary to nephrosis, CHF, or cirrhosis; chronic coughing; constipation; or pregnancy; or treatments associated with increased intra-abdominal volume, such as peritoneal dialysis or ventriculoperitoneal shunts). Umbilical hernias have been reported to develop in 7.5% to 16% of pediatric patients on continuous peritoneal dialysis.[1, 36, 37, 39] Therefore, while most umbilical hernias are "typical" and isolated, they may be indicators of or consequences of other disease entities.

NATURAL HISTORY

A number of studies have addressed the natural history of infantile umbilical hernias, and have reported rates of closure that have varied with the type of population studied. Nevertheless, it is clear that, in marked contrast to adult umbilical hernias, the vast majority of hernias in infants and children will close spontaneously.

In prospective studies, Woods[41] and Karlstrom[24] found that in predominantly white populations, more than 90% of umbilical hernias had closed by the first year. In black populations, Heifetz et al.[17] observed that 93% had closed by 3 years, and Walker[40] noted 85% closure by 6 years. Cross-sectional data show similar rates of spontaneous closure,[5, 10, 15, 22, 32, 34] and one group[15] suggested that even among hernias present at age 4 to 5 years, half would close by age 11. Only in select African populations have lower rates of closure been reported.[19, 21]

Many authors feel that the larger the size of the umbilical defect, the less the chance of spontaneous closure. Walker[40] observed that 96% of hernias less than 0.5 cm in diameter closed by age 6, while no defect larger than 1.5 cm healed spontaneously by age 6. Data from others, however, suggest that even among larger hernias, many will close by age 5 to 6.[5, 16]

CLINICAL MANIFESTATIONS

The great majority of pediatric umbilical hernias are asymptomatic, and their most common clinical manifestation is probably as a source of parental and grandparental anxiety. In one survey,[26] umbilical hernias in children caused "considerable" concern for 63% of their parents, with 33% also expressing feelings of guilt. It also seems likely that a large or protruding hernia in an older child may be a source of psychologic trauma.

Incarceration of pediatric umbilical hernias is uncommon, and strangulation is even more rare. In several large series, the incidence of incarceration was found to be less than 0.2%,[10, 16, 27, 34, 40, 41] and in recent literature reviews, only 12 previously reported cases of strangulated hernia were found.[3, 20, 29] Lassaletta et al.[25] reported that 28 of 377, or 7.4%, of umbilical hernias in children were repaired with incarceration as the indication, and only 1 of these 28 showed strangulation. They found that incarceration occurred in patients of all ages from 0 to 12 years, and that more episodes occurred with fascial defects of 0.5 to 1.5 cm diameter. These and other authors have noted that incarceration of umbilical hernias is accompanied by much less morbidity and mortality in children than in adults, and that it is much less likely to be followed by strangulation than is incarceration of inguinal hernias.[25, 28] In some cases of incarceration there has been an underlying factor such as a foreign body bezoar (e.g., newspaper or chewing gum).[18, 27] Why these complications are so infrequent is not clear, but they may be related to the relatively small and thin omentum of infants, an infant's preponderantly supine position, and the absence or relative lack of surrounding muscular components to help entrap intestine in the congenital type of umbilical hernia.

An umbilical hernia can rupture, with resultant evisceration, but this is extremely rare, being documented only by isolated case reports.[6] Umbilical hernias may also be the source of intermittent umbilical or abdominal pain.

TREATMENT

Treatment options for umbilical hernias range from simple observation to surgical repair. As noted previously, the great majority of pediatric umbilical hernias will close spontaneously, and observation with periodic followup, along with reassurance of the parents, is therefore appropriate in most cases. In the past, various methods of mechanical compression were commonly used (e.g., trusses, tape, or the application of plaster). There are no available data to suggest that strapping improves or accelerates the natural rate of closure.[16, 24, 41] Indeed, these techniques may even delay closure, and can also cause complications including skin irritation and infection. Although the clinical practice of taping has largely been abandoned, Maragos found that home remedies for pediatric umbilical hernias are still popular with parents.[26]

The central question is which, if any, umbilical hernias in children should be repaired? Clear indications for repair would include incarceration, strangulation, perforation, or recurrent pain. Relative indications would include protrusion with thinned overlying skin, and irritation of the overlying skin from frequent manipulation by the child. Extreme persistence and insistence on repair by the parents may also be a factor in a decision to operate, as may possible psychological trauma in the older child. Persistence or enlargement of a fascial defect over a period of observation should lead one to consider repair, and many authors recommend operation for defects that are greater than 1.5 cm by

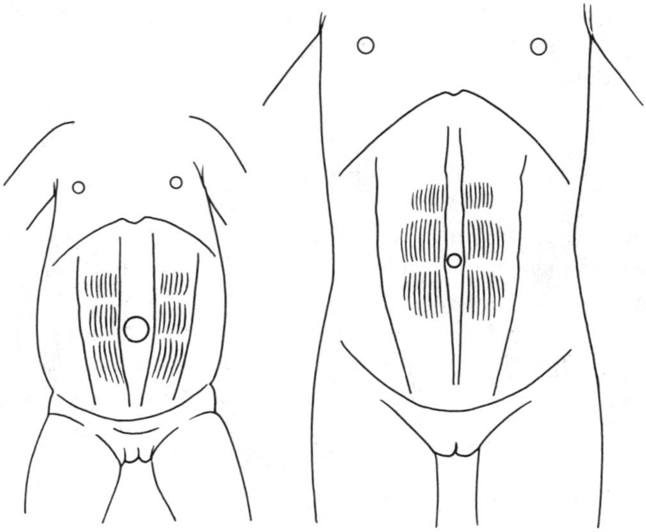

FIG 5–3.
Comparison of abdominal wall and umbilical defect in an infant and a child. As the infant grows, the defect becomes smaller (in absolute as well as relative terms), and the linea alba becomes proportionately narrower and stronger. This progression clearly favors surgical correction in the older (over 3- to 5-year) group.

age 4,[11, 25, 30] or for defects that persist at the time the child enters school.[33, 40] As long as progression of closure is observed, expectant management is warranted. On the other hand, it has been our experience that discrete supraumbilical defects are unlikely to close, and should therefore be repaired earlier.

From a practical standpoint alone, umbilical herniorrhaphies are somewhat easier to perform in the older child. As diagrammed in Fig 5–3, the infant's abdomen is proportionately larger, with a broader and weaker linea alba, and a proportionately larger incision is required. The presence of distended, air-filled loops of intestine secondary to an infant's aerophagia may also make the bowel more prone to injury, and leads to a somewhat more difficult open repair in smaller children. We believe that in the absence of complications, repair of umbilical hernias should be delayed at least until the age of 3 to 5 years.

OPERATIVE TECHNIQUE

Repair of an umbilical hernia is accomplished under general anesthesia and usually in an outpatient setting. The procedure is relatively straightforward, but several variations in technique have been proposed, including the type of incision, handling of the hernia sac, type of suture used, and closure of the defect.

An infraumbilical incision is most commonly used, although some surgeons approach the defect supraumbilically or through the umbilical cicatrix. The latter can be done either transversely[35] or vertically.[9] The hernia sac can be handled in many ways, ranging from closed methods, in which the sac is not entered but simply invaginated[33] or dissected free and ligated,[4] to open methods in which the sac is entered. Proposed benefits of the closed method include avoidance of preperitoneal vessels, decreased peritoneal irritation, and the prevention of intestinal evisceration during the procedure,[4, 33] while the open method is felt to help avoid visceral injury and allow for better definition of fascial edges. With the open method, the hernia sac may be completely excised,[30, 35] partially excised,[2] or merely incised and otherwise left intact.[9] Excellent results have been reported with each method.

The usually recommended fascial closure is done in a simple transverse fashion, using interrupted, nonabsorbable sutures, but overlapping of the fascial edges[29] or vertical closure[8] have also been used. Since most of the surrounding fascial fibers run horizontally, a transverse closure with suture placement at right angles to this direction would seem to be more appropriate, and overlapping of fascia has not been shown to improve results.[12] Running closure and the use of longer-acting, absorbable suture material, in order to avoid suture reaction, are other possible options. Specific methods for dealing with the excess and protruberant skin of large proboscoid hernias have been described,[7, 31] although skin excision is usually not necessary and may lead to unsatisfactory cosmetic results.

Our preferred method is outlined in Figs 5-4 to 5-11. A small, curved infraumbilical incision is made without excision of skin. The sac is dissected from the subcutaneous tissue and then opened and excised. The fascial edges are clearly delineated and carefully approximated transversely with interrupted, long-acting absorbable suture material (e.g., polyglactin or polydioxanone). The skin is closed with subcuticular sutures and a light dressing is applied.

COMPLICATIONS

Complications of the operative repair of umbilical hernias include those related to the anesthesia itself, local wound problems (hematoma, seroma, or infection), acute and chronic suture reactions, visceral injury, and recurrence. A poor cosmetic result, including the development of keloids, should also be considered a complication. In several of the larger reported series, no associated mortality was noted. Hematomas developed in 0.9% to 1.3%, seroma in 1.6%, wound infection in 0.8% to 1.9%, and recurrence in 0.3% to 1.3%.[2, 13, 25, 30] We have seen one recurrence, in a patient with Hurler's syndrome. No case of visceral injury has been reported, although we managed one patient in whom a

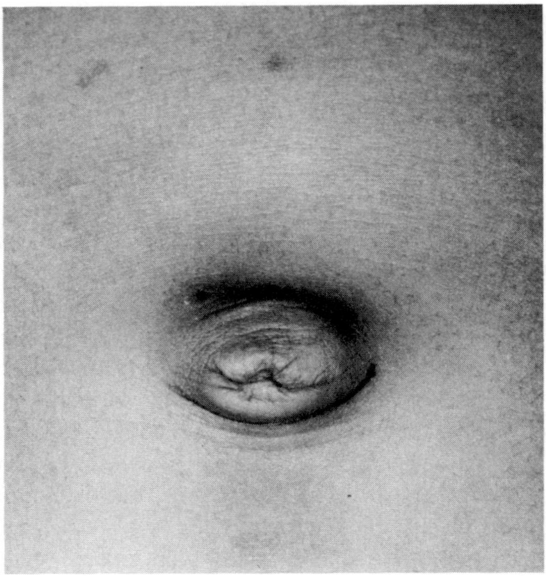

FIG 5–4.
A 2-cm umbilical hernia in a 6-year-old girl. The infraumbilical incision is marked on the skin, following one of the natural creases.

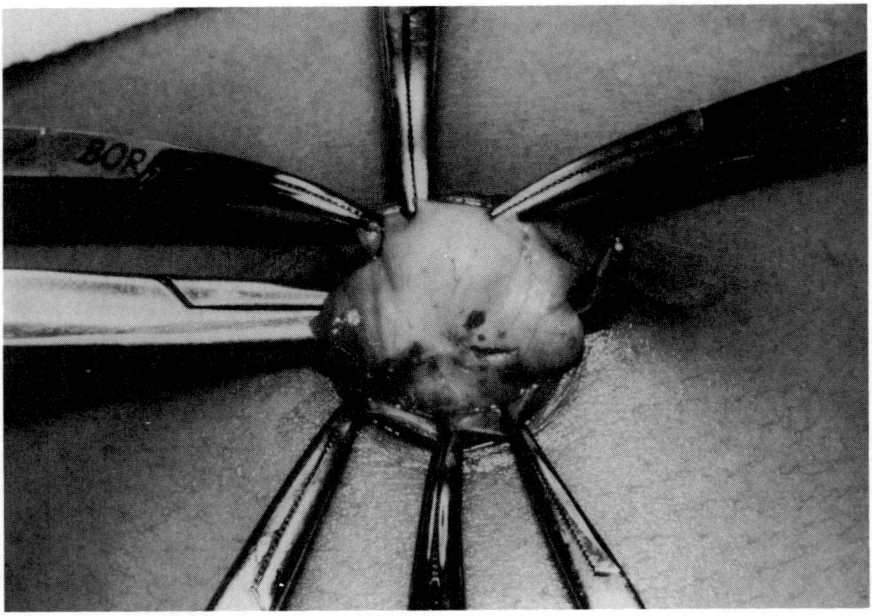

FIG 5–5.
The hernia sac has been dissected and is lifted by a right-angled clamp. The curved hemostats provide both hemostasis and exposure through gentle traction.

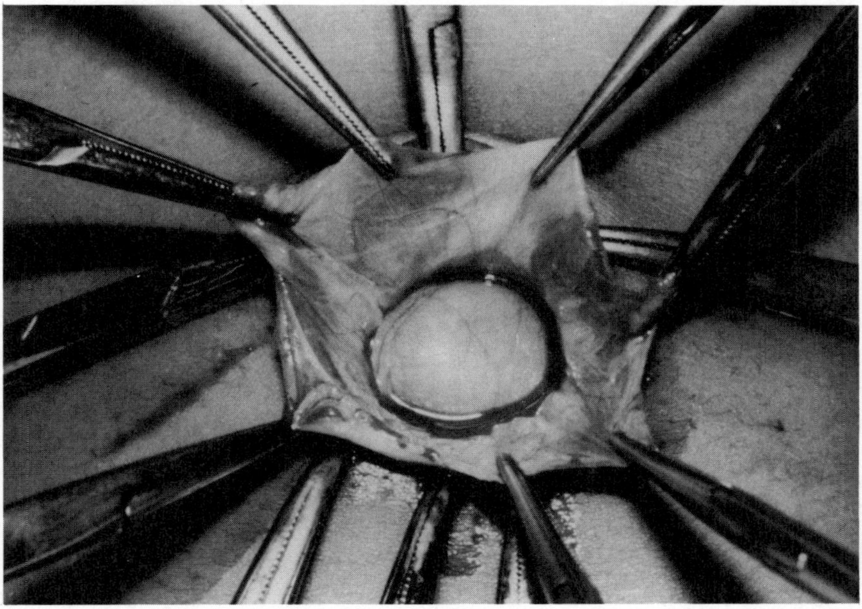

FIG 5–6.
The sac has been opened and held by straight hemostats. The fascial ring is clearly visible. The sac is then resected.

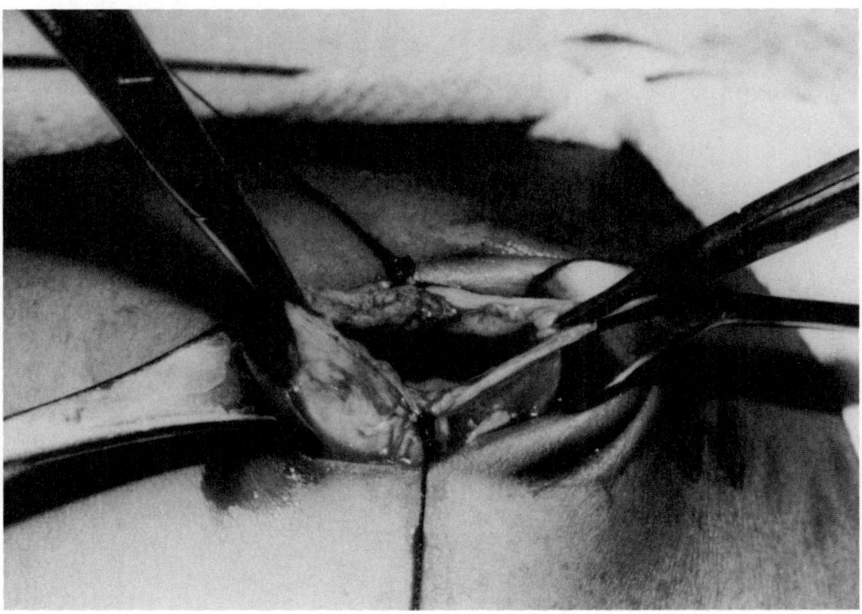

FIG 5–7.
Lateral view demonstrating the fascial edges with the corner sutures in place.

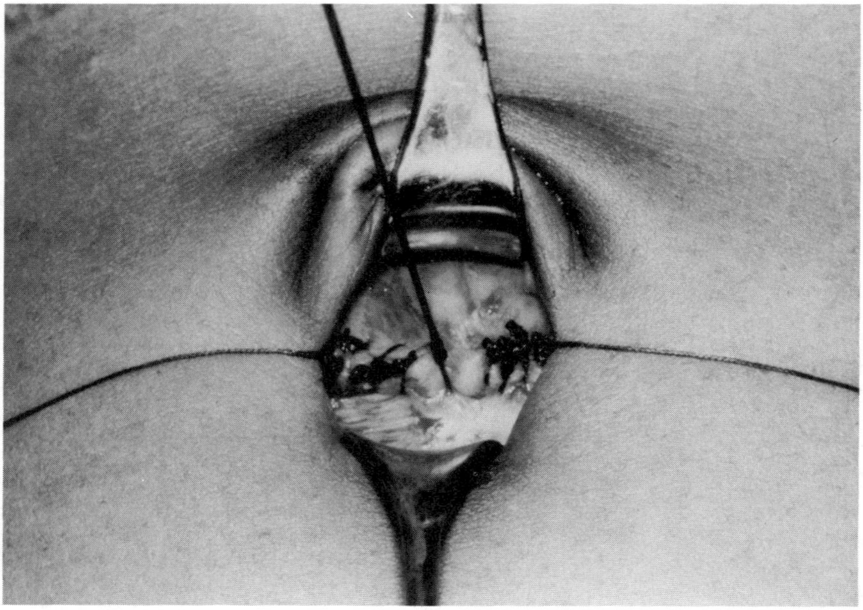

FIG 5–8.
Completed transverse fascial closure. In this instance 2-0 polyglactin sutures were used. Note the central suture, which will be used to bring the apex of the redundant skin to the level of the fascia.

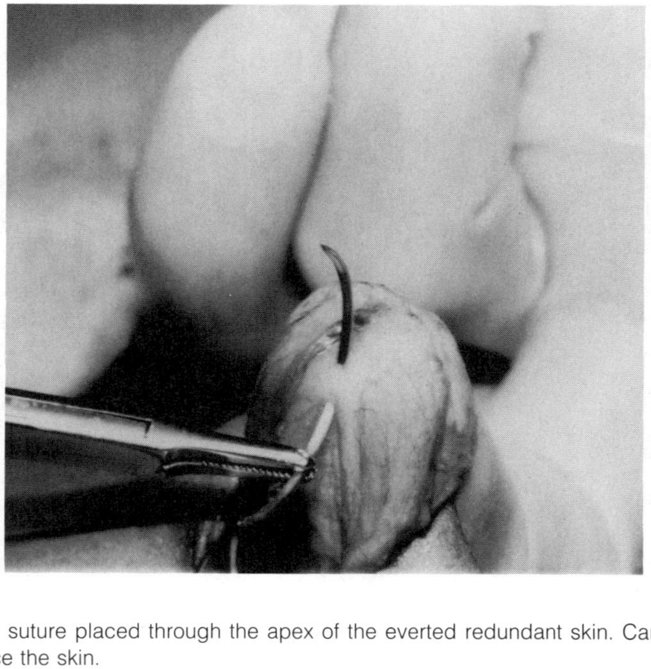

FIG 5–9.
The central suture placed through the apex of the everted redundant skin. Care is taken not to pierce the skin.

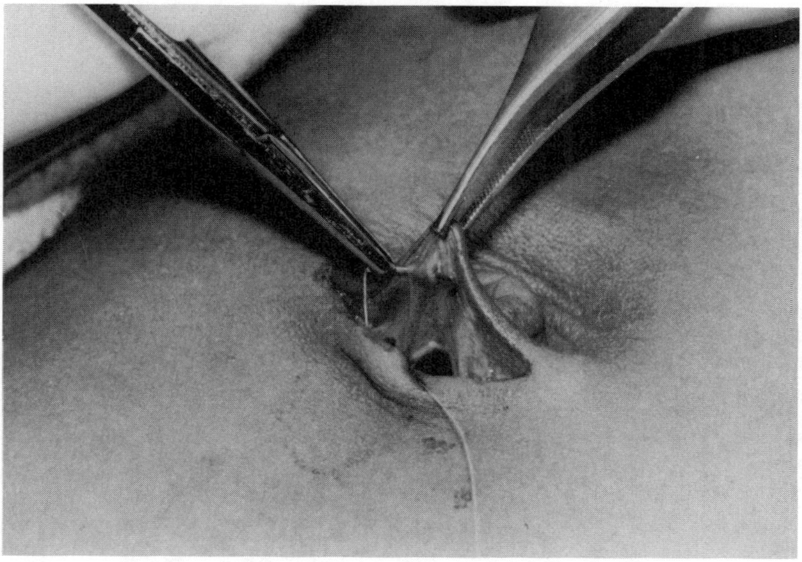

FIG 5–10.
Subcutaneous and then subcuticular sutures (5-0 polyglactin) are placed.

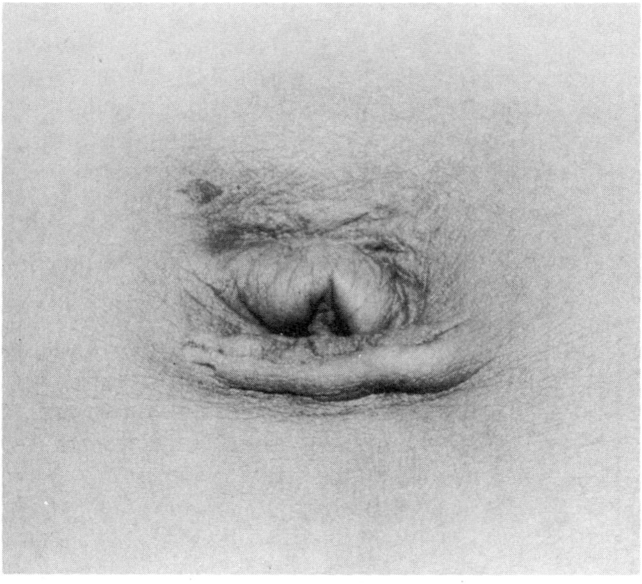

FIG 5–11.
Completed repair. Although there is skin redundancy and a small ridge at the level of the incision, both eventually disappear. A small dressing or collodion is applied.

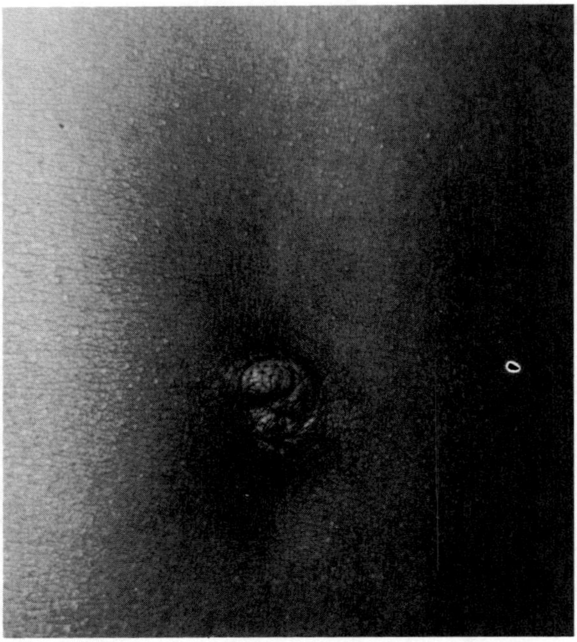

FIG 5–12.
Appearance of an umbilicus 6 months after repair.

bowel obstruction developed secondary to suture entrapment that had occurred after a closed herniorrhaphy performed at another institution. With careful technique, umbilical hernia repair in the pediatric age group can be accomplished with little morbidity and very low rates of recurrence (Fig 5–12).

SUMMARY

Umbilical hernia is a common condition among infants and children. In the great majority of cases, the natural history is one of eventual closure without treatment. The occurrence of incarceration and other complications is uncommon. Our initial approach is one of periodic office visits with measurement of the defect, along with reassurance and education of the parents. If spontaneous closure does not occur after age 3 to 5 years, operative correction can be recommended.

REFERENCES

1. Alexander SR, Tank ES: Surgical aspects of continuous ambulatory peritoneal dialysis in infants, children, and adolescents. *J Urol* 1982; 127:501–504.

2. Alvear DT, Pilling GP: Management of the sac during umbilical hernia repair in children. *Am J Surg* 1974; 127:518–520.
3. Auldist AW, Lugg P: Strangulation of an umbilical hernia in a child of six months. *Aust Paediatr J* 1982; 18:286.
4. Benjamin B, Vinocur CD, Wagner CW, et al: A closed technique for umbilical hernia repair. *Surg Gynecol Obstet* 1987; 164:473–474.
5. Blumberg NA: Infantile umbilical hernia. *Surg Gynecol Obstet* 1980; 150:187–192.
6. Brandon S, Whitehouse D: Two unusual complications of umbilical hernia in childhood. *Br Med J* 1960; 2:1935–1936.
7. Cone JB, Golladay ES: Purse-string closure of umbilical hernia repair. *J Pediatr Surg* 1983; 18:297.
8. Cresson SL, Pilling GP: Lesions about the umbilicus in infants and children. *Pediatr Clin North Am* 1959; 6:1097–1101.
9. Criado FJ: A simplified method of umbilical herniorrhaphy. *Surg Gynecol Obstet* 1981; 153:904–905.
10. Crump EP: Umbilical hernia: Occurence of the infantile type in Negro infants and children. *J Pediatr* 1952; 40:214–233.
11. Evans AG: The comparative incidence of umbilical hernia in colored and white infants. *J Natl Med Assoc* 1941; 33:158–160.
12. Farris JM, Smith GK, Beattie AS: Umbilical hernia: An inquiry into the principle of imbrication and a note on the preservation of the umbilical dimple. *Am J Surg* 1959; 98:236–242.
13. Gibson LD, Gaspar MR: A review of 606 cases of umbilical hernia. *Surg Gynecol Obstet* 1959; 109:313–322.
14. Gray SW, Skandalakis JE: *Embryology for Surgeons*. Philadelphia, WB Saunders, 1972, pp 129–132.
15. Hall DE, Roberts KB, Charney E: Umbilical hernia: What happens after age 5 years? *J Pediatr* 1981; 98:415–417.
16. Halpern LJ: Spontaneous healing of umbilical hernias. *JAMA* 1962; 182:851–852.
17. Heifetz CJ, Bilsel ZT, Gaus WW: Observations on the disappearance of umbilical hernias of infancy and childhood. *Surg Gynecol Obstet* 1963; 116:467–473.
18. Izant RJ: Personal communication.
19. James T: Umbilical hernia in Xhosa infants and children. *J R Soc Med* 1982; 75:537–541.
20. Jeans PL, Wright JE: Strangulated umbilical hernia in infancy. *Aust Paediatr J* 1984; 20:75.
21. Jelliffe DB: Racial incidence of umbilical hernia. *J Trop Med Hyg* 1954; 57:270–272.
22. Jones JW: The frequency of umbilical herniae in Negro infants. *Arch Pediatr* 1941; 58:294–300.
23. Jones KL: Abdominal wall, in Jones KL (ed): *Smith's Recognizable Patterns of Human Malformation*. WB Saunders, Philadelphia, Ed. 4, 1988, pp 753–754.
24. Karlstrom G: Should infantile umbilical hernias be treated with naval emplastras? *J Pediatr* 1961; 59:87–89.
25. Lassaletta L, Fonkalsrud EW, Tovar JA, Dudgeon D, Asch MJ: The management of umbilical hernias in infancy and childhood. *J Pediatr Surg* 1975; 10:405–409.

26. Maragos GD: Umbilical hernia in children- parental feelings and attitudes. *Nebr Med J* 1978; 64:33.
27. Mestel AL, Burns H: Incarcerated and strangulated umbilical hernias in infants and children. *Clin Pediatr* 1963; 2:368–370.
28. Morgan WW, White JJ, Stumbaugh S, et al: Prophylactic umbilical hernia repair in childhood to prevent adult incarceration. *Surg Clin North Am* 1970; 50:839–845.
29. Need AB: Obstructed umbilical hernia in children: Two case reports. *Aust Paediatr J* 1972; 8:152.
30. Ponka JL: Umbilical hernia in infants and adults and omphaloceles, in Ponka JL (ed): *Hernias of the Abdominal Wall*. Philadelphia, WB Saunders, 1980, pp 397–434.
31. Reyna TM, Hollis HW Jr., Smith SB: Surgical management of proboscoid herniae. *J Pediatr Surg* 1987; 22:911–912.
32. Riisfeldt O: Umbilical hernias in children. *Nord Med* 1945; 28:2367–2368.
33. Shaw A: Disorders of the umbilicus, in Welch KJ, Randolph JG, Ravitch MM, et al (eds): *Pediatric Surgery*, Ed. 4, vol. 2. Chicago, Year Book Medical Publishers, 1986, pp 731–739.
34. Sibley WL, Lynn HE, Harris LE: A twenty-five year study of infantile umbilical hernia. *Surgery* 1964; 55:462–468.
35. Smith-Behn J, Katz W: Transumbilical approach to umbilical hernias. *Surg Gynecol Obstet* 1988; 166:466–467.
36. Stone MM, Fonkalsrud EW, Salvsky IB, et al: Surgical management of peritoneal dialysis catheters in children; five-year experience with 1800 patient-month follow-up. *J Pediatr Surg* 1986; 21:1177–1181.
37. Tank ES, Hatch DA: Hernias complicating chronic ambulatory peritoneal dialysis in children. *J Pediatr Surg* 1986; 21:41–42.
38. Vohr BR, Rosenfield AG, Oh W: Umbilical hernia in the low birth-weight infant (less than 1500 gm). *J Pediatr* 1977; 90:807–808.
39. von Lilien T, Salusky IB, et al.: Hernias: A frequent complication in children treated with continuous peritoneal dialysis. *Am J Kidney Dis* 1987; 10:356–360.
40. Walker SH: The natural history of umbilical hernia. *Clin Pediatr* 1967; 6:29–32.
41. Woods, GE: Some observations on umbilical hernia in infants. *Arch Dis Child* 1953; 28:450–462.

6

Management of Unilateral Cryptorchid Testicle

Eric W. Fonkalsrud, M.D.

A 16-month-old boy is referred because of an empty right scrotum. The parents have never seen the right testis in the scrotal sac. The left testis is palpable in the left scrotal sac. In the frogleg position, a small mass is palpable in the right inguinal canal just above the external inguinal ring.

By the age of 16 months, both testes of the full-term and even the premature male infant should be in the low scrotum. Since retractile testes are almost invariably bilateral, it is unlikely that the patient under consideration has this condition; however, an attempt should be made to manipulate the right testicle, which has been palpated in the low inguinal canal, into the scrotum. Seating the infant on its mother's lap in the frogleg position may provide the greatest likelihood of being able to manipulate the testicle into the scrotum. Occasionally, mild sedation may be necessary to facilitate an optimal examination in a hyperactive child. The testicle must descend into the low scrotum with manipulation if one is to consider the gonad to be retractile and not truly undescended. During the manipulation, an estimate of the size of the gonad in milliliters should be recorded and compared to that on the contralateral, descended side.

In over 85% of boys with an empty scrotum, the gonad may be palpated in the inguinal canal or superficial inguinal pouch, or in an ectopic position. An undeveloped scrotum is rare and usually occurs in association with a high inguinal or abdominal testis or with atrophic or absent gonads.

Since there is no clinical or experimental evidence that orchiopexy during the first 16 months of life is more beneficial than at a slightly later age, we would recommend that surgical repair be deferred until the infant approaches 24 months of age. Surgery may be performed earlier if the child is large for its age and the scrotum is well developed. It is likely that orchiopexy at a younger age increases the risk of injury to the spermatic vessels and the lymphatics to the gonad. Only if a clinically apparent inguinal hernia is present on the ipsilateral side would an orchiopexy be recommended at an earlier time.

The higher the cryptorchid testis resides above the scrotum, the more dysgenetic the morphology is likely to be. Many studies have indicated that the undescended testis does not mature normally after the age of 2 years, and that it may produce adverse affects on the contralateral, descended testis, possibly by an autoimmune mechanism. Thus, it is very likely that the cryptorchid testis in the patient under consideration is histologically normal.

In contrast to infants with bilateral cryptorchidism, those with unilateral nondescent have a low incidence of urinary tract malformations. In the absence of urinary tract symptoms, abnormal urinalysis, or other evidence suggesting renal anomalies, urography is not believed necessary. Although occasional males are reported to have chromosomal abnormalities in association with cryptorchidism, it has been our experience that changes in the chromosomal pattern are found mainly in those with bilateral undescent, in whom intersex anomalies are more frequent, and that chromosomal evaluation is rarely necessary in cases of unilateral nondescent.

A course of treatment with human chorionic gonadotropin (HCG) for boys with low-lying, unilaterally undescended testes may produce descent in as many as 10% to 15%, and may make the technical aspects of orchiopexy easier in those who do not respond. For a 2-year-old male, hormonal treatment consists of approximately 10,000 units of HCG given over the short course of 1½ to 2 weeks by intramuscular injection in five to six doses. The response should be noted within the first week after completion of the last injection. Recent studies in which HCG has been given during the first 4 years of life suggests that subsequent function of the gonad may be better than if hormones had not been used. Nonetheless, we have not observed notable benefit from intramuscular HCG administration in a trial in young males with definite unilateral testicular undescent.

ORCHIOPEXY

The technique of orchiopexy currently in general use has been described and illustrated by several authors. The objective of the repair is to alter the course of the spermatic artery, which extends from the renal pedicle to the internal and then to the external inguinal ring, and to relocate it in a direct line from the renal pedicle to the scrotum.

An incision approximately 3 cm long is made through the lowermost abdominal skin crease. The aponeurosis of the external oblique muscle is opened in the direction of its fibers through the external ring. The testicle is usually found extending through the external ring and overlying the external oblique fascia in the superficial inguinal pouch, or in the inguinal canal above the external inguinal ring. The testis with its surrounding tunica vaginalis is mobilized from the gubernaculum and often tenacious surrounding attachments to the pubis, permitting it to be elevated with gentle traction. The cremaster muscle is mobilized gently from the spermatic vessels and the vas deferens up to the level of the internal inguinal ring. The internal oblique muscle is divided lateral to the internal ring over a distance of approximately 1 cm to obtain better exposure. The inferior epigastric artery and veins are divided, and the transversalis fascia is opened widely from the internal ring to the pubis to permit wide exposure of the retroperitoneal space.

The accompanying hernia sac, which is present in over 90% of cases, is separated from the spermatic vessels and the vas deferens, often a delicate maneuver because the structures are tenaciously adherent and the sac tears easily. This maneuver can be facilitated by injecting a small amount of saline through a small-gauge needle between the hernia sac and the cord structures, and then gently developing a plane by blunt dissection with a fine clamp. High ligation of the hernia sac is performed with a fine transfixion suture.

The gonad is inspected to note its size, consistency, and any abnormal features. Biopsy is not routinely recommended because of the risk of further injury to the delicate organ, especially in the young child, unless any unusual features are grossly apparent. Any abnormalities of the epididymis, testicle, or vestigial appendages should be noted. If the testicle is atrophic, measuring less than one-third the size of the contralateral gonad, we recommend its removal and the insertion of a small silastic scrotal prosthesis. The testicle is then replaced into the tunica, the proximal end of which is closed loosely to prevent dislodgement outside the sac. The dissection is continued into the retroperitoneal space by elevating the peritoneum, sharply dividing the lateral spermatic fascia, and bluntly mobilizing the spermatic vessels as high as is necessary to place the testicle into the low scrotum with minimal tension. Excessive mobilization of the spermatic vessels should be avoided. Similarly, tension on the spermatic vessels is likely to cause vascular spasm and injury to the gonad and should be avoided.

The scrotum is then forcibly stretched by inserting a finger through the wound into the lowermost portion of the sac. A small incision is made through the scrotal skin at this point, and a space sufficiently large to accommodate the testis is developed between the dartos muscle and the scrotal skin by blunt dissection. A small incision is then made in the dartos fascia and muscle layer through which a clamp is passed superiorly to direct the testicle downward to the lower scrotum. Twisting of the spermatic vessels must be avoided. The upper edge of the tunica is stitched to the dartos layer circumferentially with absorbable sutures, to prevent upward displacement or subsequent torsion, and the testicle is placed in the subcutaneous pouch. The scrotal skin is closed loosely with fine sutures of absorbable material. The transversalis fascia is then closed with nonabsorbable sutures, leaving a small opening just lateral to the pubis to function as the new internal inguinal ring. The internal oblique muscle is sutured to the shelving edge of the inguinal ligament, again leaving a small opening medially to serve as the new internal ring. The aponeurosis of the external oblique muscle is reapproximated. A subcuticular skin closure is performed, similar to that used for herniorrhaphy wounds.

In children without major associated anomalies, the operation is usually performed as an outpatient procedure. Despite the arrangement of the external ring almost directly over the new internal ring, which appears conducive to the occurrence of a direct hernia, this complication is extremely rare, and has not been observed in our experience.

Following orchiopexy, complications severe enough to jeopardize function of the gonad occur in less than 5% of operations performed by experienced surgeons. The most serious concerns are obstruction of the delicate vascular supply to the testicle by direct injury, compression from twisting of the vascular pedicle, or excessively tight closure of the abdominal musculature, or from narrowing the vessels by subjecting them to significant tension as the testis is placed into the scrotum. Transient testicular swelling due to partial obstruction of lymphatic and venous drainage is common, usually subsiding within 2 to 4 weeks. Injury to the vas deferens appears to be relatively rare. Retraction of the testicle up to the external inguinal ring or higher has been uncommon since the dartos pouch technique of anchoring the testicle has become standard. Recurrent direct hernia and scrotal hematoma are rare after orchiopexy.

7

Bilaterally Undescended Testes

Michael E. Mitchell, M.D.
George Ganesan, M.D.

A 6-month-old boy presents with bilateral empty scrotal sacs. The scrotal skin is flattened and without skin wrinkles. The abdominal wall musculature is sparse and weak. The overlying abdominal wall skin is severely wrinkled. An abdominal ultrasound study shows an enlarged bladder and dilated ureters.

The triad of bilaterally undescended testes, deficient abdominal musculature with lax abdominal skin, and an enlarged bladder with dilated ureters is diagnostic of the prune-belly syndrome. The severity with which it affects patients covers a spectrum ranging from severe pulmonary hypoplasia to mild with limited muscle deficiency, mild hydronephrosis, and good renal function. More severely affected infants are often detected in utero with oligohydramnios. They have a poor prognosis and usually do not survive beyond the first few days of life. Those at the other end of the spectrum have a good prognosis and require minimal or no urologic care.

Between these extremes are patients with varying degrees of involvement of the urinary and respiratory tracts. They have the potential to survive the neonatal period, but require close urologic and pediatric supervision. All have abdominal testes. The prognosis for patients in this group usually depends on the degree of renal dysplasia. Whether aggressive urinary reconstruction should be performed early, late, or not at all remains the subject of great controversy.[1, 2]

In the past, the magnitude of the urinary tract abnormality and management of its complications completely overshadowed the treatment of cryptorchidism in patients with the prune-belly syndrome. Orchiopexy was either omitted or postponed until these patients survived into late childhood. The results of delayed orchiopexy, often done in late childhood or adolescence, were far from satisfactory. The techniques employed, such as dividing the spermatic vessels (Fowler-Stephens) and standard or staged orchiopexies, resulted in significant atrophy or poorly positioned testes (high in the scrotum or inguinal canal).[3] In recent years, advances in urologic reconstruction have made it possible for boys with the prune-belly syndrome to survive childhood and puberty; a reported series of adults with the prune-belly syndrome indicate that these children have the potential to grow into mature and well-adjusted men, with normal secondary sexual characteristics and a libido similar to that of their peers.[4] Thus, it would seem that the management of the undescended testes has lagged behind that of the other components of the syndrome.

The etiology of cryptorchidism in the prune-belly syndrome may be related to the absence of the abdominal muscles (pushing force), dysfunction or absence of the gubernaculum (pulling force), a large bladder (blocking force), or an intrinsic abnormality of the testes itself. The testes in patients with the syndrome are intra-abdominal, and usually lie where the ureters cross the pelvic brim. Furthermore, these testes do not have the potential for spontaneous descent. Nor do gonadotropins have a place in their management, even though gonadotropins may be of diagnostic value in the non-prune-belly patient with impalpable testes.[5] To date, surgery offers the only means of bringing the testes into the scrotum in these patients.

The testicular vessels are exceedingly short in the prune-belly patient. Standard or staged orchiopexy is rarely successful under these circumstances. The Fowler-Stephens technique of orchiopexy has been used in patients with prune-belly syndrome with a success rate of 75%.[6] The surgery involves division of the testicular vessels intra-abdominally, as proximally as possible. This maneuver preserves the anastomotic connections between the vessels of the vas deferens and the distal spermatic vessels. Ideally, a layer of pelvic peritoneum should be left over the vas deferens to preserve these collaterals. Some surgeons have even staged this technique by clamping or dividing the spermatic vessels and then bringing the testes down on the vessels of the vas deferens at a later date.

Successful autotransplantation of the abdominal testes into the scrotum in the prune-belly syndrome was reported in 1976.[7] It has become a useful procedure to surgeons with a special expertise in microsurgery. Here the testicular vessels are anastomosed to the inferior epigastric vessels. The principles of the Fowler-Stephens technique are also observed in performing this procedure. In part, success with autotransplantation may depend on the collateral circulation provided by the vessels of the vas deferens. Since many of these patients are older, however, their spermatogenic potential may not be improved by orchiopexy. The success rate with this procedure has been reported to be 100%.[8] Most series, however, are small, with only a limited follow-up.[15–17]

Orchiopexy in patients with the prune-belly syndrome is best performed within the first few months of life.[9] The distance over which the intra-abdominal testes must be moved to place them within the scrotum becomes greater as the infant grows in length. Often the procedure can be effectively performed without division of the spermatic vessels. The vessels are mobilized transperitoneally to their origin, after which the testis is passed directly through the abdominal wall at the site of the external ring and into the scrotum. This procedure is best performed in infancy, at the time of urinary reconstruction. A high success rate has been achieved in a limited follow-up.[9] Ultimate testicular function has, however, not been ascertained in this series.

Men with the prune-belly syndrome are infertile. This is related to several factors. The bladder neck is generally felt to be incompetent, causing retrograde ejaculation. The prostatic urethra is abnormal, as are the ejaculatory ducts and the bulbus urethra. There are conflicting reports as to the histology of the testes in the prune-belly syndrome. Normal testicular histology has been noted.[10] More recent observations suggest an absence of spermatogonia.[11] Others report patients with early spermatogenesis.[4] These varied observations may reflect the timing of testicular biopsy and orchiopexy rather than an intrinsic abnormality of the testis itself. Early orchiopexy may have the potential to improve this picture.

It has been suggested that the neoplastic potential of the testes in the prune-belly syndrome may be different from that of other intra-abdominal testes. Historically, the majority of patients with the syndrome rarely survived into adulthood, and hence the tumor potential of these testes has not been established. Two cases of testicular neoplasm in patients with the prune-belly syndrome have been reported.[12, 13] While early orchiopexy may not decrease the tumor potential, it allows both the patient and the physician to easily examine for and detect abnormalities.

Adults with the prune-belly syndrome have normal secondary sex characteristics and a normal libido with normal erections and orgasms. Their serum testosterone levels are also normal. The levels of follicle stimulating hormone (FSH), however, are increased in all patients with the syndrome, indicating poor tubular function and correlating with failure of spermatogenesis. Additionally, patients with high intra-abdominal testes were noted to have high levels of luteinizing hormone (LH), correlating with the lack of gonadal tissue.[14] The production of LH is controlled by testosterone through negative feedback, so that normal testosterone levels should be associated with normal levels of LH. The high levels of LH found in patients with prune-belly syndrome suggest that a high pituitary drive may be required to induce the testes to produce adequate levels of testosterone.

Late orchiopexy in the prune-belly syndrome has produced adults with normal secondary sexual development, but with testes that are small, atrophic, and poorly functioning. Transabdominal orchiopexy in infancy has resulted in viable intrascrotal testes. Whether this will result in an improvement in overall testicular function remains to be seen.

BILATERALLY IMPALPABLE TESTES IN THE OTHERWISE NORMAL PATIENT

In many respects the model of the prune-belly patient with bilaterally impalpable testes does not fit the otherwise normal male with impalpable testes. In the patient with prune-belly syndrome it is presumed that testes are present, but this is not the case for the otherwise normal patient with impalpable testes. Hormonal stimulation was not recommended for the former group of patients because there was little doubt about the presence of testicular tissue. The presence or absence of testes and their response to hormonal stimulation is, however, an important aspect of the non-prune-belly patient with impalpable testes. Although failure to respond to hCG with an increased testosterone level would suggest the absence of normally functioning testicular tissue, particularly in the face of elevated levels of FSH and LH, it still does not rule out the presence of poorly functioning testicular tissues. In patients 10 years of age and older, nonpalpable testicular tissue would imply a low potential for fertility, and this may be true even for younger patients (aged 2 and over). Therefore, the major indication for orchiopexy in such patients is early tumor detection. Orchiopexy probably does not change the potential for tumorigenesis, and when done after the age of 2 years, may not improve the potential for fertility.

BILATERALLY IMPALPABLE TESTES WITH INTERSEX

Bilaterally impalpable testes in a patient with hypospadias requires careful evaluation for intersex. These patients should be identified while newborns, so that proper management can be instituted.

REFERENCES

1. Jeffs RD, Comisarow RH, Hanna MK: The early assessment for individualized treatment in the prune-belly syndrome. *Birth Defects* 1977; 13:97.
2. Woodhouse CRJ, Kellett MJ, Williams DI: Minimal surgical interference in prune-belly syndrome. *Br J Urol* 1979; 51:475.
3. Fowler R, Jr, Stephens FD: The role of testicular vascular anatomy in the salvage of high undescended testes. *Aust NZ J Surg* 1954; 29:92.
4. Woodhouse CRJ, McC Snyder H III: Testicular and sexual function in adults with prune-belly syndrome. *J Urol* 1984; 133:607.

5. Levitt SB, Kogan SJ, Engel RM, et al: The impalpable testis: a rational approach to management. *J Urol* 1978; 120:515.
6. Gibbons MD, Cromie WJ, Duckett JW Jr: Management of the abdominal undescended testis. *J Urol* 1979; 122:76.
7. Silber SJ, Kelly J: Successful autotransplantation of an intra-abdominal testes to the scrotum by microvascular technique. *J Urol* 1976; 115:452.
8. Wacksman J, Dinner M, Straffon RA: Techniques of testicular autotransplantation using a microvascular technique. *Surg Gynecol Obstet* 1980; 150:399.
9. Woodard JR, Parrott TS: Orchiopexy in the prune-belly syndrome. *Br J Urol* 1978; 50:348.
10. Nunn IN, Stephens FE: The triad syndrome: A complete anomaly of the abdominal wall, urinary system and testes. *J Urol* 1961; 86:782.
11. Uehling DT: Testicular histology in the triad syndrome. *Soc Pediatr Urol Newsletter,* Dec 30, 1982.
12. Woodhouse CRJ, Ransley PG: Teratoma of the testes in the prune-belly syndrome. *Br J Urol* 1983; 55:580.
13. Duckett JW Jr: The prune-belly syndrome, in Holder, TM, Ashcroft KW (eds): The Surgery of Infants and Children. Philadelphia, WB Saunders, 1980, pp 802–815.
14. Lee PA, Hoffman WH, White JJ, et al: Serum gonadotropins in cryptorchidism An indication of function of testes. *Am J Dis Child* 1976; 127:530.
15. Belker AM: Urologic microsurgery—current perspectives: II. Orchidopexy and testicular homotransplantation. *Urology* 1980; 15:103.
16. Harrison CB, Kaplan GW, Sherz HC, et al: Microvascular autotransplantation of the intra-abdominal testis. *J Urol* 1990; 144:506–507.
17. Frey P, Bianchi A: Microvascular autotransplantation of intra-abdominal testes. *Prog Pediatr Surg* 1989; 23:115–125.

8

Testicular Torsion

Robert T. Soper, M.D.

> An 11-year-old boy experiences the sudden onset of right scrotal pain. This event is followed by nausea and vomiting. Examination of the inguinoscrotal area shows edema, slight discoloration, and a partially retracted tender testis. The white blood cell count is 13,000/mm^3 and the urinalysis is normal. A radioisotope scan of the testis shows minimal flow.

Virtually every item of this case history follows that of a prototypical case of testicular torsion. The age is typical: adolescence. The sudden onset of scrotal pain is characteristic. The nausea and the vomiting, which is probably reflexive, are classical. The physical findings of a high-riding, edematous, tender, and discolored testicle testifies to the effects of vascular and lymphatic obstruction, which occur secondary to the twist. The minimal flow seen on the radioisotope scan tends to confirm the diagnosis. The mildly elevated white blood cell (WBC) count and normal urinalysis rule against a bacterial cause for the event. The only discrepant feature of the case history is involvement of the right testis: torsion occurs twice as commonly on the left as on the right side.

Given this overwhelming evidence in support of testicular torsion, I would favor taking this boy directly to the operating room for surgical exploration; if the diagnosis is confirmed, detorsion and orchiopexy for the fixation of both testes with permanent sutures is indicated. The procedure on the right (involved) testis could be performed via an incision through the interscrotal raphe. The prophylactic fixation of the left (uninvolved) testicle would be performed via the same scrotal incision. We are not privy to the time elements in this case, but if surgical detorsion were effected within 24 hours of pain onset, a viable testicle would probably result.

TYPES OF TESTICULAR TORSION

Testicular torsion is one of the few potential gonadal disasters that can be completely reversed by early treatment. It can occur at any age, from prenatally to adulthood, but characteristically tends to peak perinatally and at adolescence. Furthermore, the types of torsion are different in these two age groups. Testicular torsion that occurs prenatally, perinatally, and in early infancy is characterized by a twist that involves the distal cord *above* the gonad and its coverings; because this twist is cephalad to the tunica vaginalis, it is termed *supravaginal* (or *extravaginal*) torsion. In distinction, testicular torsion in the older child, adolescent, or young adult is *intravaginal*: the testicle is suspended freely inside the tunica vaginalis (the so-called "bell-clapper" testicle) and the twist occurs inside the tunica.

Regardless of the type of torsion, the twist of the gonadal vascular pedicle has the same effects: obstruction first of venous and lymphatic return (testicular edema, enlargement, and pain) and then of arterial inflow (testicular necrosis). The torsion itself tends to elevate the testicle in the scrotum (retraction) and also to change its orientation. Also, regardless of the type of torsion, the anatomic abnormality that allowed the torsion to occur in the first place is likely to be present on the contralateral side, thus mandating exploration and surgical fixation of the other testis. Finally, common to both types of torsion is the need for rapid derotation of the torsion in order to salvage a viable testicle.

SUPRAVAGINAL (EXTRAVAGINAL) TESTICULAR TORSION

Prenatal testicular torsion is fortunately quite rare, but is one of the causes of an empty hemiscrotum discovered on physical examination of the male newborn. More commonly, supravaginal torsion occurs perinatally, perhaps triggered by the increased pressure and activity levels associated with the labor and delivery processes. Physical examination reveals an enlarged, discolored (bluish-red), and high-riding testicle on the affected side in an otherwise normal-appearing newborn boy. Failure of the mass to transilluminate distinguishes it from an acute hydrocele. Unfortunately, even with prompt surgical detorsion it is rare to salvage a viable testicle under these circumstances; contralateral orchiopexy is mandatory in the hope of preventing the same event from later destroying the remaining testicle.

More common than either of the above scenarios is to retrospectively make the diagnosis of supravaginal torsion long after the event, when investigating an older boy because of an empty hemiscrotum. Anorchia (rare) and cryptorchidism need to be excluded by appropriate examinations. A remote torsion as the source of testicular destruction is suggested when one can palpate a firm vas deferens emerging from the external (subcutaneous) inguinal ring, which then disappears some distance above the entry point into the scrotum, often terminating in a lump of scar tissue 1 to 2 mm in size. The diagnosis can be confirmed at exploration, perhaps in concert with placement of a scrotal prosthesis as well as contralateral orchiopexy.

The precise cause of supravaginal torsion is unknown, but since the twist occurs in the lower part of the cord and necroses both the gonad and the tunica vaginalis, the gonad must lack an effective tether to the bottom of the scrotum. Without this distal anchor (gubernaculum testis), the entire mass on the end of the cord is free to participate in the twist.

INTRAVAGINAL TESTICULAR TORSION

The more common, intravaginal testicular torsion characteristically occurs during the transition years into puberty (10 to 16 years), but has been reported from the neonatal period on into middle adulthood. Intravaginal torsion occurs because of an abnormal relationship of the tunica vaginalis to the testicle. Normally, the tunica envelops only about the anterior two-thirds of the testis. The posterior surface of the testis is normally affixed to the posterior scrotal wall; this fixation discourages torsion. In contrast, patients who develop intravaginal torsion have their testes completely surrounded by the tunica vaginalis. The testicle is suspended within this space, free to twist on its vascular pedicle (Fig 8–1). Occasionally, a lengthy mesorchium (which joins the testicle to the epididymis) will allow the testis to twist on this axis.

Historically, trauma and violent physical activity or unusual movements often precede the torsion, and may give the initial impetus to the twist. The testis is perhaps further predisposed by the process of growth and increasing weight brought about by normal pubertal changes. The stage for testicular torsion is thus set by the three factors of pubertal growth of the testis, its abnormal lack of tethering to the scrotal wall, and the stage of life at which violent physical activity is the rule.

Testicular torsion is clearly not always an "all-or-none" phenomenon. Upwards of one-third of patients with confirmed torsion give a history of previous similar episodes of testicular swelling and pain which spontaneously relent after only a few minutes or hours. Further, some reports document that orchiopexy undertaken in one of these patients during an asymptomatic interval can confirm a "bell-clapper" anatomy and provide subsequent relief from these intermittent episodes. Unquestionably this is the ideal way in which to manage the problem, but unfortunately the opportunity rarely presents itself.[1, 2]

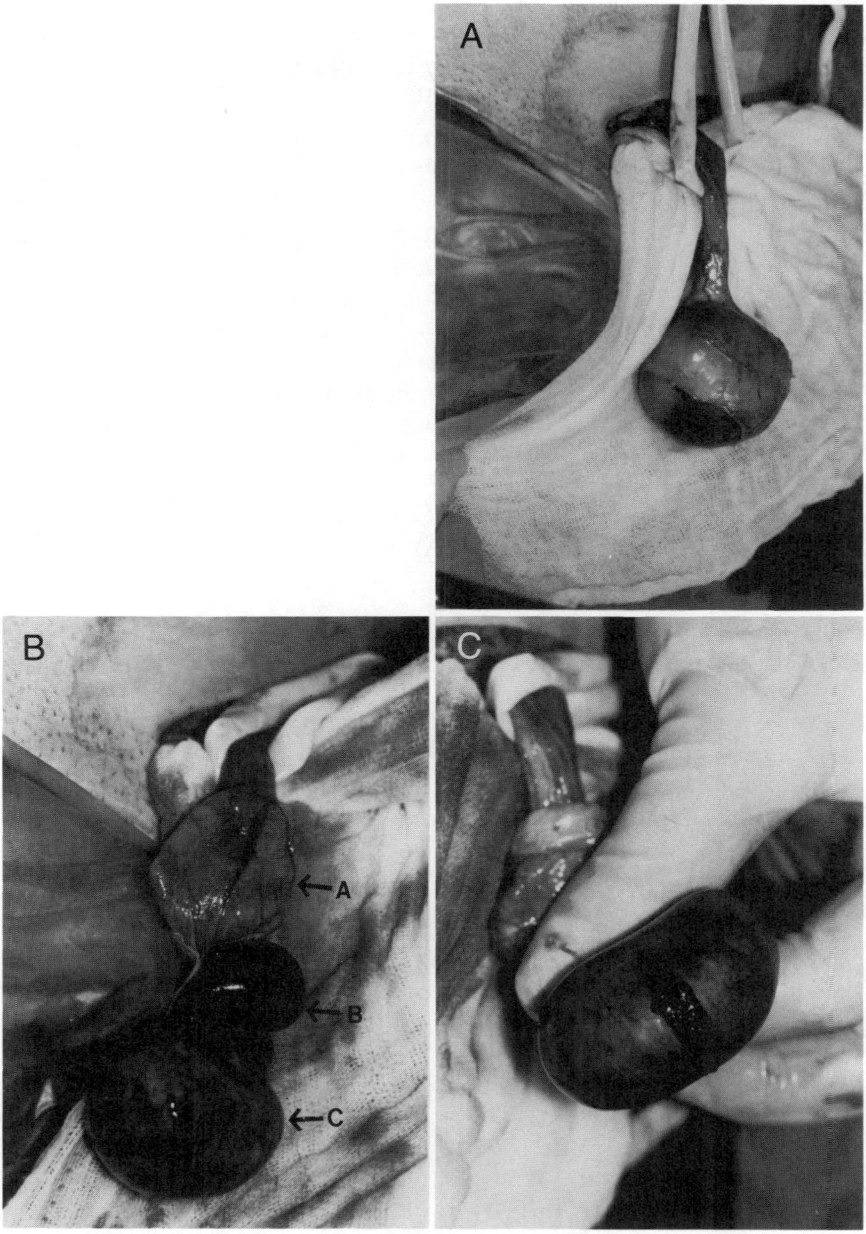

FIG 8–1.
A, the entire cord and gonad are exteriorized. There is no supravaginal torsion evident, but the tunica is suspiciously discolored. **B,** the tunica vaginalis has been opened *(arrow A)* and the dark supravaginal torsion *(arrow B)* is seen, as well as the discolored, turgid testicle *(arrow C).* **C,** an incision into the tunica albuginea confirms necrosis of the testicle.

TORSION OF THE GONADAL APPENDICES

Torsion of the appendix testis or appendix epididymis (both vestigial müllerian remnants) clinically mimics testicular torsion, and must be discussed with this subject (Fig 8–2). These tiny appendages are situated at the upper pole of the testis (or epididymis), and attain clinical significance only when they undergo torsion. Sudden onset of testicular pain (often during sleep), with enlargement and tenderness of the scrotal contents, make the distinction from testicular torsion extremely difficult. Early on, one might identify appendix torsion by noting a "blue dot" discoloration visible through the skin at the site in the upper testis where a tender pea-sized mass may be appreciated. Later in the evolution of the case, edema within the scrotal contents obliterates both of these distinctive signs, leaving a testicle that lies low in the scrotum as the only finding that tends to rule against testicular torsion.

DIFFERENTIAL DIAGNOSIS

Other causes for scrotal pain and swelling must be considered in our 11-year-old male proband. Epididymo-orchitis is numerically the next most common

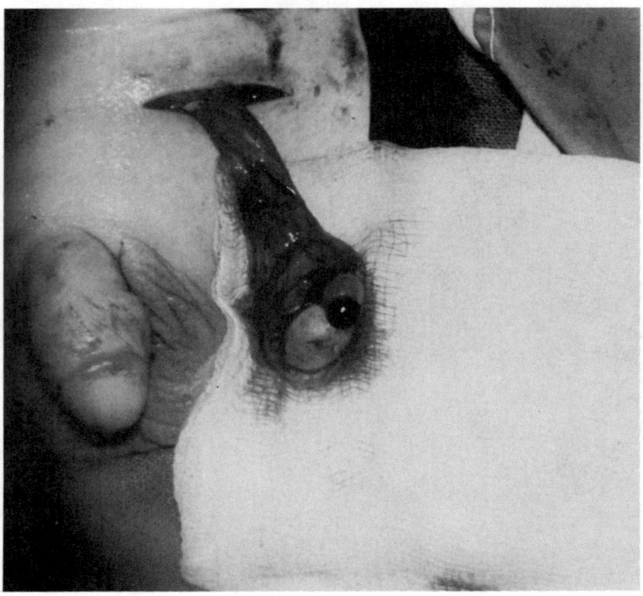

FIG 8–2.
The dark spot represents an appendix epididymis infarcted by torsion. The preoperative diagnosis was probable testicular torsion.

cause for testicular pain and swelling in adolescents after testicular torsion, with a frequency equivalent to that of torsion of the gonadal appendages. Again, examination early in the course of the disease may disclose that only the epididymis or only the testis is enlarged and tender, but these distinctions are quickly lost later in the event. However, the testis would be low-lying in the scrotum, and bilateral involvement would be common. Pyuria, a high WBC count with a left shift, and a history of recent urethral instrumentation would be helpful in making the correct diagnosis if bacteria are implicated. Viral orchitis is unlikely in this young age group. Traumatic injury to the scrotum should be evident from the history and the presence of ecchymosis, a hematoma, or other marks of physical injury.

Idiopathic scrotal edema is an unusual cause for this kind of symptom complex. The pain is not nearly so severe as in torsion or epididymo-orchitis, the condition often being heralded merely by a waddling gait. Examination reveals edema, erythema, and tenderness, which are most marked in the scrotal skin rather than in the scrotal contents, the skin changes often being bilateral and extending into the perineum. The testis is normal in location and is nontender. The event is short-lived, rarely lasting more than 24 to 48 hours; laboratory values are normal and antihistamines are helpful in treating the condition. As its name suggests, the cause of this entity is unknown.

Incarcerated inguinal hernia should not be difficult to exclude, since its discomfort is more centrally abdominal and colicky than scrotal, and its tender mass with discoloration is usually located above the scrotum rather than confined to it. Furthermore, incarceration is much more common in younger boys with hernias.

Varicocele is usually painless, and its spongy mass is palpable in the cord well above the testicle. Our patient is too young for a spermatocele and too old for the tender, enlarged testicle that occasionally complicates Henoch-Schōnlein syndrome. Moreover, scrotal and leg petechiae should confirm the latter diagnosis. A testicular tumor should have a hard, nontender mass as its distinguishing feature.

DIAGNOSIS

Testicular torsion should be the first diagnosis considered on the basis of the classic history and physical findings outlined in our prospectus. Confirmation of the diagnosis is most expediently and accurately made in the operating room. Since time is of the essence in salvaging the involved testicle, often no further workup is undertaken. However, there are noninvasive testing methods that help in the differential diagnosis. If they are immediately available, with experienced technicians and physician interpreters, and if the patient can cooperate so that a valid test can be done, then they are legitimate studies to consider having performed.

A testicular radionuclide study requires perhaps 2 hours to perform. A diminished or absent uptake in the involved testis as compared with its normal mate suggests testicular torsion, whereas trauma and epididymo-orchitis should be marked by an increased uptake. A Doppler ultrasound examination reveals blood flow to and in the testes; again, lack of flow as compared to the other normal testis suggests torsion, whereas normal or increased flow would be expected in trauma or epididymo-orchitis. Delay, inexperienced technicians or interpreters of these tests, or an uncooperative patient mandate against even considering these diagnostic undertakings.

TREATMENT

The only definitive management that we recommend for testicular torsion is surgical detorsion and suture fixation of the involved testicle, with prophylactic orchiopexy of the contralateral testis to prevent future torsion of that member. Operation should be undertaken as soon as the diagnosis is suspected. It provides accurate visual (and biopsy) evidence about the viability of the testis; permits an infarcted testis to be removed; and enables the circulation of a questionably or definitely viable testis to be restored by derotation, with fixation of its position by sutures to prevent recurrence. Surgical derotation and fixation must be considered the gold standard of treatment of this disorder.

However, the manual derotation of testicular torsion, first described by Burkitt in 1956,[3] is feasible. In 1983, Duckett et al. reported 8 successful manual derotations in 11 cases of torsion, all of which were performed under sedation (morphine sulfate, 0.1 mg/kg IV) with return of normal testicular blood flow confirmed by Doppler ultrasound examination.[4] Dramatic relief of pain and return of a soft, normal-sized testicle is further evidence of successful detorsion. Gentle rotation of the testis through one-and-a-half rotations toward the respective outer thigh is the appropriate method of manual detorsion, but Duckett is quick to emphasize that this is only a stopgap treatment. If successful, it indeed immediately restores blood flow to the testis, but surgical exploration at the earliest convenience is still needed to confirm the results and suture-fix the testis in place. Successful manual detorsion buys time to perhaps better prepare the patient for surgery.

Surgical detorsion can be accomplished either via a groin crease incision (used for hernia repairs) or directly through the scrotum. I prefer the groin route because the entire lower cord and testis can be delivered into the wound easily and the orchiopexy sutures can be placed more accurately. However, a trans-scrotal route is also accepted. An incision in the interscrotal raphe allows access to both testes.

After derotation of a supravaginal torsion, the testis is anchored in the most dependent portion of the hemiscrotum by silk sutures taken between the bottom of the tunica vaginalis and the dartos fascia; these sutures may incorporate small bites in the tunica albuginea of the testis. Disposable sutures are not recommended, since permanent fixation is desired.

In intravaginal torsion, the tunica needs to be widely opened to confirm the diagnosis, assess testicular viability, and perform a complete derotation under direct vision. Since the torsion occurs because of the free "bell-clapper" suspension of the testis inside the tunica vaginalis, successful fixation demands creating a broad area of permanent, dense adhesions between the tunica albuginea and the tunica vaginalis. We favor the "window" orchiopexy described in 1977 by Morse and Hollabaugh[5] to achieve this degree of fixation. In this technique, the edges of the opened tunica vaginalis are sutured to the tunica albuginea of the testis by six interrupted 4-0 silk sutures, leaving a substantial segment (2×2 cm in a teenager) of the testicle with no tunica covering it. This will permanently anchor the two surfaces together and eliminate the possibility of recurrence. Permanent sutures are recommended. The same "window" orchiopexy is performed prophylactically on the contralateral testis.

REFERENCES

1. Cass AS: Elective orchiopexy for recurrent testicular torsion. *J Urol* 1982; 127:253–254.
2. Chapman RH, Walton AJ: Torsion of the testis and its appendages. *Br Med J* 1972; 1:164–166.
3. Burkitt R: Torsion of the spermatic cord. A plea for manipulative reduction. *Br Med J* 1956; 2:345.
4. Betts JM, Norris M, Cromie WJ, et al: Testicular detorsion using Doppler ultrasound monitoring. *J Pediatr Surg* 1983; 18:607–610.
5. Morse TS, Hollabaugh RS: The "window" orchidopexy for prevention of testicular torsion. *J Pediatr Surg* 1977; 12:237–240.

PART TWO

Acute Abdominal Conditions

9

Acute Appendicitis

Robert M. Filler, M.D.

An 8-year-old boy developed mid-epigastric pain that was continuous in nature. He became anorexic and had nausea. The pain subsequently localized to the right side of the abdomen. The youngster refused to walk because of increasing pain. The rectal temperature was 38.1° C. The white blood cell count was 12,500/mm^3 with a slight shift to the left on the differential smear. The urinalysis was unremarkable. Physical examination showed some guarding in response to deep palpation in the right lower abdomen. Pain was also elicited by hyperextending the right leg.

HISTORY AND PATHOGENESIS

The example case presents with a classic history of appendicitis; namely, mid-abdominal pain that migrates to the right lower quadrant. Generally this transition occurs over a period of 6 to 12 hours. The periumbilical pain, which is crampy, is thought to be due to obstruction of the lumen of the appendix either by a fecalith or from lymphoid hyperplasia in the submucosal lymphatic "patches." Distention of the appendix distal to the obstruction results in mucosal ischemia, which interrupts mucosal integrity and allows bacterial invasion and transmural inflammation. Ultimately the infective process extends to the visceral and parietal peritoneum. The parietal peritoneal inflammation is responsible for the localized continuous pain noted by the patient in the region of the appendix. Untreated, the combination of obstruction and inflammation results in infarction of a portion of the appendiceal wall, and perforation. The perforation may be localized or may occur into the free peritoneal cavity, depending on the exact location of the appendix and its adherence to surrounding structures, such as the intestine and omentum. Usually, perforation of the appendix does not occur until at least 18 hours after the onset of symptoms, but in children under 4 years of age this interval is often shorter.

Vomiting is commonly associated with appendicitis. It usually begins after the onset of pain, at about the time that the pain shifts to the right lower quadrant. It is thought to be caused by peritoneal irritation. Vomiting is frequently present after perforation, owing to a paralytic ileus from peritonitis.

If all cases of appendicitis had a classic history, diagnosis of the condition would be extremely easy. However, only 50% present in this fashion. In others, the typical migration of pain to the right lower quadrant does not occur, or the pain may be felt in a different location, and gastrointestinal symptoms such as vomiting and diarrhea may suggest another etiology.

PHYSICAL EXAMINATION

In this typical case the patient was noted to have tenderness in the right lower quadrant. Persistent, reproducible, right-lower-quadrant tenderness is the most consistent feature of acute appendicitis. The decision about whether or not to operate in suspected cases is usually based on this finding. The right-lower-quadrant tenderness is often associated with involuntary guarding of the lower abdominal muscles. However, if the inflamed appendix does not lie near the anterior abdominal wall, and rests between loops of ileum or in the retrocecal space and points superiorly or inferiorly, then impressive right-lower-quadrant tenderness and muscle spasm may not be appreciated. When the appendix lies in an atypical position, aspects of the physical examination other than abdominal palpation become more important in detecting the point of inflammation. Rectal examination will reveal rectal tenderness when the tip of a retrocecal appendix extends into the cul de sac. Palpation along the flank and near the gallbladder may reveal tenderness and spasm when the appendix tip extends superiorly from its cecal origin. Hyperextension of the leg (psoas sign) evokes pain when a posteriorly located, inflamed appendix lies on the psoas muscle. Inflammation of the parietal peritoneum is associated with the presence of rebound tenderness, cough tenderness, and pain on moving. These findings indicate intra-abdominal inflammation, but are not diagnostic of acute appendicitis.

Since pneumonia may present with abdominal pain, careful examination of the chest, and especially the lower lung fields, is also essential in the evaluation of a patient with suspected appendicitis.

Typically, a low-grade fever, usually of 38° to 39° C, is seen in appendicitis. However, the presence or absence of fever and the degree of temperature elevation have minimal diagnostic significance. Some children with appendicitis are afebrile, and others present with fever as high as 40° C.

DIAGNOSTIC TESTS

To date, laboratory diagnosis has not been as accurate as clinical diagnosis in cases of acute appendicitis.

The white blood cell (WBC) count is often elevated in appendicitis, usually to between 11,000 and 20,000/mm^3. However, in our large experience with pediatric patients, many with appendicitis have a WBC below 10,000/mm^3, and many present with a WBC over 20,000/mm^3. Therefore, this test has minimal reliability.

Urinalysis is probably the most important test in children with an acute abdomen, because urinary tract infection or urinary stones may be the cause of the abdominal complaints. However, an inflamed appendix lying on a ureter or against the bladder also can cause pyuria, hematuria, or both. However, bacteria, which are often seen in the urine in urinary infections, will not be seen with appendicitis.

Roentgenograms of the abdomen are not obtained if a clinical diagnosis of acute appendicitis can be made. In doubtful cases, abdominal x-rays can be helpful. The presence of a fecalith is diagnostic. Left lumbar scoliosis suggests appendicitis, as does loss of the right psoas shadow. In some children the x-ray may indicate an alternative diagnosis such as intestinal obstruction. The finding of free peritoneal air will confirm the presence of perforation.

Abdominal ultrasound examination appears to have some value in the diagnosis of appendicitis in equivocal cases. Visualization of the appendix by ultrasound is suggestive, especially when the appendix cannot be compressed and when its diameter is greater than 6 mm. The presence of fluid around the appendix is also an important sonographic sign. Recent studies using high-resolution ultrasound have had an accuracy of about 90%, which is no better than that noted in most surgical series in which ultrasound was not used. Ultrasound examination is especially valuable in the evaluation of female pelvic structures when abnormalities of the fallopian tubes and ovaries are in the differential diagnosis.

Barium enema has been used by some to diagnose appendicitis. A positive examination comprises a partially filled appendix, indentation of the cecum by an inflammatory mass, or both. The specificity and sensitivity of this study appear to be so low that most children's centers do not employ it for this purpose.

Routine laparoscopy has been advocated by some in all equivocal cases of appendicitis. The major disadvantages of this procedure are that it requires a general anesthetic and, should it fail to reveal a cause of the acute pain, produces postoperative pain and gas in the peritoneal cavity that will hinder further evaluation. Nevertheless, laparoscopy is useful for making a specific diagnosis in a girl with a probable gynecologic abnormality.

DIFFERENTIAL DIAGNOSIS

Appendicitis is rare in children under 3 years of age, but must be considered in all children who present with a chief complaint of abdominal pain. Several common childhood conditions also present with abdominal pain and must be differentiated from appendicitis. Gastroenteritis due to viral or bacterial infection is the most common condition that presents with a syndrome often confused with appendicitis. In gastroenteritis the pain is usually colicky rather than steady. Vomiting often precedes the abdominal pain and diarrhea is often present. Unfortunately, diarrhea also occurs in appendicitis when inflamed appendix rests against the colon. With gastroenteritis, physical examination usually reveals mild and diffuse abdominal tenderness rather than localized pain. As in appendicitis, fever and an elevated WBC count may or may not be present and do not necessarily distinguish the two conditions. Further complicating the issue is that some children who end up with appendicitis start out with clinical findings typical of gastroenteritis, suggesting a viral etiology for appendicitis. In fact, it is well known that certain viral illnesses such as measles can be associated with appendicitis. Therefore, even when one is quite certain that a child's abdominal pain is due to gastroenteritis, the possibility of it evolving into appendicitis must be kept in mind until the abdominal symptoms cease.

Abdominal pain due to urinary tract infection is usually in the flank or suprapubic region. Dysuria occurs with bladder involvement. Microscopic examination of the urine is the most useful test for distinguishing urinary infection from appendicitis.

Abnormalities of the ovary, uterus, and adnexa must be considered in girls with abdominal pain, especially after puberty. A good history and careful examination, with rectal and pelvic examinations when indicated, will aid greatly in achieving a correct diagnosis. Pelvic ultrasound examination is extremely valuable in equivocal cases. Laparoscopy can also be useful in selected cases.

Upper respiratory infections commonly are associated with abdominal pain. Presumably the pain is due to inflammation of abdominal lymph nodes by the same organisms responsible for the respiratory illness. In these cases abdominal tenderness is minimal and persistent right-lower-quadrant tenderness is absent. Rarely, acute appendicitis and a respiratory infection coexist.

Constipation can be associated with crampy abdominal pain, but should not cause persistent right-lower-quadrant tenderness. One should always be wary of missing appendicitis when diagnosing constipation. In a child with steady abdominal pain in whom a large amount of stool is found in the colon on rectal examination or by abdominal x ray, a gentle saline enema can be useful. If done by a trained individual, the risk of perforation is minimal, and the procedure may have a dramatic effect on the truly constipated child.

TREATMENT AND RESULTS

Children with a clinical diagnosis of appendicitis, whether ruptured or not, are taken to the operating room as soon as they are fully hydrated. In those with a short illness, minimal preoperative fluid therapy is necessary. However, in the child with a ruptured appendix and several days of symptoms, 4 to 6 hours of fluid or colloid resuscitation or both may be required. A single dose of cefoxitin (40 mg/kg IV, 30 minutes prior to surgery) is recommended for wound prophylaxis in cases of an unruptured appendicitis. For patients with a ruptured appendix, antibiotics with superior aerobic and anaerobic coverage are indicated. We employ ampicillin (100 mg/kg/day), gentamycin (7.5 mg/kg/day), and clindamycin (50 mg/kg/day) for 5 to 7 days).

In surgery for appendicitis, a muscle-splitting right-lower-quadrant incision is used to enter the abdomen. The inflamed appendix is dissected free to its base and removed by amputating it distal to a ligature at its base. The stump is inverted into the cecum with a purse-string suture. If the appendix has ruptured, all pockets of pus are aspirated. Most surgeons at our center do not irrigate the abdominal cavity in cases of ruptured appendix, because the evidence is not convincing that it helps. In fact, such irrigation may be harmful because it can impair the function of the white cells present in the exudate. A drain is employed only to drain a local collection of pus. In the child who presents with an obvious appendiceal abscess many days after the onset of symptoms, appendectomy is usually delayed and treatment with antibiotics is started. If systemic symptoms do not subside rapidly, the abscess cavity should be drained by incision or percutaneously. In these cases an appendectomy is necessary approximately 6 weeks later, because recurrent appendicitis is likely.

About 10% of children who undergo surgery for appendicitis are found to have a normal appendix at surgery. In these cases appendectomy should be performed and the abdomen explored for inflammatory disease of the distal ileum, for Meckel's diverticulum, and for gynecologic disease in girls. In the overwhelming majority of cases, exploration will be negative and the child will experience an uneventful recovery.

Children with unruptured appendicitis usually leave the hospital within 3 days of surgery and resume normal activities within 10 days. The wound-infection rate in this group is usually under 5%. Other significant complications are rare. Those with ruptured appendicitis are kept in the hospital until the course of antibiotics is completed and fever and symptoms have subsided. Wound infection, intra-abdominal abscess, or both occur in 5% to 10% of cases. With current antibiotic therapy, complications from ruptured appendicitis have been markedly reduced and mortality virtually eliminated. Sterility due to blockage of the fallopian tubes from pelvic peritonitis is a well-recognized problem in girls who have had a ruptured appendix. However, the precise incidence of this complication is not known. Similarly, a ruptured appendix is associated with a greater risk of intra-abdominal adhesions, which can lead to late intestinal obstruction. Despite the low morbidity from acute appendicitis with current treatment, the potential long-term complications of rupture are ample reason to continue to strive for its early diagnosis and rapid treatment.

10

Intussusception

Karen W. West, MD

A 6-month-old boy developed diarrhea after two siblings in the family had gastroenteritis. Four days later, the baby was observed to draw up his legs and scream as if in pain. These episodes continued intermittently over the next few hours and the baby subsequently vomited an attempted feeding. This was followed by the passage of bloody mucus per rectum that had the appearance of "currant-jelly." The material tested positive for blood. The infant became progressively irritable and developed abdominal distention.

Intussusception is a frequent cause of bowel obstruction in infancy and childhood, and still remains one of the most common surgical emergencies in this age group. Although intussusception can occur at any age, the majority of cases (80%) are seen in children under 2 years of age (Table 10–1). Intussusception is more common in boys than girls, and most children affected with it are well-nourished and otherwise healthy babies. The clinical presentation includes the episodic abdominal pain of sudden onset characterized by screaming, irritability, and drawing the legs toward the abdomen. These episodes occur with increasing frequency and decreasing intervals between them, and may be followed by emesis. Initially the gastric content is clear, but the emesis may become bilious as the distal small-bowel obstruction progresses. The child may play or lie quietly in between the episodes of crampy pain. This may progress to lethargy, and in a few cases to unresponsiveness that can be easily confused with meningitis (until a normal spinal tap is obtained or a bloody stool is passed). The appearance of blood in the stool varies from the characteristic "currant-jelly" discharge (a combination of blood and mucous due to venous congestion) to material that is positive on a stool guaiac test, or frankly bright red blood.

The intussusception is idiopathic in 75% to 90% of cases. Sixty percent of infants with intussusception were seen by an office-based physician or evalu-

TABLE 10–1.
Age Distribution of Intussusception in 110 Patients at the James Whitcomb Riley Hospital for Children

	TOTAL CASES	
AGE	(NO.)	(%)
0–6 mo	33	(31)
6–12 mo	35	(32)
1–2 yr	20	(20)
2–4 yr	20	(10)
>4 yr	9	(7)

ated in an emergency-room setting at least once prior to their referral to our facility for treatment. There may be a history of a preceding viral illness, otitis media, or gastroenteritis in up to 30% of cases. It is possible that the lymphoid-rich tissue in the terminal ileum hypertrophies in response to viral infections and allows the Peyer's patches to act as a lead point.[1] The older child (>5 years) is more likely to have an identifiable lead point, including polyps (juvenile, Peutz-Jeghers), small bowel (B-cell) lymphomas, Meckel's diverticulum, duplication cysts, an inverted appendiceal stump, or the viscid stool associated with cystic fibrosis. Bowel-wall hematomas in children recovering from Henoch-Schönlein purpura may also act as a lead point, and are more commonly small bowel intussusceptions. Most cases of idopathic intussusception are of the ileocolic variety (Table 10–2).

On initial physical examination, a "sausage shaped" mass may be palpated in the right upper quadrant, with an empty right lower quadrant. The abdomen may be distended (depending on the duration of symptoms) and the child may appear gravely ill. Fever (>38° C) and leukocytosis (usually >10,000/mm^3) are common findings. In the last 110 children with intussusception treated at James Whitcomb Riley Hospital for Children (a tertiary care facility), the most common presenting symptoms and physical findings included vomiting (81%), pain (77%), rectal bleeding (64%), a palpable abdominal mass (60%), and lethargy or sepsis (39%). In three patients in this series the intussusception could

TABLE 10–2.
Types of Intussusception in 110 Cases

Ileocolic	98
Colocolic	5
Ileoileal	4
Jejunojejunal	3

be palpated on rectal examination. Evidence of peritonitis is a rare finding because the ischemic, potentially necrotic lead point (intussusceptum) is entirely within the lumen of the distal normal intestine (the intussuscipiens). Abdominal tenderness results from bowel distention, stretching of the highly innervated peritoneum, and the intermittent invagination of the bowel into the bowel.

DIAGNOSIS AND TREATMENT

A high index of suspicion coupled with prompt diagnostic and radiologically directed therapeutic intervention to safely reduce the intussusception may obviate the need for surgery. The barium enema has remained the mainstay of diagnosis and therapy since the early 1930s, when the technique was popularized in this country by Ravitch.[2] Few complications of this technique are reported when standard guidelines are followed. These include hydrostatic pressure with a barium column no more than 3 feet above the patient, no abdominal manipulations, and limitation of the reduction attempts to 5 minutes each. Preparation for reduction includes a nasogastric tube for gastric decompression, intravenous fluid resuscitation, and antibiotic coverage (usually ampicillin, gentamicin, and clindamycin). The surgeon observes the procedure and the operating room is alerted so that the transition from the radiology department to the operating room suite is accomplished expeditiously for irreducible cases. Sedation may be helpful during the barium study, but should not be administered until intravascular fluid deficits have been corrected (Table 10–3). Although glucagon (a relaxant of colonic smooth muscle) has been recommended as an adjunct to increase the success rate of barium reduction, its efficacy was not established in a recent radomized, multicenter study.[3]

The presence of a mass and a "coiled-spring sign" on barium contrast study usually confirms the diagnosis of intussusception. Following a hydrostatic barium enema, a complete reduction is noted when free flow of contrast material is demonstrated in at least the last 2 feet of terminal ileum (Fig 10–1,A and B). The intussusception reduction rate following hydrostatic barium enema varies

TABLE 10–3.
Sedation Prior to Reduction Attempts

Morphine (>1 yr)	0.1 mg/kg IM
Secobarbital	1 mg/kg IM
Meperidine*	1 mg/kg IM
Promethazine*	0.5 mg/kg
Chlorpromazine*	0.5 mg/kg

*These three are used in combination.

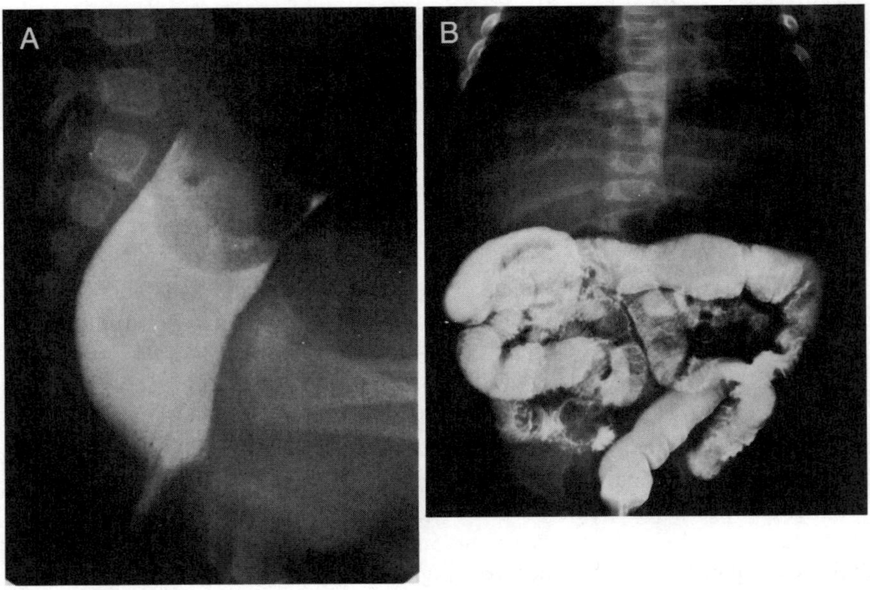

FIG 10–1.
Even though the intussusception was palpable in the rectum on initial examination **(A)**, complete hydrostatic barium reduction was possible **(B)**.

from 43% to 84%, and is related to the duration of symptoms as well as the skill of the radiologist. If symptoms have been present for more than 72 hours and a high-grade bowel obstruction is noted on plain radiographs, the chance for a successful reduction is significantly reduced. In these cases, a diagnostic barium enema procedure should be performed and prompt surgical intervention undertaken without attempting hydrostatic reduction.

Ultrasonically guided hydrostatic reduction techniques have also been reported using water-soluble contrast materials. The Chinese have reported 6,000 patients in whom air-pressure reduction has been utilized.[4] Under fluoroscopic guidence, air is carefully insufflated into the rectum to obtain reduction pressures of 80 mm Hg in infants and 110 mm Hg in children. Following initially unsuccessful attempts, efforts at reduction are repeated in 1 to 2 hours. This procedure has a reported success rate of 91% and a perforation rate of 0.14%, and requires more than one application in most children. A complete reduction occurs when there is flow of air into at least 2 feet of terminal ileum. In a recent comparative study from Toronto,[5] the rate of successful reduction of intussusception and risk of bowel perforation were similar with air or barium reduction.

The rate of bowel perforation during hydrostatic reduction varies from 0.7% to 2.0%. of reported cases.[5] Perforation most frequently occurs in the transverse colon (Fig 10–2). The blood supply to the transverse colon becomes

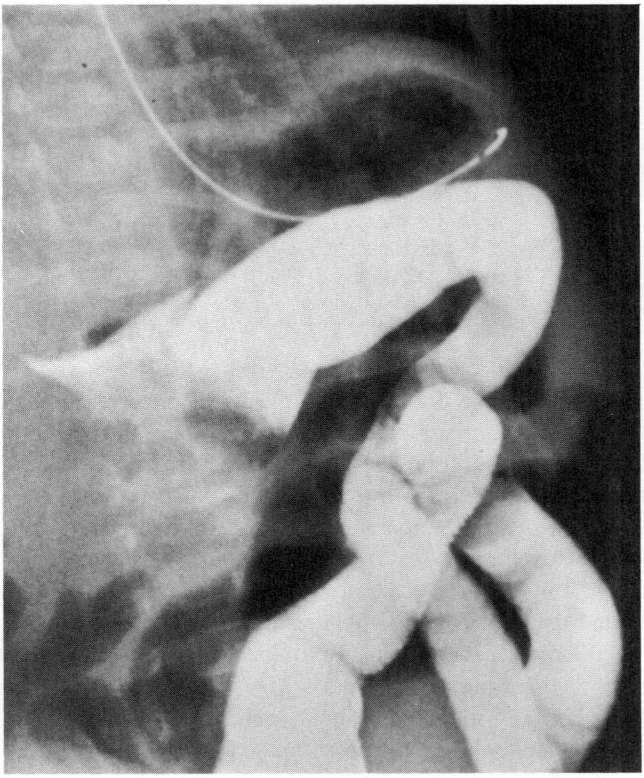

FIG 10–2.
A perforation in the transverse colon is noted on this diagnostic barium enema for intussusception.

compromised by the invagination of bowel, resulting in severe venous and lymphatic congestion. When back-pressure exceeds the arterial perfusion pressure, full-thickness tissue necrosis may occur. Most cases of perforation are not necessarily associated with attempts at excessive hydrostatic pressure reduction, but are noted in children under 6 months of age who have been ill for 3 to 4 days. Six of 110 children had a transverse colon perforation; in 3 this was observed during attempted reduction of intussusception, 2 others had perforations noted at laparotomy after attempted reduction, and 1 girl presented with free peritoneal air due to spontaneous perforation prior to any reduction attempts.[5]

Following the successful hydrostatic reduction of intussusception, an elevated temperature (above 38° C) is commonly noted. This may be due to release of bacterial toxins or intestinal bacterial translocation. Nasogastric decompression is maintained until bowel function returns (as documented by the passage of stool). Feedings may then be initiated and advanced as tolerated. Re-

TABLE 10–4.
Postoperative Complications of Surgery for Intussusception

Fever >38.5° C	70
Ileus >7 days	8
Wound infection	8
Pneumonia	4
Urinary tract infection	2
Ostomy stenosis	2
Wound dehiscence	2
Intra-abdominal abscess	2

current intussusception may follow radiologically directed hydrostatic reduction in 8% to 12% of cases, and can occur during the same hospitalization or months later. Parents should be warned of this possibility.

In patients in whom nonoperative reduction fails, prompt operative intervention is required. An intubation is performed with the patient awake, to minimize the risk of aspiration due to bowel obstruction. Laparotomy is accomplished through a right-lower-quadrant transverse incision. The intussusception is identified and the right colon is mobilized. Manual reduction is attempted as the intussusception is carefully milked proximally. Following reduction, an appendectomy is usually performed, and when present, Jackson's veil (a thick band of tissue between the cecum and terminal ileum) is divided. If serosal splitting is encountered during attempted reduction, or the lead-point mass cannot be reduced, a bowel resection is undertaken to prevent perforation and subsequent peritoneal contamination. Bowel resection may be required in 35% to 41% of patients.[6] Primary anastomosis may be safely performed in most cases; however, if there is considerable peritoneal contamination, barium peritonitis, or hemodynamic instability, a temporary enterostomy can be fashioned. Postoperative complications may be encountered, with fever, prolonged adynamic ileus, wound infection, and pneumonia being the most common (Table 10–4).

Although there were no deaths in our series of patients, significant morbidity and increased health-care costs have resulted from a delay in diagnosis, es-

TABLE 10–5.
Length of Hospitalization for Treatment of Intussusception

TREATMENT	DAYS
Barium enema reduction	1.5 (range 1–4)
Intraoperative reduction	7.2 (range 3–29)
Bowel resection	10.2 (range 4–47)

pecially in cases with bowel perforation or those requiring intestinal resection (Table 10–5). A high index of suspicion coupled with timely rehydration and prompt diagnostic measures may obviate the need for surgical reduction.

REFERENCES

1. Konno T, Suzuki H, Jutsuzawa T, et al: Human rotavirus infection in infants and young children with intussusception. *J Med Virol* 1982; 2:265.
2. Ravitch MM, McCune RM: Reduction of intussusception by hydrostatic pressure: an experimental study. *Bull Johns Hopkins Hosp* 1948; 82:550–552.
3. Franken EA, Smith WL, Chernish SM, et al: The use of glucagon in hydrostatic reduction in intussusception: A double blind study of 30 patients. *Radiology* 1983; 146:687.
4. Guo JB, Ma K, Zhou Q: Results of air pressure enema reduction of intussusception: 6,396 cases in 13 years. *J Pediatr Surg* 1986; 12:1201–1203.
5. Ein SU, Mercer S, Hymphrey A, et al: Colon perforation during attempted barium reduction of intussusception. *J Pediatr Surg* 1988; 16:313–315.
6. West KW, Stephen SB, Vane DW, et al: Intussusception: Current management in infants and children. *Surgery* 1987; 102:704–710.

11

Malrotation With Midgut Volvulus

Frederick J. Rescorla, M.D.
Jay L. Grosfeld, M.D.

A 3.1-kg term infant girl was born by normal spontaneous vaginal delivery at 38 weeks' gestation. The postpartum course was uneventful and the infant was discharged with the mother on the fourth day of life. She was well until age 17 days when she developed bilious vomiting. The infant was unable to take feedings and became listless. Bilious vomiting continued and the infant passed blood mixed with tissue per rectum. She was taken to the pediatric emergency room.

This case presentation, concerning a previously healthy infant in the first month of life who develops feeding intolerance of sudden onset and bilious vomiting with subsequent passage of blood per rectum, is a classical description of an infant with intestinal malrotation and acute midgut volvulus. Initial management of this infant would involve rapid intravenous hydration, administration of broad-spectrum antibiotics, and urgent exploration. Factors supporting the diagnosis would include abdominal distention and plain abdominal radiographs demonstrating gas in the stomach and duodenum with an otherwise gasless abdomen. At laparotomy the clockwise midgut volvulus would be detorsioned in a counterclockwise direction. The appearance of the bowel after detorsion will determine the surgical options. In order to fully understand the potentially lethal process of malrotation, one must review the basic embryologic steps that result in normal bowel rotation and fixation.

EMBRYOLOGY OF MALROTATION

The normal embryologic events of intestinal rotation and fixation occur between the 4th and 12th week of fetal life. At the fourth fetal week the entire bowel is basically a straight tube with the superior mesenteric artery (SMA) supplying the future small bowel and proximal colon (e.g., the midgut). Snyder and Chaffin[1] divided this bowel into two segments: the portion proximal to the SMA, designated the duodenojejunal loop, and the portion distal to the SMA, called the cecocolic loop. Each loop rotates 270 degrees counterclockwise around the SMA (as one faces the SMA). The duodenojejunal loop starts above the SMA and passes initially to the right and then below the SMA by the eighth fetal week. During this time the bowel is extracoelomic as it temporarily passes into the body stalk. With the return of the small bowel to the abdomen at the 10th fetal week, it completes its rotation to the left of the SMA, which is its final resting place—the ligament of Treitz. The duodenum thereby forms the normal C-sweep, with the third portion of the duodenum passing under the SMA. The distal cecocolic loop also rotates 270 degrees counterclockwise around the SMA. This loop, however, starts below the SMA, rotating initially to the left, then above, and finally to the right of the SMA. The cecum then further descends to its usual location in the right lower quadrant.

CLASSIFICATION

An interruption in the rotational events described above, or in the subsequent fixation process, gives rise to the various types of malrotation. The term malrotation is really a misnomer, but remains in the literature through longstanding common usage. Nonrotation, the proper term in the current case presentation, refers to a situation in which the duodenojejunal loop does not rotate around the SMA but remains on the right side of the abdomen. The cecocolic loop remains on the left side of the SMA. Incomplete rotation refers to an interruption prior to complete rotation of the proximal duodenojejunal loop around the SMA. In both of these instances the clinical problem, as pointed out by Ladd,[2, 3] is related to the lack of fixation of the small bowel, so that the intestine is supported by a narrow pedicle consisting of the SMA. The entire small bowel may then undergo a twist, usually in a clockwise direction, resulting in midgut volvulus (Fig 11–1). In addition, the cecum and proximal colon are located close to the duodenum, and peritoneal fixation bands form from the cecum to the right lateral abdominal wall, crossing over the duodenum (Fig 11–2). These abnormal fixation bands can cause duodenal obstruction. Abnormalities of fixation can lead to a mesocolic (paraduodenal) hernia. A right mesocolic hernia occurs when the proximal duodenojejunal loop fails to rotate and is then trapped

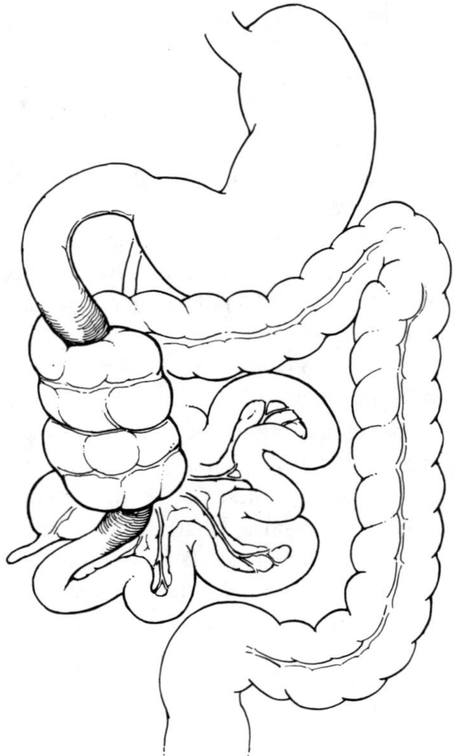

FIG 11–1.
Illustration of volvulus of the entire small bowel and proximal colon around the narrow pedicle based on the superior mesenteric artery. (From Rescorla FJ: Anomalies of rotation and fixation: Anatomy and complications. *Surg Rounds* (in press). Used by permission.)

within the mesentery of the right colon as it continues with a normal rotation and fixation. A left mesocolic hernia develops when the small bowel herniates under the inferior mesenteric vein into the mesentery of the left colon.

CLINICAL PRESENTATION AND DIAGNOSIS

Abnormalities of rotation and fixation can present in an otherwise healthy child with symptoms of duodenal obstruction from Ladd's bands, intermittent or acute volvulus, or symptoms related to intermittent obstruction with a right or left mesocolic (paraduodenal) hernia. In addition, children whose viscera are displaced by a developmental abnormality such as gastroschisis, omphalocele, or congenital diaphragmatic hernia frequently have nonrotation or incomplete

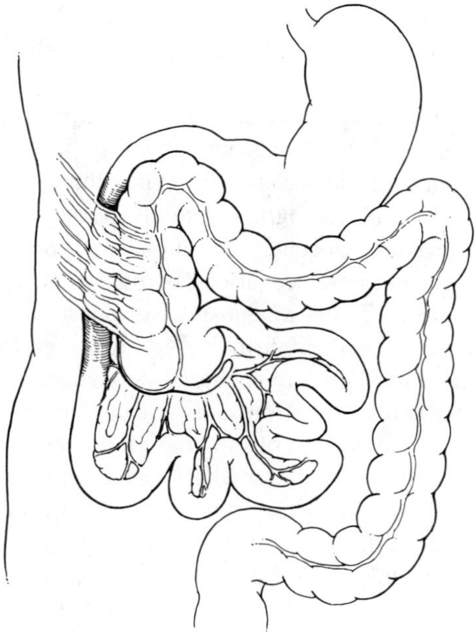

FIG 11–2.
The abnormal appearance of nonrotation. The duodenum descends on the right side of the abdomen and the cecum remains in the midabdomen, with Ladd's bands crossing obliquely from the cecum, over the duodenum, and to the right lateral abdominal wall. (From Rescorla FJ: Anomalies of rotation and fixation: Anatomy and complications. *Surg Rounds* (in press) Used by permission.)

rotation as well as lack of fixation, since the intestine resides outside the abdominal cavity. Children with these defects rarely develop midgut volvulus, probably because of adhesion formation following the neonatal surgery to correct their anomaly, which prevents the occurrence of volvulus. Malrotation is frequently also noted in infants born with duodenal and jejunoileal atresia. These infants, however, undergo surgery for bowel obstruction in the first few days of life, and their malrotation is identified and corrected at the time of their primary surgical procedure.

Malrotation with acute midgut volvulus usually occurs in an otherwise healthy infant. Presentation frequently occurs within the first month of life. In a recent review of cases involving infants with midgut volvulus at our institution, 83% were under 30 days of age.[4] Initial presenting features include abdominal pain of sudden onset followed by bilious emesis and abdominal distention. Passage of blood or in some instances sloughed mucosal tissue per rectum occurs as the process progresses, owing to vascular compromise of the intestine. The abdomen becomes progressively more tender as the ischemia involves the serosal surface of the bowel and sequestration of fluid in the abdomen results in peritoneal irritation.

Plain abdominal radiographs in cases of malrotation frequently demonstrate air in the stomach and proximal duodenum (just proximal to the neck of the volvulus) in an otherwise gasless abdomen. When the history, physical examination, and plain abdominal radiographs are consistent with midgut volvulus, these observations provide adequate indications for proceeding with surgical exploration. In the current case scenario, malrotation with volvulus would be the most likely diagnosis. If the diagnosis is in question, however, a rapidly performed contrast study will confirm it. An upper gastrointestinal contrast study will demonstrate a dilated stomach and duodenum with an abrupt cutoff at the neck of the volvulus. A barium enema can also be employed, and will frequently demonstrate obstruction of the proximal colon as it enters the volvulus, or else will demonstrate an abnormally located cecum. In a previous report from our institution, the initial history, physical examination, and plain abdominal radiographs were adequate for diagnosis in 12 of 18 cases of malrotation and midgut volvulus in infants. In six cases, contrast studies were performed (four upper gastrointestinal, two barium enema) to confirm the diagnosis.[4] Our current preference is to use the upper gastrointestinal contrast study.

TREATMENT

The patient with midgut volvulus is frequently tachycardic and hypovolemic, and requires prompt intravenous fluid resuscitation. This should be accomplished immediately upon the infant's arrival in the emergency room, and simultaneously with the clinical evaluation and preoperative preparation. A nasogastric tube is inserted to decompress the stomach and prevent aspiration. Broad-spectrum antibiotics are administered, since bacteria may be translocated through the necrotic bowel wall. Prompt laparotomy is undertaken through a generous supraumbilical transverse incision. The volvulus generally occurs in a clockwise manner, and is therefore detorsioned in a counterclockwise direction. With detorsion of the volvulus, toxins may be released into the superior mesenteric vein. After detorsion the bowel is assessed for viability. If the entire bowel becomes pink and appears completely viable, a Ladd procedure is performed by dividing the bands that pass from the cecum across the duodenum to the right side of the abdomen; duodenojejunal bands, if present, are also divided. This widens the base of the mesentery, allowing the duodenum to pass straight down the right lateral abdominal wall, with the jejunum and ileum suspended from its broad-based mesentery in the right and midabdomen. The cecum is placed in the left lower quadrant just medial to the sigmoid colon, with the right colon ascending on the left side of the abdomen to the splenic flexure, where it turns back to descend as the left and sigmoid colon (Fig 11–3). We would generally remove the appendix at this time (if the base of the cecum appeared completely normal), since it will not reside in the right lower quadrant and could lead to confusion and delay in diagnosis if the child developed appendicitis at a later date.

Occasionally, a segmental portion of the proximal small bowel at the neck of the volvulus will be necrotic. In two recent cases we have resected these segments, closing each end with an autostapling device, rather than creating a high jejunostomy. Owing to hemodynamic instability and discoloration of the bowel, an immediate anastomosis was not performed. After 24 to 48 hours a second-look procedure was performed, and since the bowel proved healthy, bowel continuity was restored with an end-to-end anastomosis. These children required several weeks of total parenteral nutrition (TPN); however, both sur-

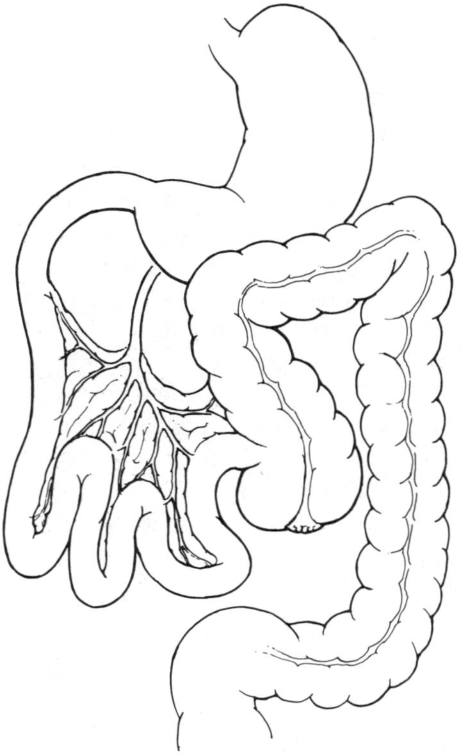

FIG 11–3.
Final position of the small bowel and colon after a Ladd procedure. (From Rescorla FJ: Anomalies of rotation and fixation: Anatomy and complications. *Surg Rounds* (in press). Used by permission.)

vived and have done well. If after detorsion, the bowel remains dusky, with poor antimesenteric pulsations observed by Doppler flow probe evaluation, we would close the abdomen and plan a second-look procedure within 24 to 48 hours, after optimization of the patient's hemodynamic status. At that time, if the bowel segments appeared nonviable, they would be resected, with exteriorization of the marginally viable ends as ostomies. If at initial exploration the entire bowel appears necrotic, the surgeon is faced with the difficult decision of either closing the abdomen and allowing the child to die or performing a complete small-bowel enterectomy with a plan of lifetime TPN or small-bowel transplantation (if this becomes an acceptable future clinical option).

OUTCOME

Malrotation with midgut volvulus is associated with significant morbidity and mortality related to bowel necrosis. Powell et al.,[5] in a review of 70 children with malrotation, noted 31 with midgut volvulus. Half of these cases (15/31), required resection of at least 50 cm of intestine, and 7 required long-term TPN. There were seven deaths, for a 23% mortality. Filston and Kirks[6] reported that 4 of 17 patients with midgut volvulus required extensive small-bowel resection, with 1 death (6%). In a recent review of 18 infants with midgut volvulus treated at our institution, 8 required small-bowel resection for necrotic bowel.[4] Two children with massive gut necrosis died within 30 days of surgery. Three other infants with massive bowel resections initially survived, but eventually died of TPN infusion-line sepsis and liver failure, resulting in an overall long-term mortality of 28%. Two other children with lesser resections also required TPN, but both are long-term survivors.

Malrotation with midgut volvulus requires prompt diagnosis and surgical intervention to preserve adequate bowel length. Any infant or child with signs and symptoms consistent with midgut volvulus should undergo immediate exploration. In addition, we would recommend that when malrotation is noted during an evaluation of gastrointestinal symptoms (or even for an unrelated problem), the patient should undergo a Ladd procedure to prevent the catastrophic occurrence of midgut volvulus.

REFERENCES

1. Snyder WH, Chaffin L: Embryology and pathology of the intestinal tract: Presentation of 48 cases of malrotation. *Ann Surg* 1954; 140:368–380.
2. Ladd WE: Congenital obstruction of the duodenum in children. *N Engl J Med* 1932; 206:277–283.

3. Ladd WE: Surgical diseases of the alimentary tract in infants. *N Engl J Med* 1936; 215:705–708.
4. Rescorla FJ, Shedd FJ, Grosfeld JL, et al: Anomalies of intestinal rotation in childhood: Analysis of 447 cases. *Surgery* (in press).
5. Powell DM, Othersen HB, Smith CD: Malrotation of the intestines in children: The effect of age on presentation and therapy. *J Pediatr Surg* 1989; 24:777–780.
6. Filston HC, Kirks DR: Malrotation—The ubiquitous anomaly. *J Pediatr Surg* 1981; 16:614–620.

12

Pelvic Inflammatory Disease

Margaret J. Blythe, M.D.

A 15-year-old girl came to the emergency room with a two-day history of lower abdominal pain and fever (38.5° C). She had nausea and vomited on two occasions. Her last menstrual period was 2 weeks prior to this illness. She admitted to previous sexual intimacy. Physical examination showed tenderness to palpation in both lower quadrants. Rectal examination elicited severe cervical tenderness. Vaginal examination detected bilateral adnexal fullness and a whitish discharge. The white blood cell count was 18,780/mm^3 with a shift to the left on differential smear. The erythrocyte sedimentation rate was 56 mm/hr.

A number of symptoms and signs have traditionally been associated with the clinical diagnosis of pelvic inflammatory disease (PID). The disease represents an acute clinical syndrome associated with ascending spread of microorganisms from the vagina or cervix to the endometrium, fallopian tubes, or contiguous structures. Salpingitis refers to infection limited to the uterus and fallopian tubes. Other areas potentially involved would be the appendix, liver capsule, and splenic capsule. Studies in Sweden and the United States have revealed the highest rate of PID to be in the sexually active adolescent female.[1] Standardized clinical criteria have been developed and verified by laparoscopy to improve the diagnostic accuracy for PID (Table 12–1). These criteria require an adequate pelvic examination which may prove difficult to perform in this age group. In young women with abdominal pain, the first step is to obtain a history in a sensitive, confidential manner that allows the determination of risk factors for PID (Table 12–2).

TABLE 12–1.
Criteria for the Diagnosis of Acute Pelvic Inflammatory Disease*

All three of the following should be present:
- Lower abdominal tenderness
- Cervical motion tenderness
- Adnexal tenderness (may be unilateral)

Plus

One of the following should be present:
- Temperature ≥38.0° C
- White blood cell count ≥10,500/mm^3
- Purulent material obtained by culdocentesis
- Inflammatory mass present on bimanual pelvic examination ± sonogram
- ESR >15 mm/hr
- Evidence of *N. gonorrhoeae* or *C. trachomatis* in the endocervix:
  - gram stain with gram-negative diplococci;
  - monoclonal antibody test for *C. trachomatis*
- Presence of >5 WBC per oil-immersion field on Gram stain of endocervical discharge

*From Sweet RL: *Infect Dis Clin North Am* 1987; 1:209. Used by permission.

TABLE 12–2.
Historical and Clinical Risk Factors Associated With Pelvic Inflammatory Disease

Age	75% of patients <25 yr old
Sexual activity	Multiple partners New partner(s) in previous 2 mo
Contraceptives	No protection Intrauterine device
Menstrual cycle	Onset of last period within 7 days of beginning symptoms History of irregular bleeding
Genitourinary symptoms	Fever and chills, nausea and vomiting, abdominal pain, dysuria, vaginal discharge
Past history of STDs/PID	
Past history of such operative procedures as legal abortions	

HISTORICAL AND CLINICAL RISK FACTORS

Age.—The risk of acquiring PID increases as age decreases among sexually experienced women. The reason for this age-dependent risk is unknown, but may be related to the immature cervix. The immature cervix, possibly because of structural and immunological factors, may be a less effective barrier to ascending infection. The risk of acquiring PID has been calculated to be 1:8 in females age 15 years old, 1:10 in those 16 years old, and 1:80 in women 24 years of age.[2]

Sexual Activity.—An increased risk of PID in sexually active women has been correlated with multiple sexual partners, with a recent history of a new partner often being elicited. For women with a history of only one partner, the risk of PID has been found to correlate with frequency of intercourse.

Contraceptives.—Use of combined estrogen/progestin contraceptive pills seems to decrease the risk that a lower genital tract infection will ascend to the upper genital tract. Recent studies have provided evidence that oral contraceptives afford protection against ascending chlamydial infection but not against gonococcal infection. Possible explanations have included progesterone-induced changes in the cervical mucus and decreased uterine myometrial activity.[3]

Menstruation.—Clinical studies suggest that symptoms of PID caused by agents of sexually transmitted disease (STD) may more often begin during or immediately after menstruation. The ascent of bacteria from the cervix to the fallopian tubes probably occurs most commonly during menses. The association between infection and menstruation is most striking among women who develop chlamydial gonococcal salpingitis. The majority of those women develop symptoms within 7 days of the onset of menses.[4]

Genitourinary Symptoms.—Lack of specificity of the symptoms associated with PID often makes its diagnosis difficult. Abdominal pain has been described as dull, bilateral, and subacute in onset. In a study of 807 women in Sweden, this pain was the most consistent symptom found in 94% with laparoscopically proven PID.[5] Approximately half the patients reported an increase in vaginal discharge. A history of irregular menstrual bleeding was reported in 35%, while 20% reported dysuria. Nausea and vomiting were infrequent symptoms, perhaps reflecting a small percentage who had developed peritonitis. Fever and chills were mentioned by over 40%, and were found significantly more often in women with laparoscopically proven PID than in those without PID.

Past History of STD/PID.—Some studies suggest that up to one third of women with PID will have a repeat infection within 1 year. Explanations given for this high recurrence rate include:

1. Noncompliance with treatment regimen.
2. Failure to examine and treat partners.

3. Tubal damage from a first infection, making the fallopian tube more vulnerable to infection.
4. Other factors, such as new partners.

Iatrogenic PID.—Operative procedures that may cause PID, such as legal abortion, must be sought in recording the patient's history.

LABORATORY ASSESSMENT

All laboratory tests described for PID are nonspecific, and discriminate poorly between cases with laparoscopically mild salpingitis and those with other diagnoses (see Table 12–1). A wet mount of vaginal secretions, microscopically demonstrating a greater number of inflammatory cells than normal epithelial cells, may suggest vaginitis, cervicitis, or PID. The presence of 5 or more white blood cells per high-power field on an endocervical smear may suggest cervicitis, PID, or both. Elevated sedimentation rates (>15mm/hr) and elevated peripheral white counts (>10,500/mm^3) are suggestive but not diagnostic of PID. A positive gram stain of endocervical secretions for gram-negative intracellular diplococci is suggestive of *Neisseria gonorrhoeae*. Positive rapid tests for chlamydia, such as enzyme immunoassay (EIA) or a direct fluorescent antibody (DFA) test, indicate this organism. Only cervical and not upper tract infection may be documented with these tests.

Serologic determinations give little information on the etiology of an upper genital tract infection, demonstrating insignificant or even no antibody change with cervical infection alone. Analyses of serial serum samples are most useful, although the results of such determinations often come too late to be of any guidance for diagnosis and therapy.

SURGICAL ASSESSMENT

Laparoscopy has become the "gold standard" for the diagnosis of acute salpingitis, and must be considered when the diagnostic problems of salpingitis, appendicitis, or ectopic pregnancy exist. The differentiation at laparoscopy between slight inflammatory changes in the tubes and normal conditions may be difficult to assess. Reddening and slight edema of the tubes can be seen at menstruation and in early pregnancy, but an inflammatory exudate is never seen under normal conditions. Culture specimens have been obtained by swabbing the tubal mucosa with cotton-tipped sticks or brushes, or by aspirating tubal contents with thin plastic catheters. The puncture of closed cavities and abscesses, as well as biopsy of the fimbriated ends of the fallopian tubes, has occurred at laparoscopy.

For the diagnosis of acute salpingitis, cul-de-sac puncture has been advocated by some investigators. Samples for culture obtained from this procedure have been less conclusive, with contamination from the vagina and bowel often occurring. Specimens sent for evidence of chlamydial infection are less reliable whether submitted for rapid tests or tissue culture. Furthermore, cul-de-sac puncture is often very difficult and unduly traumatic to perform in a frightened, uncooperative adolescent female patient.

Endometrial biopsy has been suggested as a less invasive alternative to laparscopy for diagnosing salpingitis, and has revealed a high correlation between histologic endometritis and laparoscopically confirmed salpingitis.[8] The usefulness of this procedure remains to be confirmed by additional clinical studies.

ULTRASONOGRAPHY

One study utilizing transabdominal ultrasound to diagnose PID in the adolescent population suggests that it is useful.[9] Hyperemia of the fallopian tube in early salpingitis may not be visualized by ultrasound examination. Ultrasound may identify adnexal enlargement with distention of the tubal lumen with salpingitis. As the disease progresses, purulent material exudes from the fimbria and may cause localized peritonitis. A tubo-ovarian abscess (TOA) may be present and distinguished from adnexal enlargement. An abscess appears as a large, complex mass with varying areas of echogenicity. The diagnosis of TOA may influence patient management in terms of inpatient or outpatient treatment plans, antibiotics to cover anaerobes, and the possibility of surgery. In this study of 100 hospitalized adolescent patients with the diagnosis of PID, 19.3% (17/88) had TOAs; in 12 (70.6%) the abscesses were diagnosed by transabdominal ultrasound before being suspected clinically.[9]

TREATMENT AND MANAGEMENT

The physician making the diagnosis of PID in an adolescent patient has to make the decision to treat on an outpatient basis with oral antibiotics or on an inpatient basis with parenteral antibiotics. No well-controlled clinical trials have been done to determine the efficacy of outpatient versus inpatient treatment in controlling the sequelae of such infections. Suggested treatment regimens for PID are designed to provide broad-spectrum coverage. In young women with clinically mild or moderately severe PID, the disease is most often associated with a sexually transmitted infection. Initial treatment may be on an outpatient basis and selected to eradicate *Neisseria gonorrhoeae, Chlamydia trachomatis,* and *Mycoplasma hominus* (Table 12–3).

TABLE 12–3.

Recommended Treatment for Acute Pelvic Inflammatory Disease, Centers for Disease Control, 1989

Ambulatory treatment
Cefoxitin 2 gm IM plus probenecid 1 gm PO
or
Ceftriaxone 250 mg IM
plus
Doxycycline 100 mg PO twice a day for 10–14 days
or
Tetracycline 500 mg PO four times a day for 10–14 days
Alternative for doxycycline/tetracycline intolerance
Erythromycin 500 mg PO q.i.d. for 10–14 days

TABLE 12–4.

Recommended Treatment for Acute Pelvic Inflammatory Disease, Centers for Disease Control, 1989

Inpatient treatment
Regimen A
Cefoxitin 2 gm IV every 6 hr
or
Cefotetan 2 gm IV every 12 hr
plus
Doxycycline 100 mg every 12 hr PO or IV*
Regimen B
Clindamycin 900 mg IV every 8 hr
plus
Gentamycin (2 mg/kg) loading dose IV or IM
then 1.5 mg/kg every 8 hr*

*Either regimen should be given until the patient improves and is afebrile for at least 48 hours. After discharge, antibiotics should be continued as doxycycline 100 mg PO b.i.d. for a total 10 to 14 days, clindamycin 450 mg PO four times a day for a total 10 to 14 days.

In febrile cases with palpable adnexal swelling, hospitalization for parenteral therapy is clearly preferable. Intravenous antibiotic coverage should cover sexually transmitted organisms as well as anaerobic and gram-negative enteric pathogens and streptococci (Table 12–4). Hospitalization should be considered in other situations, especially where diagnosis, compliance, and severity of ill-

TABLE 12–5.

Guidelines for Hospitalization of Adolescent Patients*

Hospitalization considered for each adolescent with suspected/proven PID.
Pelvic abscess suspected or documented.
Patient with pregnancy.
Severe illness as with temperature ≥38.5° C.
Patient unable to tolerate outpatient treatment (i.e., nausea and vomiting).
Patient failed to respond within 48 hours to outpatient therapy.
Intrauterine device in place.

*Adapted from Sweet RL: *Infect Dis Clin North Amer* 1987; 1:199–215.

ness are questioned (Table 12–5). Surgical procedures may be necessary in cases of life-threatening disease, failure of medical treatment, and abscess.

SUMMARY

Hospitalization with parenteral fluid and antibiotic therapy is warranted for the adolescent patient in the case report presented here. Hospitalization ensures compliance with antibiotic therapy and allows observation. Temperature elevation may indicate gonococcal PID or more serious complications of anaerobic infection. Other emergent surgical diagnoses, such as a ruptured appendix, must be considered, but seem less likely when vomiting is absent and there is a history of normal bowel function. Ectopic pregnancy must be ruled out with a pregnancy test that detects human chorionic gonadotropin (HCG) at less than 50 mIU/ml. As fluids and antibiotics are initiated, a pelvic ultrasound examination would be desirable to delineate the possibility of tubo-ovarian abscess. If the latter is found, the decision must be made to continue antibiotics and to follow up with ultrasound or to intervene surgically. Antibiotics providing better coverage for anaerobes should be administered if an abscess is detected (Regimen B, Table 12–4). If the diagnosis still seems uncertain, laparotomy rather than laparoscopy may be indicated. Once afebrile for 48 hours, and with evidence of healing, the patient may be discharged and continued on oral antibiotics for 10 to 14 additional days (Table 12–4). Her sexual partner(s) must be evaluated and treated empirically for STDs.

The goals for treatment of PID include preservation of fertility and prevention of ectopic pregnancy and other long-term sequelae. Women with a history of one or more episodes of PID have involuntary infertility rates of 21% compared to 3% of a control population, and a sixfold increase in ectopic pregnancies.[11] Early recognition with appropriate treatment of both the patient and the patient's partner(s) may minimize risk for such long-term sequelae.

REFERENCES

1. Sweet RC: Pelvic inflammatory disease and infertility in women. *Infect Dis Clin North Am* 1987; 1:199–215.
2. Weström L: Incidence, prevalence, and trends of acute pelvic inflammatory disease and its consequences in industrialized countries. *Am J Obstet Gynecol* 1980; 138:880–892.
3. Wolner-Hanssen P, Eschenbach DA, Paavonen J, et al: Chlamydial pelvic inflammatory disease associated with oral contraceptive use. *JAMA* 1990; 263:54–59.
4. Sweet RL, Blankfort-Doyle M, Robbie MO, et al: The occurrence of chlamydial and gonococcal salpingitis during the menstrual cycle. *JAMA* 1986; 255:2062–2064.
5. Jacobson L, Weström L: Objectivized diagnosis of acute pelvic inflammatory disease on fertility. *Am J Obstet Gynecol* 1969; 105:1088–1096.
6. Jacobson L: Differential diagnosis of acute pelvic inflammatory disease. *Am J Obstet Gynecol* 1980; 138:1006–1011.
7. Svensson L, Weström L, Ripa KT, et al: Differences in some clinical and laboratory parameters in acute salpingitis related to culture and serologic findings. *Am J Obstet Gynecol* 1980; 138:1017–1021.
8. Paavonen J, Kiviat N, Brunham RC, et al: Prevalence and manifestation of endometritis among women with cervicitis. *Am J Obstet Gynecol* 1985; 152:280–286.
9. Golden N, Neuhoff S, Cohen H: Pelvic inflammatory disease in adolescents. *J Pediatr* 1989; 144:138–143.
10. Centers for Disease Control: Sexually transmitted disease treatment guidelines, 1989. *MMWR* 1989; suppl 38, no. S-8.
11. Weström L: Effect of acute pelvic inflammatory disease on fertility. *Am J Obstet Gynecol* 1975; 122:707–713.

13

Torsion of the Ovary

Neil R. Feins, M.D.

A 12-year-old girl experienced the sudden onset of sharp lower left quadrant pain. This was followed by nausea and vomiting. The pain persisted and was unremitting. She developed fever (38.3° C), and her pulse rate was 110 beats/minute. On physical examination, pain and guarding were elicited on palpation of the left lower abdomen. Rectal examination showed left-sided fullness and tenderness. The white blood cell count was 14,000/mm^3 with 6% band forms and 80% polymorphonuclear leukocytes. The urinalysis was normal. Erect and recumbent abdominal roentgenograms showed nonspecific bowel loops in the lower abdomen. Pelvic ultrasound examination, however, showed a mass in the left side of the pelvis.

Sudden, acute abdominal pain occuring in infants and children demands a rapid, safe, and essentially simple management plan. A complete history and physical examination are essential as is a family history. Insight into the differential diagnosis can be helped by knowing if youngsters in the immediate family have required surgical intervention.

After the history and physical examination, the essential indicated studies that will correspond with the differential diagnosis should be requested. In the case described here, involving a 12-year-old girl, the sudden onset of pain without a history of a change in bowel habits rules out chronic enteritis or colitis. The characteristics and location of the pain, tenderness, and fullness are poor for appendicitis, but this diagnosis must be kept in mind. The tip of the appendix could be in the lower left quadrant, or incomplete rotation of the gut could exist with the appendix on the left side. A midgut volvulus is ruled out by the mass seen on the subsequent ultrasound examination.

The minimal studies indicated by the history and physical findings for rapid diagnosis in this case would be a complete blood cell count, erythrocyte sedimentation rate, urinalysis, pregnancy test, and erect and recumbent abdominal roentgenograms. A rapidly performed pelvic ultrasound examination would be important in light of the findings.[1] A normal sedimentation rate would rule out tubo-ovarian abscess or appendiceal abscess, and a negative pregnancy test would rule out an ectopic pregnancy. The mass seen on ultrasound examination points toward the diagnosis of a left adnexal problem. An obstructed left ectopic ureter could present in this fashion, but previous symptoms should have been present and the ultrasound examination should reveal a dilated ureter. If this possibility exists, an intravenous pyelogram is diagnostic. A uterine fusion abnormality may appear as a pelvic mass on ultrasound examination. This anomaly usually presents at puberty, but rarely has an acute onset and may be accompanied by other embryologic problems such as an absent kidney.

Torsion of an abnormal ovary containing a mass or tumor is a well-known phenomenon in pediatric patients. Torsion of a normal ovary, however, occurs more frequently than is generally appreciated.[2] Some large pediatric series have reported that one out of four oophorectomies resulted from the torsion of a normal adnexa. The right adnexa is more frequently involved than the left, by a 3:2 ratio. Most likely the sigmoid colon's mass effect helps prevent left adnexal twisting. The signs and symptoms of adnexal torsion are those of an acute abdomen due to lower abdominal disease. If the pain is cramplike it results from twisting of the tube and its sympathetic nerve supply in the ovarian pedicle. Vomiting accompanies the pain and is related to peritoneal irritation. In an acute situation the patient becomes extremely ill within a short period of time. Tachycardia and leukocytosis are usually present, and if adnexal necrosis has occurred the temperature is elevated.

Twisting of an abnormal, solid- or cystic mass-containing ovary on its relatively narrow pedicle can be readily understood. Torsion of a normal adnexa may be due to excessive mobility resulting from congenitally long supportive ligaments, mesovarium, or mesosalpinx. The ligament of the ovary, the gubernaculum in the female, may also be abnormally long and poorly fixated to the lower pole of the ovary in a situation similar to the undescended testes in the male.

The symptom complex in our patient is quite diagnostic of adnexal torsion, which can be a challenging entity to pinpoint, especially if it occurs on the right side.[3] However, a high index of suspicion should lead to the operating room in a rapid but deliberate fashion. An intravenous infusion should be started, a nasogastric tube passed, and a broad-spectrum antibiotic begun, since these steps increase the viability of a borderline salvagable ovary. After the patient has received general endotracheal anesthesia, a Foley catheter should be placed and a gentle bimanual rectal and abdominal examination done to help confirm the other findings and delineate the mass. The Pfannenstiel incision is ideal for surgical evaluation of adnexal masses, and leaves an imperceptible scar; if one is not familiar with the infraumbilical curved incision, a paramedian incision will suffice.

The abdomen is entered, serosanquinous fluid is noted, and some is collected for culture. If a clearly necrotic, swollen ovary is found, it should be excised without untwisting the torsed pedicle. Usually the fallopian tube is twisted and infarcted, necessitating a unilateral salpingo-oophorectomy. Torsion of the tube and ovary occurs more often than torsion of the ovary alone, because the broad ligament acts as a fulcrum. The infarcted ovary may be quite large due to venous and lymphatic obstruction with continuous arterial inflow. The torsed mass should be inspected carefully before it is excised; it may represent torsion of a parovarian cyst, which usually involves the broad ligament and tube and can leave the ovary uninvolved and salvagable. Parovarian cysts originate in the broad ligament and are Wolffian-duct remnants. Torsion of the fallopian tube alone is rare, but I have seen one case. If the left ovary has been removed the right ovary should be inspected for abnormalities including fixation. If a cyst or mass is present it should be enucleated or wedge resected. Asynchronous torsion of normal and abnormal adnexa in female children has been reported.[4]

It appears that the remaining ovary should have some type of oophoropexy. The ovary can be fixed to the broad ligament, the uterine serosa, or the lateral part of the pelvic wall or the ovarian ligament can be plicated. The efficacy of oophoropexy has not been established, but it appears to be a practical step. Theoretically this procedure could hinder fertility by distorting normal spatial relationships and promoting adhesion formation. Since an appendectomy is indicated as well, future right-lower-quadrant pain would signal possible ovarian pathology demanding a rapid work-up and exploration to salvage the remaining functional ovary.

If the ovary appears mottled, brown, gray, or even edematous at exploration, it may be salvagable. Since the ultrasound examination showed a mass but no fluid in the cul-de-sac—a late sign of torsion—the situation in this case may be fortunate. Untwisting of the ovarian pedicle carries the risk of releasing thrombi from vascular stasis and must be evaluated on an individual basis. If the color improves, an attempt to save the ovary should be undertaken. A Doppler ultrasound study may help in determining whether any vascular flow is present. Oophoropexy should be performed. The methods used can be one of the previously described procedures, depending on the surgeon's perception of the anatomic defect. A wedge-resection biopsy of the ovary with a frozen section must be done to rule out neoplastic involvement. A wedge resection can also help reduce the size of ovarian edema and allow for proper fixation. Any evident cyst or mass must be removed. The patient requires 72 hours of antibiotic coverage. An ultrasound examination in 3 months will reveal whether any part of the ovary has been saved. The right ovary should be evaluated for cysts and neoplasms and fixated. As noted above, the appendix should be removed.

The absence in adulthood of an ovary and tube without evidence of any anomaly may be the result of undetected torsion in childhood. Physicians evaluating girls with abdominal pain should always consider the diagnosis of ovarian torsion. Preoperative ultrasonography is noninvasive and could lead to early operative intervention, resulting in salvage of ovarian tissue. Laparoscopy in our patient would only have delayed the open exploration. I feel there is little need for laparoscopy in acute situations in which the ultrasound examination and physical findings demand rapid laparotomy. The efficacy of oophoropexy has not been proven, but I feel that it could prevent repeat torsion and contralateral torsion.

REFERENCES

1. Bower A: Ovarian torsion by ultrasonography. *So Med J* 1985; 78:1376–1378.
2. Bower R, Adkins J: Surgical ovarian lesions in children. *Am Surg* 1981; 47:474–478.
3. Case Records of The Massachusetts General Hospital (Case 9-1971) *N Engl J Med* 1971; 284:491–496.
4. Davis AJ, Feins NR: Subsequent asynchronous torsion of normal adnexa in children. *J Pediatr Surg* 1990; 25:687–689.

14

Hydrometrocolpos

John G. Raffensperger, M.D.

A 3-day-old infant girl is admitted to the neonatal unit because of fever, decreased urine output, and a midline lower abdominal mass. Physical examination demonstrates lower abdominal distention and a mass ascending up to the level of the umbilicus. The abdomen is tender to palpation. Examination of the introitus shows a bulging membrane in the lower third of the vagina. The white blood cell count is 15,000/mm^3 with a shift to the left on differential smear. The blood urea nitrogen is 29 mg/dl and the creatinine 1.8 mg/dL. Ultrasound examination of the pelvis shows a lower abdominal midline mass anterior to the rectum and posterior to the bladder, associated with hydroureter and hydronephrosis.

This infant has a hydrometrocolpos with an imperforate hymen, secondary to failure of the fused mullerian ducts to join with the urogenital sinus. The mother's high estrogen levels normally stimulate the infant's cervical and vaginal glands to secrete mucus. This secretion, together with vaginal obstruction, distends the vagina, which in turn obstructs the ureters and displaces the intestines upward. The vagina may be so enlarged that it puts upward pressure on the diaphragm, causing severe respiratory distress.

The diagnosis is easily made on the basis of a physical examination that demonstrates the mass rising from the pelvis. An ultrasound examination proves that the cystic mass lies between the bladder and bowel. The only other diagnosis to be considered would be an ovarian cyst. An ovarian mass, however, is movable and would not displace the bladder on ultrasound examination.

This infant should be given intravenous fluids and antibiotics; when she is hydrated and afebrile she should be taken to the operating room and examined under anaesthesia. The presence of the bulging hymen should be confirmed and the position of the urethra noted. A Foley catheter is inserted and the membrane is simply incised to drain the vaginal fluid. The cut edges of the hymen may be approximated with absorbable sutures. While the infant is under anaesthesia, it is important to perform a vaginal examination with a speculum or cystoscope in order to rule out a septated vagina or a double cervix and uterus.

When the vaginal septum is higher because the fused mullerian ducts did not descend, there is an opening in the perineum that may resemble a vagina on external inspection, but which is in reality, a persistent urogenital sinus. The urogenital sinus communicates with the urethra and bladder, but the vagina is completely obstructed. These infants also have a large abdominal mass rising up from the pelvis to the costal arch. They often have intestinal adhesions secondary to the spillage of vaginal contents from the fallopian tubes, and a higher incidence of urinary tract anomalies. An ultrasound examination of the abdomen will demonstrate the dilated vagina, and is used to search for associated defects.

If the infant is premature, has associated anomalies, or is in respiratory distress severe enough to require ventilation, the vagina can be drained through a small abdominal incision under local anesthesia. Ideally, however, the infant should have a corrective operation. After the infant is under general anesthesia and in the lithotomy position, the perineum is carefully examined. Catheterization or endoscopic examination of the urogenital sinus reveals the urethra high on the anterior wall, but there is no opening into the vagina. The abdomen and perineum are then prepared and, through a low transverse incision, the vagina is identified and opened. Its contents are drained and cultured, after which a posteriorly based perineal skin flap is raised and, with blunt dissection posterior to the urogenital sinus, the back wall of the vagina is found, mobilized, and brought down to the skin flap, which is sutured to the vaginal wall.[1] This operation leaves the urogenital sinus as the urethra and provides drainage for the vagina at its normal location on the perineum.

Vaginal obstruction may not become evident until the pubertal girl reaches the time of menstruation. Instead of having normal menstrual periods, she has recurrent bouts of lower abdominal pain that may simulate appendicitis or torsion of an ovary. Examination reveals a lower abdominal mass. The diagnosis is easily confirmed with an ultrasound examination, which reveals the distended vagina displacing the bladder forward. If there is a bulging hymen, the diagnosis is confirmed and the condition treated by simple incision.

On the other hand, the vaginal septum may be higher and treatment more complicated. A careful ultrasound examination will demonstrate the distance from the distended vagina to the perineum, as well as associated problems such as a septated vagina, uterine duplication, or other mullerian anomalies (Fig 14–1). These children must always be studied for associated urinary tract anomalies, since ectopic ureters and renal problems are common. A computed tomographic (CT) scan is helpful in revealing cross-sectional anatomy and demonstrating the distance from the vagina to the perineum (Fig 14–2). The

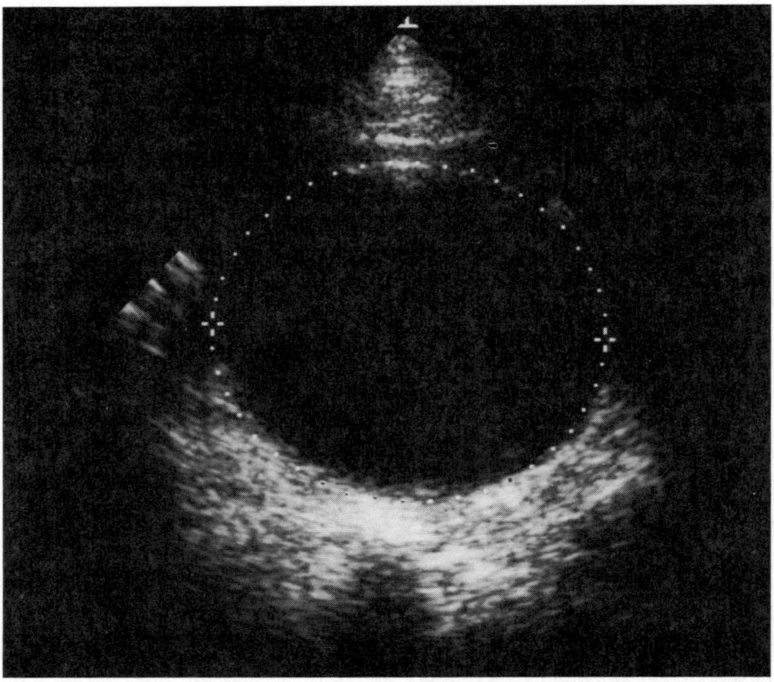

FIG 14–1.
Ultrasound demonstrating echogenic-free distended vagina.

position of the vagina is further verified by a pelvic and rectal examination under anaesthesia immediately prior to the operation. Endoscopy may be helpful in demonstrating the urethra if it is within a urogenital sinus. A simple imperforate hymen is incised and the edges approximated with absorbable sutures. If a thick, higher obstruction is identified, it too may be opened from a perineal approach. The CT scan in Figure 14–2 is of a 13-year-old girl who had recurrent pain, a lower abdominal mass, and only a shallow dimple on her perineum behind a normally located urethra; there was a 6-cm gap between the lower vagina and the perineal skin. The vagina was identified through a midline perineal incision between the urethra and anus, after which skin flaps were made from the labia minora and adjacent perineal skin. The flaps were then sutured to the vaginal mucosa to create a skin-lined lower third of the vagina. If the vagina can't be reached from a perineal incision, a combined abdominal and perineal approach is necessary to locate and mobilize the vagina so that it will reach the perineal skin flaps.

Total absence or agenesis of the vagina is often associated with an absent uterus; this is termed the Mayer-Rokitansky syndrome.[2] Even though there is

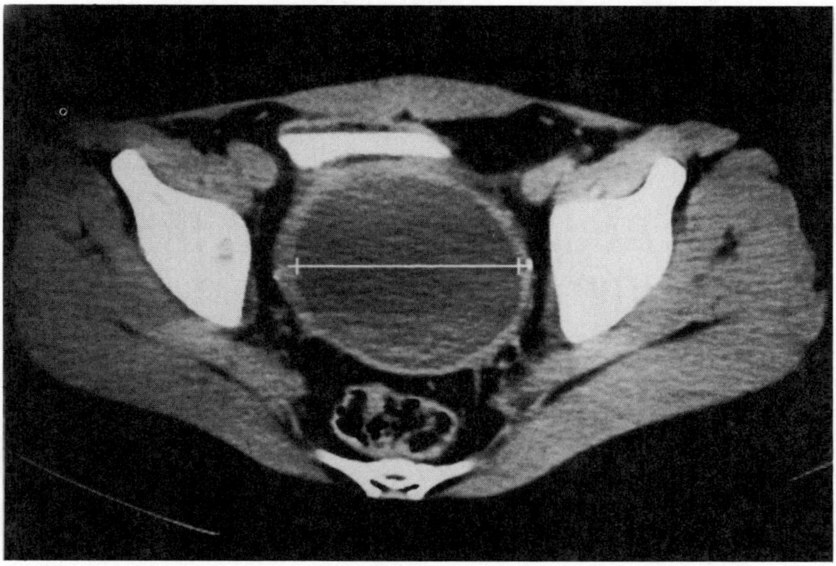

FIG 14–2.
Computed tomographic scan of a 13-year-old girl with hydrometrocolpos. The bladder, compressed anteriorly, is filled with contrast material. This study rules out a septate or duplicated vagina.

no menstrual secretion, a vagina must be created for normal sexual function. This procedure is postponed until the girl is old enough to wear a tampon or stent to keep the artificial vagina open.

These forms of vaginal obstruction should not be confused with simple fusion of the labia, which may be observed in baby girls during their first year or so. This is a perfectly harmless condition that may be treated with gentle separation of the labia and the application of estrogen cream.

REFERENCES

1. Ramenofsky, ML, Raffensperger, JG: An abdominoperineal-vaginal pullthrough for definitive treatment of hydrometrocolpos. *J Pediatr Surg* 1971; 6:381.
2. Griffen J, Edwards C, Madden J, et al: Congenital absence of the vagina: the Mayer-Rokitansky-Kuster-Hauser syndrome. *Ann Intern Med* 1974; 85:224.

15

Abdominal Pain in the Immunosuppressed Patient

Marc I. Rowe, M.D.
Edward P. Tagge, M.D.

A 13-year-old white female with acute myeloblastic leukemia (AML) developed abdominal pain and fever. She was in the induction phase of chemotherapy, and her last treatment was 11 days ago. Her body temperature was 39.6° C, and she had right lower quadrant tenderness and guarding. Her white blood cell count was $1400/cc^3$, with an absolute neutrophil count (ANC) of 0. Plain x-ray films showed several dilated loops of small intestine, and a dilated right colon. Ultrasound examination demonstrated a thick-walled loop of intestine in the right lower quadrant.

The major indication for the use of immunosuppressant agents in the pediatric patient is malignant disease. Antineoplastic agents produce cytotoxic effects by interfering with DNA. Actively proliferating cells, such as those of the bone marrow and gastrointestinal mucosa, are particularly susceptible. All leukocytes are affected, but granulocytes, with a 6-hour half life, are most severely reduced in number. Myelosuppression results in the reduction of specific and nonspecific immunity, and increases the patient's vulnerability to infection.

Abdominal pain often develops in the immunosuppressed child. The pain can be a result of conditions common to all children, such as appendicitis or gastroenteritis. The abdominal pain can also be directly related to the malignant disease itself or the effects of the antineoplastic drugs. In a study of 400 young patients with leukemia, 32% had episodes of abdominal pain and 16 patients required operation. Appendicitis was found in 8 patients, typhlitis was found in 7 patients, and mesenteric adenitis was found in 1 patient. Other causes of abdominal pain identified at autopsy or clinically diagnosed included gut perforation, leukemic infiltration of the intestine, graft vs. host disease, and parasite infestation. Since typhlitis and appendicitis are the most common abdominal conditions in the immunosuppressed child that require specific treatment, differentiating the two conditions is essential. Most physicians are familiar with the diagnostic features of appendicitis, but are not familiar with those of typhlitis.

Wagner[1] in 1970 coined the term typhlitis, taken from the Greek word *typhlon,* meaning cecum. Typhlitis is a colitis, primarily affecting the cecum. Typhlitis occurs principally in the treated leukemic patient who is neutropenic. Recent studies indicate that the incidence of typhlitis is increasing. Katz et al,[2] in a 1990 review of autopsy findings, found typhlitis in 24% of patients with acute leukemia. Shamberger et al[3] found 32% of 77 AML patients had developed typhlitis, and a Vancouver study reported a 26% incidence of typhlitis in AML patients. The high rate of occurrence in this form of leukemia is attributed to aggressive chemotherapy and increased patient survival.

PATHOGENESIS

Invasion of the intestinal wall by microorganisms is a key feature in the pathogenesis of typhlitis. The mechanism that allows bacteria to pass through the gut barrier is not known. Cytosine arabinoside, an antimetabolite that inhibits DNA synthesis, induces mucosal ulcerations. Vincristine, a plant alkaloid that interferes with microtubule and spindle protein function, produces mucosal cell alterations. Both drugs have been associated with typhlitis. However, no particular drug, or combination of agents, has been consistently associated with the development of typhlitis.

Sepsis is a predominant feature of typhlitis. In a series of 37 children with typhlitis, 84% had positive premortem blood cultures. The predominant organisms were bacteria (84%), usually the *Pseudomonas* species. In 16% of the patients fungus was cultured. Ninety-seven percent of the patients had positive postmortem cultures, and the incidence of fungus was increased to 47%. However, no one microorganism has been identified as the etiologic agent.

Most authors believe that alterations of the local and systemic host defense play a major role in the development of typhlitis. Neutropenia is a consistent finding in typhlitis. In a series of 37 patients with typhlitis, all had an ANC of less than 1500/cc^3 and 80% had an ANC of less than 500/cc^3. In the Vancouver series, an ANC of less than 100/cc^3 was found in all typhlitis patients.

PATHOLOGY

Grossly, the cecum is dilated, edematous, and frequently hemorrhagic. The bowel wall is thickened and there are mucosal ulcerations and hemorrhage. Microscopically, there is submucosal edema, minimal inflammation, and loss of mucosa. Neoplastic infiltration is usually absent. Bacterial and/or fungal wall invasion is frequent.

CLINICAL PRESENTATION

The vast majority of patients with typhlitis have leukemia, usually AML. Typhlitis occasionally develops in children with lymphoma, aplastic anemia, and cyclic neutropenia. The presenting symptom is abdominal pain and the location is variable, most commonly on the right side. Diffuse pain is less common. Diarrhea is frequent and the stool is usually grossly bloody. Vomiting occurs in from 8% to 45% of cases, but nausea is frequent. Almost all patients have a fever.

A right lower quadrant mass is felt in 11% of cases. Tenderness is usually in the right lower quadrant, and in advanced cases there is rebound and muscle rigidity. Laboratory findings include an ANC of less than $500/cc^3$, and thrombocytopenia ranging from 4,000 to $120{,}000/cc^3$.

IMAGING

An abdominal x-ray demonstrates cecal distention and bowel wall edema. Pneumotosis intestinalis is infrequently found. Barium enema findings are nonspecific, thumbprinting of the bowel and irregular mucosal folds. Because of the risk of cecal perforation, this study is now rarely utilized. Arteriography, although seldom performed, shows increased cecal vascularity, mucosal staining, and arterial-venous shunting.

Computerized tomography clearly demonstrates the changes associated with typhlitis, bowel wall edema, and spiculation of the pericolic fat. Ultrasonography shows the same processes. In addition, the density of the bowel wall shadowing on ultrasound can be used to differentiate disease processes. A hyperechoic bowel wall suggests typhilitis, while hypoechoic shadows are seen in other diseases such as granulomatous colitis and appendicitis.[6] Ultrasound is preferred over CT scanning because it can be done as a bedside procedure, does not require sedation, eliminates x-ray exposure, and can be done repeatedly so that serial evaluations can be performed.

TREATMENT

The initial therapeutic approach to typhlitis is nonoperative. Dehydration and electrolyte abnormalities are corrected by intravenous infusion. The gastrointestinal tract is decompressed by nasogastric suction. Broad spectrum antibiotic coverage with an aminoglycoside and antipseudomonal penicillin are recommended. Antifungal agents are added if there is no clinical improvement within 72 hours. The effectiveness of granulocyte transfusions, or granulocyte stimulating factor has not been determined.

Generally three criteria are agreed upon indications for operation: (1) persistent gastrointestinal bleeding after correction of clotting abnormalities, (2) evidence of free intraperitoneal perforation, (3) clinical deterioration requiring support with vasopressors, or large volumes of fluids suggesting uncontrolled sepsis. The role of surgery in the leukemic patient with localized right lower quadrant peritoneal findings is more controversial. Skeiber et al[4] reported that there was an equal incidence of appendicitis and typhlitis in patients with localized right lower quadrant tenderness. The authors believe that there are no preoperative factors that differentiate appendicitis from typhlitis. In order to avoid missing the diagnosis of appendicitis, they advocate operation. However, most clinicians manage these patients nonoperatively with serial physical and ultrasound examinations. The decision for operation is individualized and based on progression of symptoms, physical and x-ray findings.

Operative treatment of typhlitis necessitates a right hemicolectomy. Appendectomy should be reserved for patients with appendicitis. Primary anastomosis is not recommended, but an ileostomy and mucous fistula are usually done. A divided ileostomy, without resection, is reserved for patients with pancolitis without perforation.

OUTCOME

There was an initial lack of support for surgical therapy, based on the patients' overall poor prognosis, and high operative mortality (50% to 100%). More effective chemotherapy has now greatly improved the prognosis of leukemic patients. Likewise, the operative morbidity and mortality rates for typhlitis are improving. Shamberger et al[3] reported a nonoperative mortality rate of 5%, and an operative mortality rate of 20% in typhlitis patients with AML.

REFERENCES

1. Wagner M, Rosenberg H, Fernbach D, et al: Typhlitis: A complication of leukemia in childhood. *AJR* 1970; 109:341–350.
2. Katz J, Wagner M, Gresik M, et al: Typhlitis: An 18-year experience and postmortem review. *Cancer* 1990; 65:1041–1047.
3. Shamberger R, Weinstein H, Delorey M, et al: The medical and surgical manage-

ment of typhlitis in children with acute nonlymphocytic (myelogenous) leukemia. *Cancer* 1986; 57:603–609.
4. Skibber J, Matter G, Pizzo P, et al: Right lower quadrant pain in young patients with leukemia-A surgical perspective. *Ann Surg* 1987; 206:711–716.
5. Moir C, Scadamore C, Benny W: Typhlitis: Selective surgical management. *Am J Surg* 1986; 151:563–566.
6. Alexander J, Williamson S, Siebert J, et al: The ultrasonographic diagnosis of typhlitis (neutropenic colitis). *Pediatr Radiol* 1988; 18:200–204.

16

Inflammatory Bowel Disease

Robert L. Telander, M.D.

A 14-year-old boy was referred because of multiple perianal fistulae unresponsive to previous fistulectomy. The youngster also complained of intermittent crampy abdominal pain and frequent episodes of diarrhea. He was relatively short in stature for his age (<5th percentile) and lost 5 lb over a period of 4 weeks. On abdominal examination, palpation elicited tenderness in the right lower abdomen. The white blood cell count was 12,000/mm^3, the platelet count 500,000/mm^3, and the serum albumin 2.5 g/dL.

The striking features of this 14-year-old boy's history include the persistent perianal disease combined with the abdominal pain and diarrhea. The child's short stature suggests a more chronic nature to the illness, as does the hypoalbuminemia. Findings of this sort must always suggest possible inflammatory bowel disease, and in this boy's situation particularly, Crohn's disease (CD). As the initial workup begins, blood studies may promptly suggest CD. An elevated erythrocyte sedimentation rate (ESR) is more commonly elevated in CD than chronic ulcerative colitis (CUC), and anemia and hypoalbuminemia are often present in CD. It is essential to rule out infectious agents that may cause cramping abdominal pain and diarrhea, such as *Salmonella enteritides, Yersinia enterocolitica, Shigella, Campylobacter jejuni,* and *Clostridium difficile.* Crohn's disease in a child is diagnosed by consideration of the clinical history, physical findings, and especially endoscopic and radiologic findings. The diagnostic accuracy approaches 90% when the history, radiologic, and endoscopic findings are combined.

CLINICAL PRESENTATION

This patient's history suggests CD because of his crampy abdominal pain and diarrhea combined with severe perianal disease. Abdominal pain is the most common manifestation (79%) of CD, followed by diarrhea (68%), anorexia (51%), fever (41%), and fatigability (35%) (Table 16–1). A right lower quadrant mass is present in only 11% of patients. Perianal disease strongly suggests CD rather than CUC, since CUC rarely includes perianal disease of any magnitude. The perianal disease seen with CD often consists of indurated, dusky skin with edematous hyperplastic skin tags and linear ulcers. Short stature itself was present in approximately one quarter of our patients, and is often attributed to poor nutrition, chronic illness, and the use of steroids.

ENDOSCOPY

Endoscopy is very helpful in the evaluation of children with CD. While involvement of the esophagus, stomach, and duodenum is uncommon, it has

TABLE 16–1.
Clinical Features at Diagnosis in 177 Patients 15 Years of Age or Less at the Mayo Clinic*

MANIFESTATION	NO. (%) OF PATIENTS
Abdominal pain	140 (79)
Diarrhea	120 (68)
Asthenic body habitus	109 (62)
Weight loss	90 (51)
Anorexia	75 (42)
Fever	73 (41)
Fatigability	62 (35)
Growth failure (patient's assessment)	46 (26)
Vomiting	43 (24)
Joint symptoms	28 (16)
Perineal inflammation	27 (15)
Hematochezia	24 (14)
Digital clubbing	20 (11)
Right lower quadrant mass	20 (11)
Fistula	18 (10)
Stomatitis	7 (4)

*From Castile RG, Telander RL, Cooney DR, et al: *J Pediatr Surg* 1980; 15:462–469. Used by permission.

been noted in 5% to 20% and is often best demonstrated by endoscopy.[4, 5] The earliest mucosal lesion seen is an aphthoid ulcer. The small oval mucosal ulcerations are made up of a small central microabscess within a lymphoid follicle. The small ulcers extend and give rise to a longitudinal penetrating ulcer. Aphthoid ulcers may be seen in the mouth and throughout the entire gastrointestinal tract. The longitudinal defect often extends to the serosa and is transmural rather than mucosal. The ulcerations have been referred to as rake ulcers or "bear-claw" lesions. The mucosa between lesions may appear normal. Biopsy is often of little benefit because of the frequent absence of granulomas.

Endoscopic examination of the rectum and colon in CD usually reveals discontinuous involvement of the gut. A normal anal canal is common. Colorectal ulcerations in CD range from the small aphthoid to the extensive linear ulcers noted above. This contrasts to CUC, in which there is characteristically diffuse granularity of the mucosa beginning at the anus and extending proximally for varying distances, often involving the entire colon. Unfortunately, 5% to 10% of patients with CD fall into a category referred to as indeterminate colitis because the disease has not progressed to a more classic appearance.

ROENTGENOGRAPHIC STUDIES

X-ray examination is extremely helpful in aiding the diagnosis. Flat and upright views of the abdomen can demonstrate the presence of a toxic megacolon in CUC and complete or partial bowel obstruction in CD.

Barium studies of the upper gastrointestinal tract can include the enteroclysis technique to provide finer detail. Lesions of the esophagus, stomach, and duodenum are usually better seen by endoscopy, but may be demonstrated by a barium study. The findings often resemble those in peptic ulcer disease with mucosal thickening. Biopsy of suspected areas occasionally demonstrates a granuloma, but often does not. Most reports describe ileocolitis in 40% to 50% of patients with CD, small-bowel involvement alone in 30% to 50%, and involvement of the colon alone in 10%.[5]

This patient would probably demonstrate disease of the distal small bowel, which is the most common region of the gastrointestinal tract involved by CD. Perianal disease that does not heal is often present in patients with CD of the rectosigmoid colon. Thickening and induration of the terminal ileum, often extending 15 to 20 cm proximal to the cecum, is the usual finding. The ulcerations of the bowel may penetrate through the bowel wall to the serosa, resulting in an abscess that can be contained or can penetrate into adjacent loops of bowel or any organ. Internal fistulae and bowel obstruction may result with an inflammatory mass. A "string sign" represents a long stenosis. If resolution occurs, it is assumed that edema was responsible for the narrowing. Fibrosis and scarring are suggested by chronicity and proximal dilation.

THERAPY

Medical therapy for CD is initially aimed at relieving the diarrhea and cramps. Prednisone, sulfasalazine, and metronidazole appear to be beneficial. Numerous studies have also upheld the beneficial effects of nutritional support, both by the parenteral route and by continuous tube feedings.

The indications for surgery in CD are well established, but the specific timing can be difficult. Surgery is necessary when bowel obstruction, internal fistulas, or free perforation occur. When partial obstruction with a poor response to medical therapy is present, surgical resection of the diseased bowel can restore the patient to health. The patient described here would appear to be a candidate for surgery if he did not respond promptly to medical therapy. The surgical management is determined by the nature of the patient's disease. If the disease is localized to the terminal ileum and ileocecal region, a resection of that portion of bowel with an ileo–ascending colon anastomosis is appropriate. Internal fistulae can be managed without resection of the secondary portion of the fistula, but usually the primary diseased portion of the small bowel is resected and closure of the secondary opening to the adjacent organ is carried out.[1, 3] All gross disease manifested by thickened, edematous bowel with "creeping fat" is usually resected, along with several centimeters of normal bowel. The removal of all microscopic residua is not necessary. Excision of asymptomatic distant "skip areas" is not beneficial. Urgent complications requiring prompt surgery include Crohn's colitis with toxic megacolon or massive hemorrhage, or both. A free perforation is another urgent indication for surgery.

Perianal disease in patients with CD is notoriously difficult to treat, having a tendency to slow healing and recurrence of disease. Nevertheless, patients with anorectal fistulae may successfully undergo fistulotomy or fistulectomy. Through the careful trimming of overlying edges and maintenance of clean lesions, healing often occurs, albeit slowly. Patients with severe CD involving the rectosigmoid colon have a particularly poor prognosis and often require removal of the diseased bowel to permit healing of severe perianal disease.[1, 2]

Strictureplasties have been beneficial in patients who have numerous strictures. This eliminates the obstructing lesion and at the same time minimizes the amount of bowel resected. Growth failure is a relative indication for surgery, since without good nutritional support, growth will not occur.

Approximately 50% of children undergoing surgery for CD require additional surgery by the age of 10 years (Fig 16–1). Nevertheless, patients with complications of CD can often be restored to good health and a near-normal lifestyle during the important teen years. Long-term follow-up of such patients often reveals a surprisingly satisfied group of patients.[1, 5] From 50% to 80% of persons with childhood CD who are followed into adulthood state that their health is good to excellent. We observed that 76% of children who had CD had

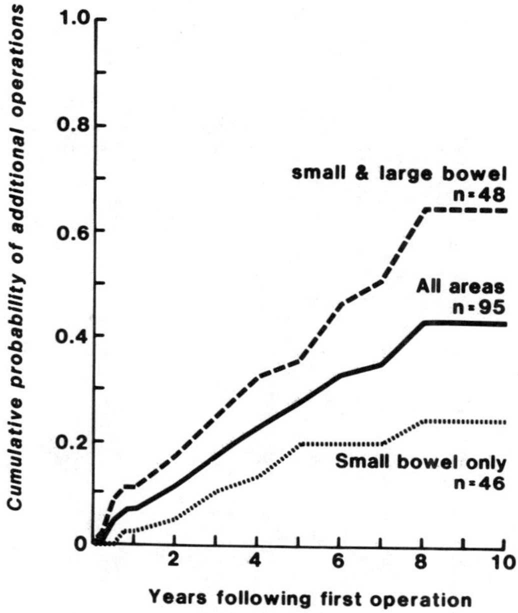

FIG 16–1.
Cumulative probability of additional operation. (From Castile RG, Telander RL, Cooney DR, et al: *J Pediatr Surg* 1980; 15:462–469. Used by permission.)

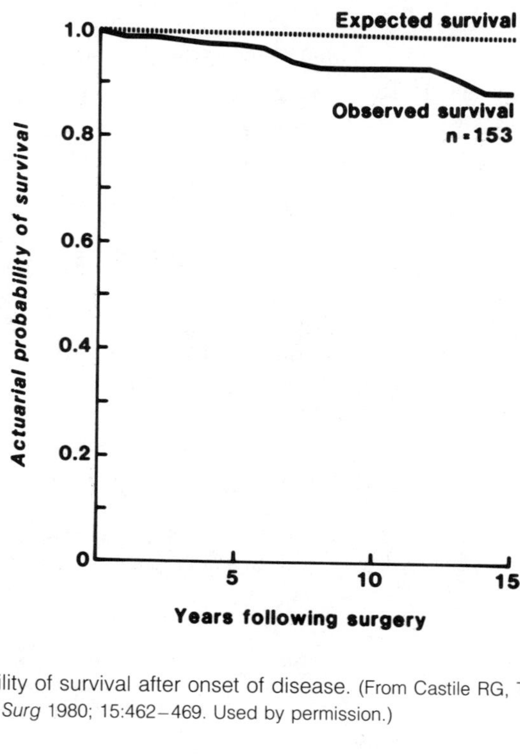

FIG 16–2.
Actuarial probability of survival after onset of disease. (From Castile RG, Telander RL, Cooney DR, et al: *J Pediatr Surg* 1980; 15:462–469. Used by permission.)

TABLE 16–2.
Patient Assessment of Status at Follow-up (160 Patients)*

PATIENT STATUS	NO. (%) OF PATIENTS
Current state of health	
Excellent	61 (38)
Good	67 (42)
Fair	23 (14)
Poor	7 (4)
Very ill	2 (1)
Patient assessment of disease	
Cured	69 (43)
Present but not an active problem	65 (41)
Currently an active problem	27 (17)
Limitation of daily activities	
Not at all	113 (71)
Moderate	41 (26)
Severe	6 (4)

*From Castile RG, Telander RL, Cooney DR, et al: *J Pediatr Surg* 1980; 15:462–469. Used by permission.

no limitation of activities as adults, while 26% had some limitation, often related to an ostomy (Table 16–2). The life expectancy of patients who developed CD in childhood is near normal (Fig 16–2).[5]

REFERENCES

1. Welch K, Randolph J, Ravitch M, et al: Crohn's Disease in *Pediatric Surgery,* ed 4. Chicago, Year Book Medical Publishers, Inc., 1986, pp 958–969.
2. Leven DH, Surrell J, Mazier WP: Surgical treatment of anorectal fistula in patients with Crohn's disease. *Surg Gynecol Obstet* 1989; 169:133–136.
3. Pettit SH, Irving MH: The operative management of fistulous Crohn's disease. *Surg Gynecol Obstet* 1988; 167:223–228.
4. Lenaerts C, Roy CC, Vaillancourt M, et al: High incidence of upper gastrointestinal tract involvement in children with Crohn's disease. *Pediatrics* 1989; 83:777–781.
5. Castile RG, Telander RL, Cooney DR, et al: Crohn's disease in children: Assessment of the progression of disease, growth and prognosis. *J Pediatr Surg* 1980; 15:462–469.

17

Hirschsprung's Disease With Superimposed Enterocolitis

Lester W. Martin, M.D.

A 1-month-old male infant was referred because of fever (38.5° C), abdominal distention, explosive episodes of diarrhea alternating with constipation, and failure to thrive. The infant vomited bilious material on two occasions. The infant was full term and weighed 3.2 kg at birth. Meconium was passed on the second day of life after a glycerine suppository was inserted in the rectum. On physical examination the abdomen was distended. Dilated loops of intestine were visibly outlined on the abdominal wall. Rectal examination showed an empty rectal vault, but an explosive discharge of watery fluid followed removal of the examining finger. Flat and recumbent abdominal roentgenograms demonstrated many loops of dilated intestine and air–fluid levels in both the small bowel and colon.

This case presentation is classic for Hirschsprung's disease with superimposed enterocolitis.

Since Hirschsprung's disease is a congenital malformation, the symptoms almost always date from birth, beginning with delay in the initial passage of meconium and followed by symptoms of varying degree suggesting partial obstruction (i.e., abdominal distention, infrequent stools, inanition, loss of appetite, failure to thrive, occasional vomiting, and varying degrees of malnutrition).

The basic abnormality consists of an absence of the parasympathetic innervation of the rectum. By microscopic examination, the parasympathetic plexuses of Meissner and Auerbach are missing in the submucosal and muscular layers of the rectum. This aganglionic segment usually involves the rectum only, but may extend further into the colon. In about 5% of cases it involves the entire colon, and sometimes a part of the small bowel. In rare instances the entire gastrointestinal tract has been found to be aganglionic. It is unknown why the severity of symptoms correlates only somewhat with the length of the aganglionic segment. Some infants with involvement only of the rectum will present with complete bowel obstruction in the first day or two of life, whereas others will have only minor complaints until several months of age. Thus, for example, a case was reported of a child 14 years of age with total colonic aganglionosis. She had been managed at home with nonoperative measures for 14 years. When an infant with Hirschsprung's disease is breast fed, its bowel habits are often reported as having been entirely normal until it is weaned from the breast; then, within only a few days, the symptoms progress rapidly to a picture of complete obstruction.

It is more common, however, for symptoms of Hirschsprung's disease to present during the first few weeks of life, as in the case report above. In such a situation, the working diagnosis is noted and lifesaving measures, directed at treatment of the enterocolitis, are initiated. When the condition of the infant has improved sufficiently, the diagnosis can be confirmed by microscopic or histochemical studies of a biopsy from the rectum.

ENTEROCOLITIS

Enterocolitis is the most frequent cause of death in untreated Hirschsprung's disease. It is caused primarily by incomplete functional obstruction of the rectum with proximal dilatation, stasis, and bacterial overgrowth, which in turn leads to infection, epithelial destruction, and ulceration with subsequent bacterial invasion and sepsis as well as protein loss from the ulcerated surface. Clinically, the incomplete obstruction causes abdominal distention and voluminous, watery diarrhea leading to electrolyte depletion, dehydration, and intravascular volume depletion, with eventual death from sepsis and shock. The condition can be rapidly progressive and fulminant with explosive liquid, foul-smelling, diarrhea stools; listlessness; fever; and prostration leading to shock and death within a matter of a few hours. In the more chronic forms, it may masquerade as a troublesome, unexplained diarrhea over a period of several weeks, with failure to thrive, malnutrition, hypoproteinemia, and a slow but progressive clinical deterioration.

The treatment of enterocolitis is directed at: (1) relief of the obstruction, (2) combating the infection, (3) correction of the electrolyte imbalance, and (4) restoration of hydration. The initial relief of obstruction can generally be accomplished by digital rectal examination with anal sphincter dilatation. Following this initial decompression, a large-bore (32 or 34 F) rectal tube can be inserted and left in position, with its continued patency assured by periodic irrigation with a normal saline solution. Following stabilization of the child's overall condition, and within a period of several days, a more permanent decompression is accomplished by diversion of the fecal stream proximal to the diseased segment of colon.

The most appropriate intravenous antibiotic for use in enterocolitis is subject to some debate, but should provide broad-spectrum coverage, should be effective against anaerobic as well as gram-negative organisms, and should be chosen on the basis of the results of blood culture studies. Appropriate intravenous fluids and electrolytes are administered immediately to correct the dehydration and electrolyte imbalance.

DIAGNOSIS

After the condition of the infant has been stabilized, attention can be directed to confirming the diagnosis. Roentgenographic examination with barium enema will confirm the clinical impression that the abnormality involves the colon, and will provide an indication of the length of the aganglionic segment. The diagnosis is confirmed by rectal biopsy which, in the infant, can be obtained by the suction technique at the bedside. It requires no anesthesia, and the discomfort to the infant is limited to that of a digital rectal examination. In our institution, we routinely examine the biopsy specimen by both histologic and histochemical methods. Histologic examination characteristically demonstrates the absence of ganglion cells and hypertrophy of nerve fibers, whereas histochemical studies demonstrate a characteristic pattern of acetylcholinesterase. By using both methods, the chances of error are essentially eliminated.

COLOSTOMY

For the infant with symptomatic short-segment Hirschsprung's disease, the initial operative procedure should be establishment of a colostomy. This provides diversion of the fecal stream, permits healing of the enterocolitis, gives complete decompression, and stops the loss of serum proteins from the ulcerated bowel. The infant returns to a normal state of health and nutrition prior to the time of the definitive operation.

The colostomy should be located sufficiently proximal to the transition zone so that the definitive operation can be performed at a subsequent date without the need to disturb the colostomy. This permits healing of the extraperitoneal rectal anastomosis without fecal contamination, and avoids the risk of catastrophic pelvic sepsis. Our preference is usually a right transverse diverting-loop colostomy, after the method of Turnbull. A vertical, 1-inch incision is made over the midportion of the rectus muscle midway between the level of the umbilicus and the costal margin. The rectus muscle fibers are separated and the peritoneum opened vertically. Care is taken to make the wound just large enough to accommodate the colostomy, utilizing the entire incision. The omentum is detached from the portion of colon selected for the stoma. A temporary rubber catheter is passed through the colonic mesentery immediately adjacent to the colon and is used to withdraw the colon through the incision. Care must be taken not to injure colonic marginal vessels. The colon is sutured to the peritoneum and the rectus fascia with absorbable sutures and the catheter is removed. The distal limb of colon is then transected through four-fifths of its circumference at the skin level, and the full-thickness colon is folded back to immediately "mature" the proximal stoma with a significant protruding nipple. Subcuticular absorbable sutures are then used to fix the colon to the skin. This method permits decompression of the distal colon segment, allows its manual irrigation if necessary, and yet permits ready placement of a colostomy bag appliance with complete diversion of the fecal stream. A glass rod or other support is not necessary.

The rapid improvement in the infant's nutritional status is dramatic. The definitive operation is much better tolerated when performed at a later date on a healthy infant.

DEFINITIVE OPERATION

There are several advantages to selecting the age of 1 year for the definitive operation for Hirschsprung's disease: (1) the pelvis is large enough to accommodate the surgeon's hands as well as the mechanical stapling device, (2) the critical level for transecting the aganglionic internal sphincter can be more accurately determined, (3) general anesthesia is well tolerated with no additional risk at this age, and (4) all surgery can be completed to permit toilet training at the usual age of 18 to 24 months. Complete bowel rest with a diverting colostomy for at least 6 months prior to the definitive operation appears to decrease the incidence of postoperative enterocolitis.

Our preference is for our own modification of the Duhamel procedure (Fig 17–1). It preserves the normal proprioceptive nerves of the anterior rectal wall, does not disturb the delicate nerves to the bladder and ejaculatory mechanism, permits removal of the posterior half of an appropriate amount of the aganglionic internal sphincter, preserves the sensory transitional epithelium overlying the anorectal columns of Morgagni, relieves the obstructive process, and if carefully performed, practically eliminates blood loss from the operation. Technically, this operation may be more difficult to perform than either the Soave or the Swenson procedures, but we believe this factor is overcome by its many advantages.

The operation is performed with the child in the lithotomy position. The

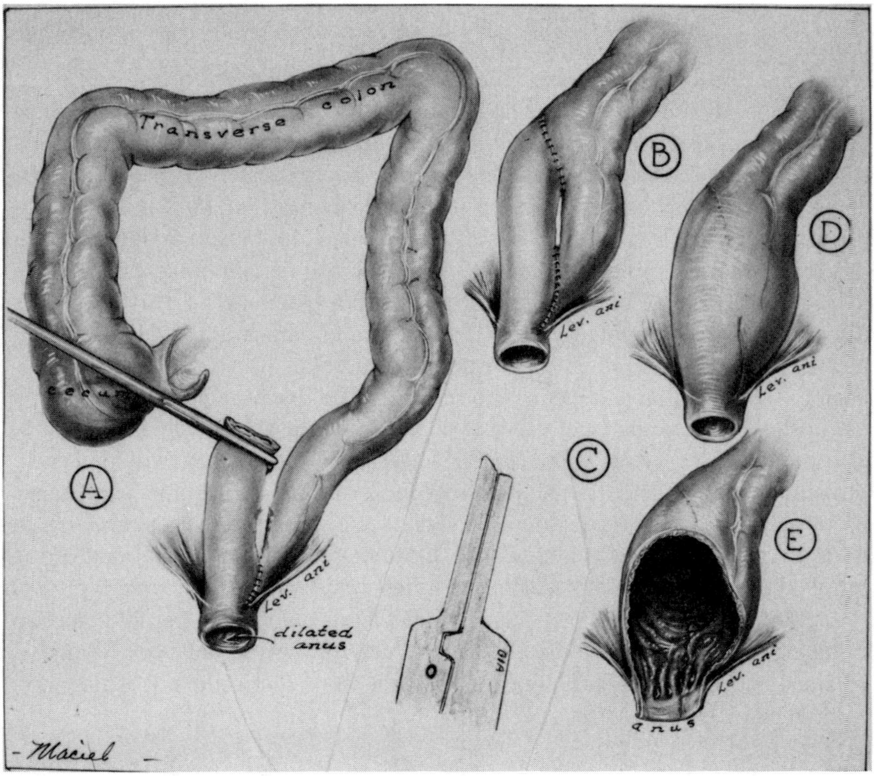

FIG 17–1.
Diagram of definitive operation as performed by the author.

distal colon is irrigated with normal saline through the mucous fistula as well as through the rectum until completely clear. A long, transverse, skin crease incision below the umbilicus provides adequate exposure and leaves minimal subsequent scar tissue. It is important to resect the dilated, thickened segment of colon proximal to the transition zone, since the damaged, thickened segment will never function as normal bowel. Confirmation of the presence of ganglia at the level selected for transection is accomplished by frozen-section microscopic examination. The rectum is transected distally at the level of the pelvic peritoneal reflection, which has been incised in order to permit adequate mobilization for subsequent anastomosis. Blunt dissection of the avascular presacral space down to the level of the levator muscles is accomplished with the index finger, and if performed carefully is a completely bloodless maneuver. It is often necessary to mobilize the splenic flexure of the colon so that the resected end of colon will reach the anal canal without tension.

At this point the surgeon proceeds to the perineal portion of the operation and an assistant remains at the abdominal field. The perineum is cleansed and draped and the rectum further irrigated. Retraction sutures are placed in the anal canal to provide exposure. The posterior 180 degrees of rectal wall is incised at the level of the top of the columns of Morgagni, incising the mucosa only. The mucosa is then retracted distally and the internal sphincter is incised at the level of the dentate line, thus leaving approximately 1 cm of mucosa above the level of transection of the internal sphincter (Fig 17–2). The transitional epithelium is necessary for sensation, but if the muscle is transected at this level, enough aganglionic internal sphincter will remain to increase the risk of postoperative enterocolitis as well as residual symptoms of Hirschsprung's disease. The GIA stapling device is then placed on either side, with one prong in the rectum and the other in the pulled-down colon. By this method the opposing walls of colon and rectum are resected. The mucosal anastomosis across the posterior distal anorectal canal is completed with absorbable sutures. It is also advisable to oversew the lateral staple lines, since they will otherwise sometimes grow together, creating a septum across the neorectum, particularly if colostomy closure is delayed for several weeks. The surgeon then returns to the abdominal field and completes the anastomosis of the proximal end of the rectal stump to the side of the adjacent colon.

Colostomy closure is best delayed for at least 3 months to permit complete healing of the rectal anastomosis. Closure may be further delayed if blood is obtained on rectal examination or if extravasation of contrast media is observed radiographically.

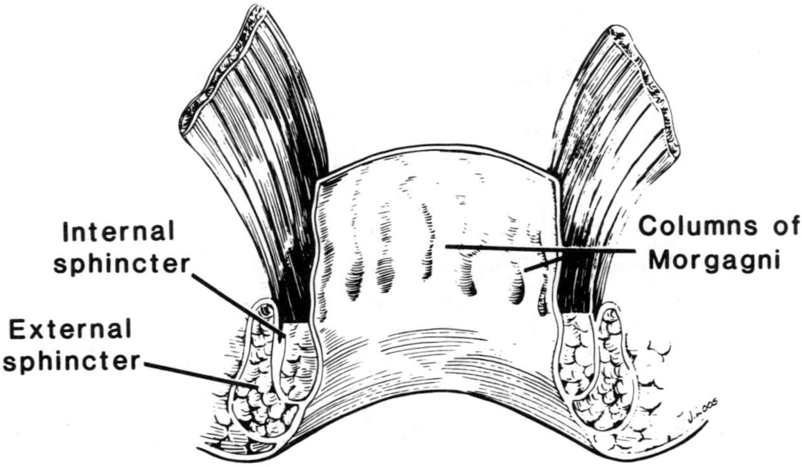

FIG 17–2.
Illustration of the level for the anorectal anastomosis. Note the preservation of transitional (sensory) epithelium by transecting the rectal wall at the level of the top of the columns of Morgagni. The muscular layer (internal sphincter) is transected at the level of the dentate line.

COLOSTOMY CLOSURE

For closure of the colostomy, it is preferable to completely mobilize and resect the colostomy site and perform an accurate end-to-end anastomosis. Care must be taken, however, not to injure the vascular arcade, which lies near the colon and may represent the only blood supply to the entire distal, pulled-through colon. Injury to this vessel could result in necrosis of the distal colon with catastrophic results.

ASSOCIATED CONDITIONS

Several conditions are found in association with Hirschsprung's disease. Down's syndrome occurs in about 10% of most reported series and in 12% of our own. In addition, another 8% to 10% of patients have other neurologic syndromes variously labeled as cerebral palsy or other unexplained varieties of psychomotor developmental delay. Waardenburg's syndrome, with or without mental retardation and with or without nerve deafness, has been observed in our patients as well as being reported in other series (Cohen, oral communication, 1990).

Congenital deafness has been observed in six of our patients. One was from a family with Waardenburg's syndrome and another was born to parents of whom both were congenitally deaf. One of our patients was the focus of a medical malpractice suit, the deafness having been attributed to an excess dose of aminoglycoside antibiotic, which is known to be ototoxic. This was the only one of the six who had received an aminoglycoside. At our institution, we have adopted a policy of performing an evoked potential hearing evaluation on any infant with Hirschsprung's disease prior to prescribing aminoglycosides.

POSTOPERATIVE COMPLICATIONS

Enterocolitis occurring in the postoperative period has been attributed to some mysterious etiology. Many theories have been proposed. This complication has been virtually eliminated in my experience by observing two principles: first, in the event of preoperative enterocolitis, a totally diverting colostomy is done to put the colon at complete rest for at least 6 months prior to the definitive operation, with an additional 3 months after the definitive operation before closure of the colostomy. The second principle is removal of the internal sphincter to the level of the dentate line at the time of the definitive operation. It is our firm belief that enterocolitis, whether preoperative or postoperative, is caused by a persistent distal obstruction (i.e., persistent aganglionic internal sphincter).

Night-time stooling sometimes occurs following colostomy closure. We have been aware of this in 6 of 250 patients. In each instance it was disturbing in that the only bowel movement occurred at night in the diaper. In each instance the problem was self-limiting, with daytime bowel movements beginning after several months and complete bowel training with continence developing spontaneously. In one instance, a psychiatrist was consulted by the family. He was intrigued but claimed no credit for the subsequent satisfactory outcome.

RESULTS

The results of my experience with over 250 cases of aganglionosis have been gratifying, with no deaths and no complete failures. Numerous complications were, however, encountered early in the experience when other operations were attempted. The technique described above has been followed in the last 75 patients, with no serious infections, no permanent residual constipation, and no incontinence. Nevertheless, it is a long and technically demanding operation. Initially the bowel habits may be abnormal, with either constipation or diarrhea sometimes lasting for as long as 2 years. This, together with the frequently associated malformations, which are sometimes initially overlooked, leads to patient dissatisfaction, primarily through lack of understanding or miscommunication. Over the past 6 years, I have been asked for expert opinion in 13 instances of alleged medical malpractice throughout the United States involving patients who have undergone surgery for Hirschsprung's disease. The potential for significant complications following this complicated operation cannot be overemphasized when discussing the condition with the family prior to surgery.

In general, however, the long-term results are most gratifying. Any complications seem to occur in the early postoperative period. When the patients are seen a number of years later, their growth, development, and bowel habits are invariably normal. Three of my earlier patients have returned a number of years later with their own infants with Hirschsprung's disease.

18

Meckel's Diverticulum

Dennis W. Vane, M.D.

> A 4-year-old boy presents with a 24-hour history of passing maroon-colored stools. He is listless and appears pale, but has not complained of abdominal pain. The abdomen is soft, flat, and nontender on physical examination. Rectal examination is normal except for the presence of obvious dark blood on the examiner's gloved digit. The pulse rate is 160/min and the hemoglobin is 7.0 g with a hematocrit of 23%.

The scenario presented above, of a 4-year-old boy with painless bleeding per rectum, a nontender abdomen, anemia, and physical signs of hypovolemia, is almost pathognomonic of a bleeding Meckel's diverticulum. Children with anemia and physical signs of hypovolemia require urgent resuscitation to prevent profound shock. Once resuscitation has been completed, diagnosis of the problem must be made expeditiously. Placement of a nasogastric tube with the observation of clear gastric material virtually eliminates a peptic ulcer or unrecognized esophageal varices as the source of hemorrhage. Other conditions in the differential diagnosis of rectal bleeding include polyps, unrecognized trauma, arteriovenous (AV) malformation of the gut, hemangioma, or intestinal duplication. Anemia and hypotension are infrequently associated with bleeding from rectal polyps. The most common cause of this type of lower intestinal bleeding in young children is a persistent vitelline-duct remnant (Meckel's diverticulum).

DESCRIPTION

Meckel's diverticulum was first noted by Ruysch in 1730, and more fully described by Johann Freidrich Meckel in 1808. Under normal circumstances, the vitelline duct obliterates in the fifth to ninth week of intrauterine life, with complete dissolution of intestinal attachment to the umbilicus. In approximately 2% of the population, however, some remnant of the duct remains (in males more commonly than in females). This remnant may persist as a patent vitelline duct with a fistula at the umbilicus, a fibrous band extending from the ileum to the undersurface of the umbilicus, a vitelline sinus not attached to the bowel, or a rare cyst, but more commonly remains as a diverticulum on the antimesenteric border of the small intestine, approximately 2 ft proximal to the ileocecal valve. The Meckel's diverticulum may contain ectopic tissue from the stomach, pancreas, or duodenum. Although the exact incidence of ectopic tissue varies in reported studies, it is generally accepted that bleeding or inflammation from the diverticulum requires the presence of ectopic gastric mucosa.

Symptoms of a Meckel's diverticulum vary with age, and are by far more common in the pediatric population, with 45% of symptomatic lesions presenting before the patient reaches 2 years of age.[1] Intestinal obstruction develops in infants and young children, either from volvulus around an attachment of the diverticulum to the umbilicus, or from an internal hernia through a space between a persistent vitelline artery and the diverticulum itself. Bleeding occurs in somewhat older children, usually over the age of 3 years. Hemorrhage is caused by ulceration of the intestinal mucosa in juxtaposition to ectopic gastric mucosa. Often the ulcer erodes into an artery in the submucosa, producing profuse bleeding frequently resulting in anemia (hemoglobin usually <8.0 g), and occasionally hypotension. The bleeding will be painless. The consistency and appearance of the stool is an indication of the volume of blood loss. Melena indicates a slow loss of blood and may often be present for some days or weeks prior to a severe hemorrhage. Frank blood and current-jelly, maroon, or brick-red stool all indicate brisk bleeding and may precipitate shock. The third, somewhat less common presentation, is inflammation, which occurs in a slightly older population about 7 to 8 years of age. These children often present with a history and examination findings similar to those in acute appendicitis. In these cases the inflamed diverticulum often contains ectopic tissue or is occluded by a foreign body. Most commonly the neck of the diverticulum is wide, but in cases of inflammation the neck is often described as narrowed, allowing for obstruction of the lumen. The diverticulum may even perforate from distension or ulceration. Most series indicate the presence of ectopic tissue in cases with this presentation.

DIAGNOSIS

Some surgeons, presented with the case scenario given above, would proceed directly to the operating room for laparotomy. Today, with the rapid availability of state-of-the-art diagnostic equipment in most pediatric centers, most surgeons would prefer to arrive at a diagnosis prior to laparotomy, as long as the child's condition remains stable.

A ^{99m}Tc-pertechnetate radionuclide scan is the first test ordered.[2] Isotope dosage is calculated by body weight at 20 megabequerelles (MBq) + 3 MBq/kg. Sequential images are obtained at 5-minute cuts for 1 hour. Administration of pentagastrin and glucagon prior to the scan has given improved results. Pentagastrin is injected at 6 μg/kg body weight 20 minutes before injection of the ^{99m}Tc isotope, and the glucagon is given at 5 μg/kg body weight 10 minutes after the ^{99m}Tc-pertechnetate is administered. The specificity of this examination in identifying a Meckel's diverticulum is reported to be 95%, with a sensitivity of 85% and an overall diagnostic accuracy of 90%. Recently, cimetidine has been advocated as an additive agent for enhancing the scan by causing retention of the radioactive material in the secreting cells. Although no large clinical trials have been done with this methodology, retention of the isotope appears to persist for about 2 hours, which may allow for increased diagnostic accuracy. Positive scans demonstrate uptake of the radioactive material in the lower right abdomen. A Foley catheter may be required to eliminate dye collected in the bladder, which may obscure the uptake from the Meckel's diverticulum. A positive scan may be observed in cases of intestinal duplication (ectopic gastric mucosa is often present), and false-negative findings may be related to instances in which the gastric mucosa is insufficient in quantity to be appreciated on the scintillation camera. Although several articles in the radiology literature have suggested the routine use of barium enema and angiography for the diagnosis of Meckel's diverticulum, contrast studies are generally unrewarding. The rationale for these examinations is somewhat circumspect, given the safety and accuracy of the ^{99m}Tc-pertechnetate scan and its general availability in most hospitals.

If the scan is negative and the child continues to bleed, a labeled-red-cell scan may be employed, and if this is negative one may have to resort to angiography to identify the bleeding source. In some cases barium enema has identified multiple polyposis as an unrecognized source of this type of bleeding, but the low incidence of this problem makes this diagnosis highly unlikely in a patient with the clinical presentation described above.

TREATMENT

The treatment for a symptomatic Meckel's diverticulum is surgical excision. Although bleeding requires prompt evaluation, most children stop bleeding and emergency laparotomy is not always necessary. Patients with intestinal hemorrhage are best resuscitated initially with 20 cc/kg of crystalloid, followed by blood products and colloid as necessary. In most children with rectal bleeding as the presenting symptom, the bleeding will usually stop spontaneously, allowing for adequate preoperative preparation and diagnostic work-up. Children presenting with peritonitis due to a ruptured Meckel's diverticulum will require fluid resuscitation and preoperative antibiotic therapy. When these guidelines are followed, the expeditious treatment of Meckel's diverticulum should be accompanied by low morbidity and virtually no mortality.

Surgical resection of a Meckel's diverticulum can be accomplished in several ways. Most recent reports describe excellent success with simple amputation of the diverticulum with a stapling device, either transversely or longitudinally along the axis of the intestine. Transverse resection appears preferential in cases of young infants with a broad-based diverticulum, in whom longitudinal resection may narrow the intestinal lumen. Imbricating sutures may be placed over the staple line, although this is unnecessary if a double-line stapling device is utilized. Suture closure of the defect after amputation is similarly effective and allows the surgeon to inspect the intestine for a bleeding ulcer prior to closure. It is probably unnecessary to explore the diverticulum in cases in which bleeding has stopped preoperatively.

Simple amputation of the diverticulum constitutes effective treatment in most cases, without the need for opening the bowel or for intestinal anastomosis. Resection of the intestine is occasionally necessary because of necrotic bowel related to volvulus, or in the presence of gross inflammation and perforation. Resection may be required in instances in which the diverticulum has a very wide base and simple amputation of the diverticulum may result in stricture. Bowel resection can always be considered in instances of uncontrolled bleeding, and provides an immediate solution to the problem of the ulcer bed.

PROPHYLACTIC DIVERTICULECTOMY

The question of prophylactic removal of an asymptomatic Meckel's diverticulum has frequently been raised. The problem with arriving at an answer to this query on a purely scientific basis is that data from historical reviews have come from different patient populations, making it difficult to draw any solid conclusions. Some series indicate an incidence of symptoms of as high as 27% to 34% in the projected patient population (2% of the general population).[4] These numbers are clearly too high, and a more appropriate lifetime incidence of symptoms appears to be about 4%. What is clear, however, is that the incidence of symptoms is significantly higher in children than in adults, and that approximately 45% of symptomatic Meckel's diverticula occur in patients under 2 years of age. In reports describing only young children, the overall incidence of symptoms appears to be quite high (>40%). These latter data suggest that incidental Meckel's diverticulectomy is probably indicated in infants and young children (<8 years). In older children and adults, statistics indicate that elective incidental diverticulectomy may be unnecessary as long as there has been no prior history of symptoms. Incidental diverticulectomy can be done safely and effectively by using careful surgical technique, especially when the closed technique of surgical stapling is employed.

REFERENCES

1. Vane DW, West KW, Grosfeld JL: Vitelline duct anomalies: Experience with 217 childhood cases. *Arch Surg* 1987; 122:542–547.
2. Dutro JA, Santanello SA, Unger F, et al: Rectal bleeding in a 4-month-old boy. *JAMA* 1986; 256:2239–2240.
3. Dixon PM, Nolan DJ: The diagnosis of Meckel's diverticulum: A continuing challenge. *Clin Radiol* 1987; 38:615–619.
4. Amory RA: Meckel's diverticulum, in Welch KJ (ed): *Pediatric Surgery,* ed 4. Chicago, Year Book Medical Publishers, Inc., 1986, pp 859–867.

19

Necrotizing Enterocolitis

James A. O'Neill, Jr., M.D.

An 800-g premature male infant of 30 weeks' gestation had Apgar scores of 2 and 6 at 1 and 5 minutes. He required ventilator support because of respiratory distress ($Pa{O_2}$ = 58 torr on $F{IO_2}$ of 1.0) for 3 days. He was successfully extubated and premature feedings were started. At 6 days of age, increased gastric residuals were observed on attempted gavage feeding. The stool guaiac test was positive. The abdomen was distended and abdominal radiographs demonstrated dilated intestine with pneumatosis intestinalis in the right lower quadrant. The arterial pH was 7.22, the WBC count was 31,000/mm^3 with a shift to the left on differential smear, and the platelet count was 38,500/mm^3.

This case history details the typical presentation of a low-birth-weight, premature newborn who sustains a critical event that triggers the development of intestinal necrosis related to bowel ischemia. The first clear-cut description of the clinical and diagnostic findings of necrotizing enterocolitis in the low-birth-weight infant was published by Berdon and co-workers in 1964.[1] It would appear that various factors may be responsible for the initiation of a process that results in the clinical picture of necrotizing enterocolitis. The precise cause is unknown, but it is most likely that the disorder requires a host who is susceptible and one or more contributing factors. First, necrotizing enterocolitis is encountered primarily in the premature and low-birth-weight newborn as in this case, and the younger the infant the higher the incidence of this problem. Necrotizing enterocolitis only occasionally affects term infants. It has been suggested that mucosal injury, occurring in the presence of pathogenic bacteria and intraluminal feeding, sets the stage for the development of necrotizing enterocolitis.

Numerous other factors are also thought to contribute to mucosal injury. Kliegman and Fanaroff reported that when immature animals are subjected to stress such as hypoxemia or shock, there is redistribution of blood flow favoring vital organs at the expense of the vascular beds of the splanchnic system and peripheral musculature.[2] Various experimental studies have demonstrated that low cardiac output and hypoxemia decrease intestinal blood flow in the fetus and newborn. The case described above is typical in that the subject is a very small, high-risk, low-birth-weight, premature newborn, and the low Apgar scores indicate the high initial probability of low cardiac output or shock. Second, respiratory distress syndrome and hypoxemia lasting for 72 hours are additional major factors promoting the development of necrotizing enterocolitis. Respiratory distress syndrome, shock, asphyxia, hypothermia, and congestive heart failure related to patent ductus arteriosis have all been reported to be contributory factors. Additionally, polycythemia and hyperviscosity have been indicted as additive factors expected to lead to diminished blood flow to the intestinal vascular bed, something often seen in association with intestinal infarction in the newborn infant.

In addition to these and many other natural events that may occur in the low-birth-weight newborn, a number of iatrogenic factors related to treatment of the neonate have been shown to be associated with diminished intestinal flow, either directly or through generalized decreases in cardiac output. The use of umbilical artery catheters has been associated with intestinal infarction, but peripheral embolization is probably responsible for segmental intestinal compromise under those circumstances. Exchange transfusion via an umbilical venous catheter has also been associated with necrotizing enterocolitis; it is thought that exchange transfusion performed via this route may produce intestinal ischemia by sumping portal blood away from the splanchnic bed; additionally, hypotension associated with this procedure may well be a contributing factor. It has been suggested that a number of drugs may be related to the etiology of necrotizing enterocolitis, including vitamin E, indomethacin, and theophylline. However, we have not been able to confirm these associations, and no mention is made of this in the case history.

Santulli and his group were the first to implicate early feedings as another possible factor in either producing or extending intestinal mucosal injury.[3] Early feeding has been considered detrimental since it may provide a substrate for bacterial growth, and since hyperosmolar formulas could cause mucosal damage by producing a process like the dumping syndrome, whereby intestinal flow is redistributed on a segmental basis. It is now accepted by most neonatologists that early feedings and too rapid advancement of volume are undesirable in infants with the risk factors mentioned above as being associated with diminished cardiac output and hypoxemia in the perinatal period. Currently, it is our practice to avoid feedings of any type for at least 1 to 3 weeks in susceptible infants, depending on how sick they appear to be. When feeding is possible, breast milk from the baby's own mother is utilized for feeding because of the potential advantage of providing protection in the form of IgA and immunocompetent cells.

This infant was fed at 3 days of life immediately after withdrawal of respiratory support. This would appear to have been imprudent, since 3 days later the infant presented with findings suggestive of necrotizing enterocolitis. Additionally, since it is known that bacteria are essential for the development of this process once mucosal damage has occurred, clinical signs of the disease often suggest sepsis, which is certainly the situation in this case.

CLINICAL PRESENTATION

The infant described above had onset of symptoms at 6 days of age. The average age at onset of symptoms related to necrotizing enterocolitis 20 years ago was 3 or 4 days, but this has gradually been increasing, so that it is now about 10 to 12 days of age. In our experience, the average patient who has presented with hypoxemia, lung disease, and low cardiac output has generally stabilized without any signs of intestinal problems during the first few days of life. However, as with the infant described here, a clinical picture of sepsis has developed from 7 to 10 days after birth, with gastric retention and bilious vomiting, ileus, abdominal distension, and bloody stools. Lethargy, bradycardia, hypothermia, apneic spells, and hypotension have generally followed. Progressive clinical deterioration has unfortunately occurred in most such cases. In this regard, late findings have been abnormal bleeding, hyperbilirubinemia, and oliguria. Occasional infants have had circulatory collapse and intestinal perforation as their first presenting sign.

Physical signs have included lack of responsiveness, abdominal distension, patterning of intestinal loops visible through the abdominal wall, redness of the abdominal wall, and occasionally a palpable, fixed, firm loop of intestine. Physical findings have not always been reliable indicators that an intestinal catastrophe has occurred, because many infants have been so lethargic that abdominal examination has not been reliable.

DIAGNOSIS

Infants with postnatal necrotizing enterocolitis generally have serial laboratory determinations, including a complete blood count, pH and blood gas measurements, and electrolyte assays. Anemia, a sudden decrease in the serum sodium concentration, and metabolic acidosis have been characteristic, indicating advanced sepsis. In our experience, a sudden decline in platelet count, unexplained by any other finding such as an intraventricular hemorrhage has been one of the most reliable indications of intestinal gangrene.[4] Such significant declines in the platelet count are probably based on aggregation induced by the presence of endotoxin in the serum. The infant presented in the case history described above had findings of severe metabolic acidosis, a high white cell count with a shift to the left, and significant thrombocytopenia. The last finding, taken together with severe metabolic acidosis and pneumatosis intestinalis, is a strong indication that surgery is in order.

We generally perform abdominal radiography every 8 hours during the acute phase of necrotizing enterocolitis. The characteristic radiographic findings on plain films of the abdomen include intestinal distension with varying amounts of intramural gas. It is important to realize that the x-ray picture may vary according to the chronology of the disease state, and that x-rays must accordingly be interpreted in terms of when the process is believed to have begun. For example, we have noted that pneumatosis generally clears within 72 hours of its first being noted in patients who respond to treatment. Usually, intestinal distension remains for a longer period, even if pneumatosis clears. At times, the radiologic picture changes from one of intestinal distension and pneumatosis to one of abdominal distension and opacity suggesting the presence of free fluid. We have used diagnostic paracentesis, either with or without saline lavage, in patients whose abdominal x-rays show apparent free fluid, in order to make an early diagnosis of bacterial peritonitis, which is always related to either intestinal perforation or gangrene. In fulminant cases of necrotizing enterocolitis, portal vein gas may be seen in addition to pneumatosis intestinalis on the abdominal radiograph. This usually indicates fulminant disease, and when portal venous gas has been noted, only rarely do patients recover without the need for surgery. Since the intestine in such patients is extremely fragile, we have not used radiographic contrast studies such as barium enema in such cases, and consider them to be contraindicated.

TREATMENT

In general terms, the treatment of neonates with necrotizing enterocolitis takes two forms: supportive therapy and surgical intervention. The first report to suggest that vigorous physiologic support might be helpful in the care of desperately ill infants with necrotizing enterocolitis was presented in 1971 by Stevenson and co-workers, who used an aggressive regimen of supportive treatment.[5] These workers were actually able to demonstrate that such an aggressive approach to physiologic support might avoid the need for surgery even though it defied the generally accepted surgical dictum that surgery should be performed in patients with generalized peritonitis. Prophetically, Stevenson advised that surgery should not be avoided when necessary, and suggested that no infant should die having received supportive therapy alone. This recommendation has been borne out by subsequent experience.

Since supportive therapy for neonates with severe necrotizing enterocolitis is directed at reversing the pathophysiology of the disease, its success is measured by demonstrating normalization of physiologic function. Supportive therapy includes replenishment of the circulating blood volume using appropriate monitoring techniques, correction of electrolyte and acid-base imbalances and anemia, vigorous respiratory support designed to correct hypoxemia and hypercarbia, gastrointestinal rest and decompression, and broad-spectrum, systemic antibiotic therapy. Since intestinal distension accentuates the problem of intestinal ischemia, gastric suction should be initiated early in the course of treatment. Generally speaking, infants of low birth weight are born malnourished, and intensive parenteral nutritional support is therefore provided, either by peripheral vein or via a centrally placed intravenous catheter. We have used the guideline that if nutritional support is expected to be required for only a week or so, peripheral techniques of administration are used, but if the required interval of intravenous nutritional therapy and gastrointestinal rest is anticipated to be longer than that, a central venous Broviac catheter or "long line" is placed for full nutritional support.

During the period of intensive supportive care, serial diagnostic studies are performed, every eight hours at first and then at increasing intervals thereafter, depending on the infant's progress. We have found that if surgery is going to be required, it is usually necessary within the first 5 days of initial diagnosis. The most helpful studies have been serial abdominal radiographs, white blood and platelet counts, and pH and blood gas measurements. If this vigorous approach to supportive physiologic therapy is successful, all of the various monitoring parameters will improve, as will the clinical condition of the infant.

The main indication for surgery is clinical deterioration despite what would be thought to be adequate support. Usually, there is no single indication that surgery is in order, but rather a constellation of findings suggesting that the infant is not showing improvement.

The main purpose for obtaining serial abdominal x-rays is to demonstrate pneumoperitoneum. The latter finding is occasionally extensive and easily recognized, but is more often initially subtle on a supine film, with only small amounts of free air visible under the right diaphragm or liver or anteriorly in the midabdomen. We have found that a left lateral decubitus film is particularly helpful, since it may reveal relatively small amounts of free air along the lateral border of the liver. However, since it is far better to determine the need for surgery before intestinal perforation has occurred, we have put more emphasis on other studies that demonstrate continued clinical deterioration despite adequate supportive treatment. One such finding is irreversible metabolic acidosis, as seen in the patient described above. More importantly, we have found that a significant decrease in the platelet count in patients who have no other reason for such a decrease has reliably indicated the presence of gangrenous bowel. Over the years, we have found that every patient who has such a finding also has other indications of clinical deterioration. While we have found that many patients whose platelet counts decrease to the range of 100,000/mm^3 may improve with supportive therapy, we have never seen a patient with a platelet count as low as 38,500/mm^3, as in the case described above, avoid surgery. For this reason, surgery would be appropriate for this patient, although the severe metabolic acidosis and high white blood count also strongly indicate that irreversible bowel damage has occurred.

Although no mention of physical findings is given in the preceding protocol, we have found physical signs of severe peritonitis on examination of the abdomen to be another reliable indicator of the need for surgery. All patients in whom paracentesis has yielded bacteria upon gram staining have been operated on and found to have irreversible intestinal pathology. Other reliable indicators of the need for surgery are the radiographic presence of a sentinel intestinal loop for over 24 hours, the radiographic finding of portal vein gas associated with extensive pneumatosis intestinalis, and abdominal-wall cellulitis.

The safest approach to surgical therapy is resection of the gangrenous intestine with exteriorization of the proximal and distal bowel.[5] Although there have been some reports of successful primary anastomosis, particularly when the necrotic intestine has been in the proximal small intestine, this technique requires a great deal of experience and judgement, and most surgeons advocate a staged approach to this problem.

Another reason for exteriorization resection and delayed anastomosis being the safest approach in patients with necrotizing enterocolitis relates to the scattered areas of intestinal ischemia in many patients. Somewhere between 5% and 10% of patients treated supportively for necrotizing enterocolitis develop late strictures related to localized areas of gangrene that did not result in perforation. The timing of anastomosis following exteriorization resection has been based on the fact that these strictures generally form within 4 weeks of the onset of disease. While in the past, patients were allowed to grow and develop for as long as 3 to 6 months prior to anastomosis, many did not thrive during this interval, and our current preference is to close ostomies after 4 weeks, surveying the intestinal tract beforehand through contrast studies in order to determine whether any intestinal strictures are present, particularly in the distal, defunctionalized bowel.

Postoperatively it is essential to continue the same intensive level of supportive care that was provided preoperatively. Particularly important is nutritional supportive therapy using intravenous techniques. Although enteral nutrition is more desirable than intravenous nutrition, it is usually not possible to begin enteral feedings sooner than 7 days postoperatively, and it is often 2 to 3 weeks before any appreciable enteral nutrition can be provided. Since recurrent necrotizing enterocolitis is a distinct possibility in patients who have been treated either medically or surgically for necrotizing enterocolitis, enteral feedings are begun in a dilute form in low volume, and are gradually advanced. Another reason why intravenous nutritional therapy may be required is that many patients require extensive resection, and even in those who do not, extensive mucosal damage may result in severe carbohydrate and fat malabsorption that can last several months. Much depends on whether or not the ileocecal valve is present, although the degree of involvement of the remaining small bowel is probably the main determinant of the severity of malabsorption. Reconstitution of gastrointestinal continuity is clearly helpful in promoting the resumption of normal gastrointestinal absorption and function. Using these techniques, a long-term survival of approximately 80% has been achieved. In the absence of short-bowel syndrome, we have not seen any detectable long-term effect on growth and development, intestinal function, or nutritional status in low-birth-weight infants in our series. Additionally, the incidence of central nervous system complications appears to be no higher than that noted in a population of seriously ill low-birth-weight newborns who have not had necrotizing enterocolitis. This is probably a reflection of the aggressive supportive therapy given to all of these infants.

REFERENCES

1. Berdon WE, Grossman H, Baker DH, et al: Necrotizing enterocolitis in the premature infant. *Radiology* 1964; 83:879–887.
2. Kliegman RM, Fanaroff AA: Necrotizing enterocolitis. *N Engl J Med* 1984; 310:1093–1103.
3. Santulli TV, Schullinger JN, Heird WC, et al: Acute necrotizing enterocolitis in infancy: A review of 64 cases. *Pediatrics* 1975; 55:376–387.
4. O'Neill JA, Stahlman MT, Meng HC: Necrotizing enterocolitis in the newborn: Operative indications. *Ann Surg* 1975; 182:274–279.
5. Stevenson JK, Oliver TK, Graham CB, et al: Aggressive treatment of necrotizing enterocolitis and analysis of 45 consecutive cases. *J Pediatr Surg* 1971; 6:28–35.

PART THREE

Gastroesophageal Disorders

20

Esophageal Atresia With Tracheoesophageal Fistula

Thomas M. Holder, M.D.
Peter B. Manning, M.D.

A 2.5-kg female infant was born at 34 weeks' gestation by uneventful vaginal delivery. The infant was noted to have excessive salivation in the nursery requiring frequent oropharyngeal suctioning. Difficulty was encountered during attempts at passing an orogastric tube into the stomach. A chest roentgenogram was obtained and showed the orogastric tube coiled in the upper mediastinum, air in the viscera beneath the diaphragm, and right-upper-lobe atelectasis.

Fifty years ago, esophageal atresia (EA) was a uniformly fatal anomaly.[1, 2] Through improvements in surgical technique, and more importantly in newborn intensive-care management, survival rates of greater than 90% are now expected.

Current management schemes focus on a tailored approach to each infant,[2] based as much on the respiratory status and magnitude of associated anomalies (particularly cardiac anomalies) as on the esophageal anatomy itself.[1]

PRESENTATION

Drooling, the need for frequent suctioning, and coughing or cyanosis with oral intake are the most common presentations of esophageal atresia in infants. The inability to pass a nasogastric tube and its coiled appearance in the upper esophagus on chest x-ray confirms the diagnosis of atresia. The presence of air in the gastrointestinal (GI) tract documents the coexistence of a distal tracheoesophageal fistula (TEF).

Many aspects of the initial management of an infant with esophageal atresia and tracheoesophageal fistula (EA/TEF) are the same, regardless of the presence of associated anomalies or pulmonary compromise. The need for secure intravenous access and initiation of dextrose-containing fluids is obvious.

Other aspects of the initial management focus on preventing the aspiration of oral secretions and preventing gastroesophagotracheal reflux, both of which threaten stable pulmonary function. Constant nasopharyngeal or oropharyngeal suctioning of the upper esophageal pouch with a sump suction catheter must be instituted to avoid spillover aspiration of oral secretions into the lungs. Elevation of the head of the bed, and the avoidance, if feasible, of positive pressure ventilation (which, via the TEF, will distend the stomach) are important measures for preventing acid reflux into the airway via the TEF.

The initiation of broad-spectrum antibiotics is also recommended during the early management of the infant. We prefer ampicillin (50 mg/kg every 12 hours) and gentamicin (2.5 mg/kg every 12 hours; levels should be closely monitored during therapy).

Continuous monitoring of the electrocardiogram (ECG) and respiratory pattern is routine, as should be oxygen-saturation monitoring. In the premature infant, particularly with any evidence of pulmonary compromise or suspicion of cardiac anomaly, placement of an umbilical artery catheter is recommended for frequent blood gas determinations.

ASSESSMENT

In the early 1960s the major causes of death in infants with EA/TEF were found to be pulmonary complications, prematurity, and severe associated congenital anomalies. The classification of patients into high- and low-risk categories, based on the presence of these factors, is important in tailoring the surgical approach to an individual infant. Currently, we use an assessment of the infant's cardiac and pulmonary condition as the main indicator of risk status. Congenital heart defects and sepsis are the major contributors to cardiovascular instability in these infants, while pneumonitis (secondary to aspiration or reflux) or prematurity are prime etiologies of pulmonary compromise. Gestational age and birthweight do not appear to be significant independent risk factors.

The sequence of events in the definitive management of the infant with EA/TEF therefore depends more on the severity of associated anomalies and the physiologic status of the infant than on the esophageal anomaly itself. The presence of respiratory compromise or of another anomaly requiring more urgent intervention may require delay in performing the esophageal repair (Fig 20–1). A thorough evaluation of the infant is imperative in planning an operative strategy.

The initial assessment of the infant with EA/TEF therefore has three main

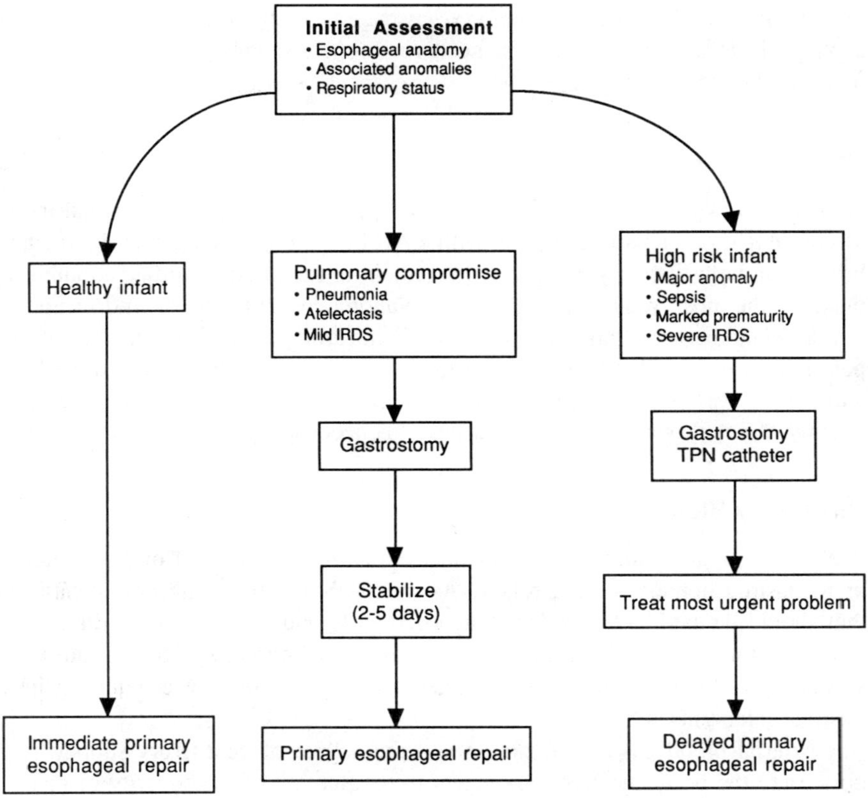

FIG 20–1.
Management algorithm for infants with esophageal atresia and tracheoesophageal fistula, based on assessment of risk status. (IRDS = infant respiratory distress syndrome).

areas of focus: (1) evaluation of the tracheoesophageal anomaly itself; (2) identification of associated anomalies, some of which may present a more immediate threat to life and require treatment prior to correction of the esophageal anomaly; and (3) Assessment of the respiratory status of the infant.

Esophageal

As noted earlier, the findings of a nasogastric tube coiled in the proximal pouch and air-filled bowel in the abdomen are classic for EA with distal TEF. This is the most commonly anatomic variant of EA, representing 85% of cases.

Confirmation of the proximal atresia is done via a "pouch-o-gram" using a small volume (0.5 cc) of barium instilled through the nasoesophageal tube. It is important not to overfill the pouch and cause aspiration. Any barium noted in the airway should raise the suspicion of a second, proximal fistula or laryngoesophageal cleft, and indicates the need for bronchoscopy when the patient is first anesthetized.

Other Anomalies

Anomalies of other systems or more distal segments of the gastrointestinal tract are present in over half of infants with EA/TEF. They may have a significant bearing on both the early and late management of the infant. Cardiac anomalies make up the most frequent group of severe anomalies and have the most important association with long-term survival. Echocardiography has become indispensable in the rapid, noninvasive evaluation of infants with suspected cardiac anomalies. The term "VACTERL" constellation refers to the systems most frequently affected: *v*ertebral, *a*nal, *c*ardiac, *t*racheoesophageal, *r*enal, and *l*imb.

Pulmonary Status

Atelectasis or pneumonia are most often related to aspiration of oral secretions or to gastroesophagotracheal reflux. As noted above, these are complications that should be avoidable if EA is diagnosed early and proper attention is given to protecting the airway. In the premature infant, respiratory distress syndrome secondary to lung immaturity may cause significant compromise requiring immediate intervention.

Arterial blood gas determination and the degree of ventilatory support required are the best objective parameters for evaluation of the severity of respiratory compromise.

Evaluation

Infants in the low-risk category (those without major associated anomalies or significant pulmonary compromise) undergo immediate primary repair of the esophagus and division of the TEF. In the case of the high-risk neonate (with a major associated anomaly, severe respiratory distress, sepsis, or marked prematurity), tube gastrostomy and central venous catheter insertion are performed, upper-pouch suction is continued, and parenteral alimentation is begun. Direct management of the EA/TEF is deferred until the patient's condition has stabilized. Generally, decompression of the stomach and constant upper-pouch suction will prevent pulmonary complications related to the presence of the EA/TEF. With this management, esophageal repair can be delayed for as long as required to treat concomitant disease. Those infants without severe associated anomalies but with pulmonary compromise from pneumonia, severe atelectasis, or prematurity make up an intermediate group. A gastrostomy is created initially, the lung disease is managed, and primary esophageal repair is then performed, usually at 2 to 5 days of age. Cervical esophagostomy is unnecessary and undesirable.

SURGICAL MANAGEMENT

As mentioned previously, if contrast medium is seen in the trachea during the pouch-o-gram study, bronchoscopy should be performed after induction of anesthesia, to identify a possible proximal fistula or laryngoesophageal cleft.

A posterolateral, fourth-interspace thoracotomy is performed on the side of the chest opposite the aortic arch, typically the right side. The pleural space is not entered, but a retropleural plane is developed around to the mediastinum. The azygous vein need not be divided, but may be reflected inferiorly after dividing its highest intercostal branches. This maneuver lessens the chance of entering the pleura. Such an approach allows generous exposure of the tracheoesophageal region and protects the pleural space from infection should an anastomotic leak occur.

The dissection of the mediastinum begins with the TEF and distal esophagus, because control of the fistula means control of the airway for the anesthesiologist, both for preventing reflux and stopping any ventilatory air leak. The vagus nerve is an important landmark for identification of the distal esophagus. Only the immediate region of the fistula should be dissected, since extensive mobilization of the distal esophageal segment may increase the risk of later gastroesophageal reflux, or may compromise the blood supply to this segment.

The TEF is divided so as to leave a thin rim of esophageal tissue on the tracheal side to allow closure of the trachea without narrowing it. Too generous a rim of tissue can produce a diverticulum. Following tracheal closure, the upper esophageal pouch is dissected. Its identification is aided by the passage of a nasoesophageal tube by the anesthesiologist. The proximal pouch is dissected as needed to allow it to reach to the distal esophageal segment with minimal tension for anastomoses. Various techniques for increasing the pouch length, if needed, have been described. Circular myotomy is used most frequently, but in general these methods are unnecessary.

The technique of anastomosis is subject to individual variation. Initially a two-layer, telescoping anastomosis was most frequently employed, but most pediatric surgeons now prefer a single-layer technique. Most surgeons use silk suture, although some advocate the use of absorbable material, believing that it decreases the rate of anastomotic complications.[3]

A small chest tube is left in the retropleural space near the anastomosis as a drain, should an anastomotic leak occur. If a tube gastrostomy was not performed as the initial procedure in a delayed repair, it may be performed concomitantly with the esophageal repair. The current trend, however, is to avoid tube gastrostomy if it has not already been done, because of a possibly increased risk of gastroesophageal reflux that some sources feel is associated with this procedure.

Postoperative Management

The general postoperative support of the infant with EA/TEF continues as in the preoperative period. If pulmonary support is required, it is generally more easily accomplished after the TEF has been divided. Parenteral nutrition is continued, or if a gastrostomy has been created, enteral feeding may be initiated. A more thorough search for less severe associated anomalies is pursued. Oral feedings are begun between the third and seventh postoperative day, depending on the patient's cardiorespiratory status. The chest tube is observed for output of saliva, which would indicate an anastomotic leak. A routine postoperative upper GI is not generally necessary. The drain is removed on the tenth postoperative day if there is no evidence of a leak, and feedings are advanced as tolerated. Anastomotic leakage does occur in approximately 15% of cases, but the anastomosis in nearly all will close with time and continued, adequate drainage. Because of the extrapleural approach, a leak does not lead to empyema, which would require more aggressive intervention.

Symptomatic gastroesophageal reflux is present in nearly half of all patients and often requires fundoplication. Anastomotic stricture is noted at a rate similar to that of anastomotic leakage. Strictures generally respond to serial dilations, but indicate a need to evaluate for the presence of gastroesophageal reflux. There is evidence that the severity of postoperative strictures is related to reflux, an additional reason for aggressive detection and management of the latter problem.

Feeding difficulties are common in infants with EA/TEF, in part due to the high frequency of reflux, but also to esophageal dysmotility, which has been demonstrated to persist for life. Tracheomalacia and recurrent TEF each have about a 2% to 5% incidence.

Results

In the past 15 years, we have cared for 114 infants with EA or TEF or both. Fifty-eight (51%) were healthy babies in whom the abnormality was repaired immediately. Eighteen (16%) infants required treatment of pulmonary compromise prior to esophageal repair. The early survival rate was 100% in both groups. Thirty-eight (33%) infants required delayed management of their EA because of severe associated conditions. Twenty of these underwent surgical management of another problem prior to esophageal repair. Hospital survival in this high-risk group was 84% (4 infants died from associated anomalies prior to esophageal repair, and 2 others died in the postoperative period).

In summary, excellent results are achieved in the management of this complex anomaly, through the use of a tailored approach to each infant based on a thorough evaluation and aggressive management of any severe associated anomalies and respiratory compromise. Utilizing such an approach, we have achieved a 95% hospital survival rate in the past 15 years.

REFERENCES

1. Holder TM, Ashcraft KW, Sharp RJ, et al: Care of infants with esophageal atresia, tracheoesophageal fistula and associated anomalies. *J Thorac Cardiovasc Surg* 1987; 94:828–835.
2. Randolf JG, Newman KD, Anderson KD: Current results in repair of esophageal atresia with tracheoesophageal fistula using physiologic status as a guide to therapy. *Ann Surg* 1989; 209:526–531.
3. Spitz L, Kiely E, Bereton RJ: Esophageal atresia: A five year experience with 148 cases. *J Pediatr Surg* 1987; 22:103–108.

21

Type A Esophageal Atresia

Morton M. Woolley, M.D.

A 1.8-kg male was born at 32 weeks' gestation by vaginal delivery. The pregnancy was associated with polyhydramnios. The initial Apgar score was 4 at 1 minute but improved to 8 at 5 minutes. The baby was cyanotic with a PaO_2 of 45 torr with an FIO_2 of 0.8. The infant also had excessive salivation. An orogastric tube could not be passed into the stomach. A chest roentgenogram was obtained and showed the tube in the upper mediastinum and no air beneath the diaphragm.

This prematurely born infant has the usual findings of proximal and distal esophageal atresia without a distal tracheoesophageal fistula. The presence or absence of a fistula between the proximal esophagus and the trachea must be determined, but at a later date. The most pressing matter, which must be addressed immediately, is the respiratory distress. The patient is described as clinically cyanotic and has less than an ideal PaO_2. Endotracheal intubation, followed by mechanical ventilatory support with an appropriate FIO_2, should be accomplished with alacrity and without fear of abdominal distension, since there is no distal tracheoesophageal fistula. The blood gases are best monitored through an umbilical arterial cannula, the tip of which should be positioned above the renal arteries. Prior to its removal, the arterial cannula can be used for a retrograde aortogram to determine the locus of the aorta. If the aorta is located on the left side, the eventual definitive thoracotomy can be accomplished through a right extrapleural thoracotomy. Alternatively, if the aorta is on the right a left thoracotomy would be preferable.

Once the infant has been intubated and given ventilatory support, and the arterial monitoring has been implemented, a cardiac ultrasound examination should be performed to exclude congenital heart disease. This is particularly important in this infant, who is clinically cyanotic. The cyanosis could be due to cyanotic heart disease rather than respiratory distress. It is important to differentiate between the two at an early time. If the infant does not have life-threatening heart disease and if the ventilatory support is successful in correcting the blood gas abnormalities, a Stamm gastrostomy can be performed for gastrointestinal alimentation. The surgeon will find the stomach to be quite small in this infant because it has never contained any significant amount of gas or fluid. The usual purse-string suture around the gastrostomy catheter will not be possible. The anterior gastric wall is approximated to the gastrostomy tube by folding the anterior wall proximally and distally with nonabsorbable sutures (Fig 21–1). Prior to using the gastrostomy for feedings, an upper gastrointestinal study is performed to exclude the possibility of distal intestinal atresia. If an associated intestinal atresia is present and the infant is fed through the gastrostomy, the gastrostomy will leak, resulting in serious if not lethal peritonitis. The upper gastrointestinal study will show a very small stomach (Fig 21–2). With a gradually increased volume of formula, the stomach will grow to normal or near-normal size (Fig 21–3).

Since the infant is unable to swallow, the oronasopharyngeal secretions must be constantly suctioned from the upper esophageal segment. A double-lumen Replogle tube is quite satisfactory for this purpose. The tube can be attached to a low-pressure intermittent suction pump. Manual suctioning may be necessary and is readily accomplished by a well-trained neonatal intensive-care nurse.

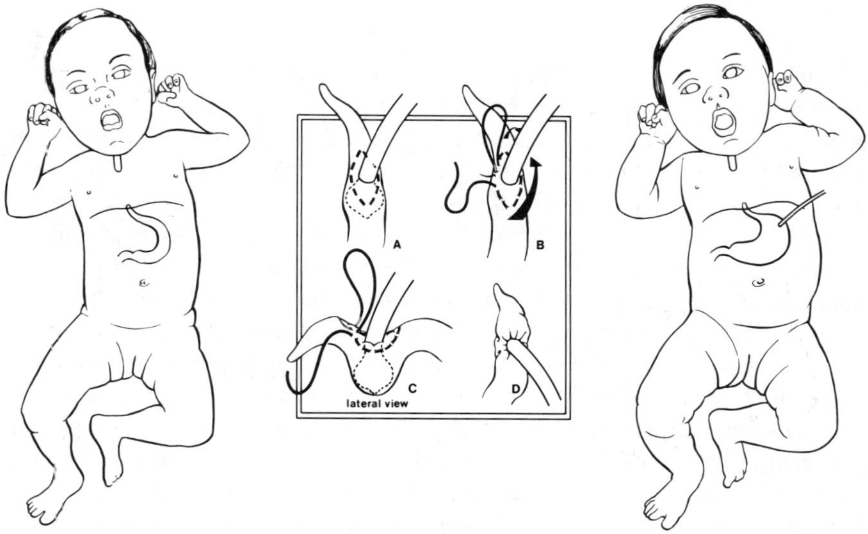

FIG 21–1.
Because of the narrow configuration of the stomach, the anterior gastric wall must be plicated in a longitudinal fashion in performing the gastrostomy.

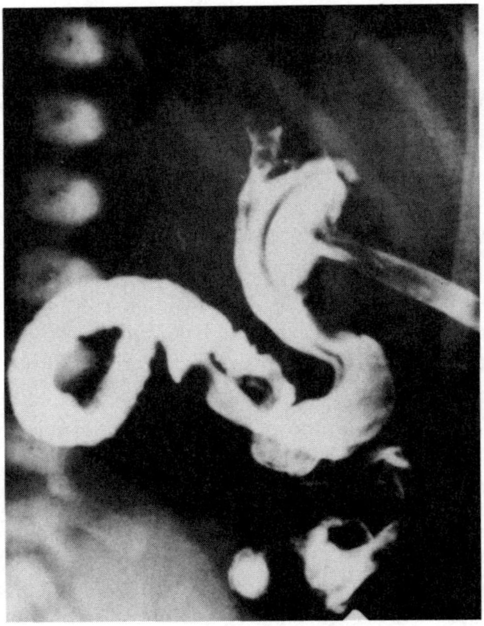

FIG 21–2.
X-ray of the stomach, showing a very small gastric lumen soon after the gastrostomy is performed.

Once the infant's ventilatory status has been stabilized and the infant is being fed via the gastrostomy, it has been our policy to gently stretch the upper esophageal segment using a mercury-weighted, size-20 Bougie. This stretching can be accomplished once or twice per day. If one measures the distance from the gum line to the pouch, it will be found to gain 3 cm in length in approximately 3 weeks (Fig 21–4). Beyond 3 weeks there is usually no additional measurable lengthening; however, the thickness of the upper esophageal segment is increased, making it a more stretchable conduit. Approximately half of infants will have a fistula between the upper esophagus and trachea, and in one of our patients two fistulae were present. If there is any problem with the initial intubation of the trachea, the surgeon should be alerted to the possibility of a laryngotracheoesophageal cleft, which is readily diagnosed by endoscopy.

Some infants with proximal and distal esophageal atresia do not have enough esophageal substance to allow for eventual esophageal reconstruction. The majority of infants, however, do have adequate esophageal tissue to eventually allow for reconstruction of the esophagus.[1, 2] If there is any radiographically demonstrable distal esophagus, one is justified in attempting to stretch the upper esophageal segment. Doing this generally makes it eventually possi-

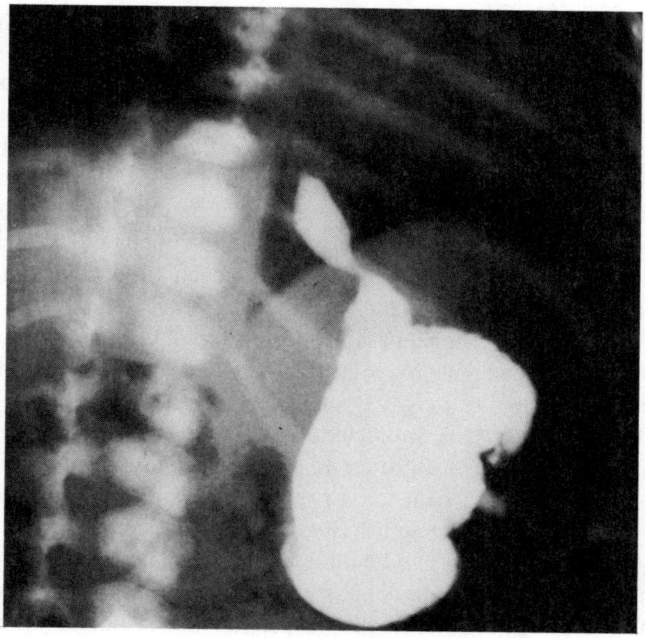

FIG 21–3.
Same infant in Fig 21–1, two weeks after gastrostomy. After feeding of the infant through the gastrostomy tube, the gastric volume increases rapidly to normal or near-normal size.

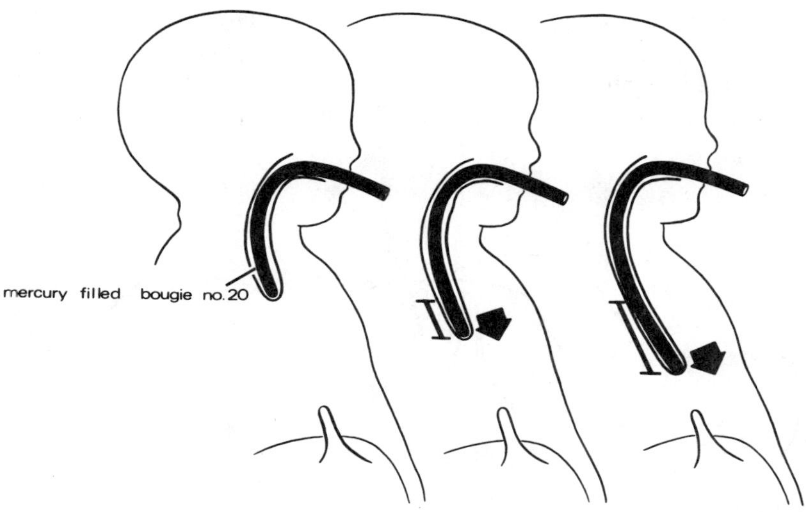

FIG 21–4.
By gentle stretching with a mercury bougie, one can generally elongate the upper esophageal segment by a distance of 3 cm.

ble to anastomose the esophageal segments so that an anatomic esophagus is reconstructed. If there is no distal esophagus, the likelihood of an anatomic esophageal reconstruction is remote. I am aware of one infant whose esophageal atresia was within 1 cm of the diaphragm. In this infant an esophagogastrostomy could be readily performed. This is a unique anatomic abnormality. With this exception, if there is no demonstrable distal esophagus, one is justified in performing a cervical esophagostomy early in the clinical course, under which circumstances a colon interposition will be the method of creating a conduit between the upper esophagus and the stomach. The colon interposition would be performed at approximately 18 months of age.

The timing of the esophagoesophagostomy will depend on the patient's general condition and weight. It can generally be done when the infant is 3 to 6 weeks of age, provided its weight is approximately 2,500 g.

In patients with type A esophageal atresia, the distal esophagus is frequently difficult to locate at the time of the thoracotomy. I would recommend placing a foreign body (a catheter) in the distal esophagus through the gastrostomy prior to the thoracotomy (Fig 21–5). The catheter may be taped loosely to the skin so that it can be pulled out under the drapes after the distal esophagus has been located. In contrast to the case of an infant with proximal esophageal atresia and a distal tracheoesophageal fistula, under which circumstances the upper segment is short and the distal segment is longer and we use the third interspace for the thoracotomy, we use the fifth interspace in infants with proximal and distal atresia because the distal segment is the shorter. The operation is performed through an extrapleural dissection. If the two esophageal segments can be approximated without a myotomy, this is done. If there is inadequate length, a Levaditis myotomy is performed on the upper segment. I have found it helpful to use Potts ductus clamps to help coapt the two ends of the esophagus as they are being sutured. The surgeon must look carefully for a

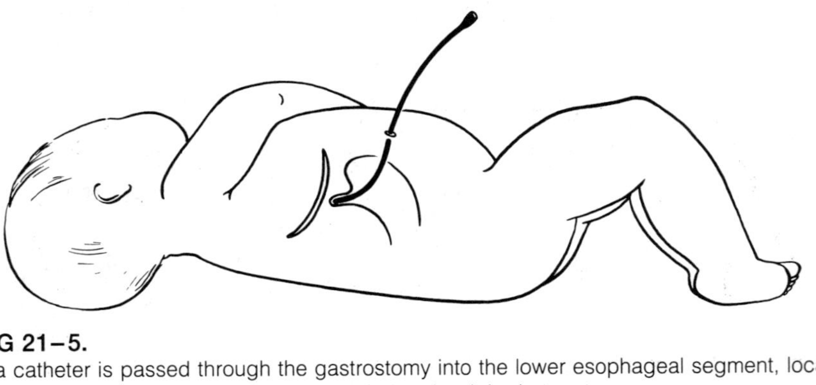

FIG 21–5.
If a catheter is passed through the gastrostomy into the lower esophageal segment, location of the esophagus will be facilitated during the right thoracotomy.

proximal tracheoesophageal fistula during the dissection. It is easier to isolate and ligate the fistula than to cut into it and then attempt to define the upper portion of the fistula.

In our experience, most patients with type A esophageal atresia have had a leak from the esophagoesophagostomy. With appropriate extrapleural drainage, the leaks closed spontaneously.

Gastroesophageal reflux is common, and the patient may require an antireflux procedure. Strictures also commonly occur, and are best treated by esophageal dilatation through the gastrostomy using Tucker dilators.

Long-term follow-up of these patients has shown that they are able to eat table food and have maintained normal nutrition, normal growth, and weight gain. As adults they will discover that if they do not chew their food satisfactorily, they will have some midsternal discomfort, and will occasionally have a piece of solid food incarcerate at the anastomotic site.

If the two segments of the esophagus cannot be anastomosed, then the proximal esophagus is exteriorized in the neck, and a colon interposition is performed when the patient reaches approximately 1 year of age.

REFERENCES

1. Howard R, Myers NA: Esophageal atresia: A technique for elongating the upper pouch. *Surgery* 1965; 58:725.
2. Johnston PW: Elongation of the upper segment in esophageal atresia: Report of a case. *Surgery* 1965; 58:741.

22

Esophageal Replacement Procedures

Kathryn D. Anderson, M.D.

A 10-year-old boy was referred because of difficulty in swallowing. He had suffered an alkaline burn of the esophagus at 16 months of age, which resulted in a stricture that was dilated three or four times annually. The youngster tolerated liquids; however, attempts at solid intake resulted in three instances of a foreign body lodging in the esophagus, requiring esophagoscopy and retrieval. A barium-contrast swallow showed a long, narrow, and rigid stricture of the mid and distal esophagus. There was limited peristaltic activity.

Once investigations have proceeded to the point at which it can be said that an esophageal stricture is truly undilatable, esophageal replacement can be performed electively. The barium esophagogram is carefully reviewed to define the stricture length, and esophagoscopy is performed to ascertain the upper level of the stricture. Gastrostomy feedings may be necessary to ensure good nutritional status. Removal of the damaged native esophagus is planned to reduce the future risk of carcinoma. Simultaneous removal and reconstruction of the esophagus in the native esophageal bed can be done, or esophagectomy can be done separately via a right thoracotomy, establishing a left cervical esophagostomy. The next decision to be made is which portion of the bowel to use in the esophageal reconstruction. There are several highly acceptable methods of esophageal replacement, all of which have their vigorous supporters. The truth is that there is very little difference between different methods, each type of replacement serving as a conduit of food to the stomach, each supporting nutrition and growth, and each having its own set of complications. Four options will be discussed in this chapter: (1) use of the right or left colon; use of a reversed gastric tube; and use of the whole stomach and jejunum. Three routes through the thorax will be outlined: substernal, left retrohilar, and transmediastinal.

THE COLON

The colon remains the most popular organ for esophageal replacement in North America. Both the right and the left colon are used with equal facility. Both depend on a good marginal artery for vascular supply, the segment between the right and middle colic artery being taken in the former case and between the middle and left colic artery in the latter. It matters little whether the segment is placed in isoperistaltic or antiperistaltic fashion, the choice depending on personal preference. The precise length needed can be selected, avoiding overshortening of the remaining colon. The disadvantage of using the colon is that its use foreshortens the absorptive surface of the remaining bowel, which is sometimes a problem, at least in the short term. Furthermore, the vascular supply is not always ideal, and submucosal collateral vessels are sparse. However, vascular adequacy can be assessed by temporary clamping of the artery to be sacrificed before the segment of bowel is committed. A disadvantage of using the right colon is that it tends to become redundant over the long term, although this is rarely a problem clinically. A major disadvantage of using the colon is that its mucosa does not have a natural barrier to acid produced by the stomach, and ulceration from acid reflux has been reported. The operation itself is quite difficult and requires considerable experience with the technique.

THE GASTRIC TUBE

The stomach has an extensive vascular supply from four arteries. The left and right gastroepiploic arcade provides the greater curvature, and gives an excellent blood supply as well as extensive submucosal collaterals that assure abundant vascularity. Because of these extensive collateral vessels, however, it is not possible to test whether the arcade is satisfactory by temporary clamping of the right gastroepiploic vessels. Although the procedure reduces the size of the stomach by about one third, the remainder grows to "normal" size in about 3 months. Redundancy of the tube has been infrequently observed, occurring in my experience only when it is placed substernally. The absence of peristalsis is of no consequence. Perhaps the greatest advantage of the gastric tube is that its mucosal lining has a natural barrier to acid. Ulceration has been recorded when there is stasis or outlet obstruction in the tube, but careful attention to technique should avoid this. Finally, the operation itself is not very difficult.

THE STOMACH

In adults, the entire stomach is often used to replace the esophagus. Several decades ago it was also used in children, but fell into disfavor because of complications of reflux and also because the large space occupied by the stomach in the chest was poorly tolerated by young children. Recently, however, use of the stomach has returned as an alternative to the more usual methods of esophageal replacement. The advantages and disadvantages are much the same as with the gastric tube. To these must be added the caution of introducing a "space-occupying mass" in small children, which has the potential of undergoing rather large changes in size during meals. The question of whether the stomach retains its digestive function in its new position has not been answered. We have no experience of this procedure in our institution, but the technique will be described for completeness.

THE JEJUNUM

Use of the jejunum for esophageal replacement has never been popular. The vascular arcades of the small bowel are very short compared with the length of intestine they support. This makes it difficult to establish a precise length of neo-esophagus without redundancy. Additionally, the small bowel has no barrier to acid digestion, relying in its normal position on the addition of bile to neutralize the stomach acid, a protective mechanism that is lost in its transposed state. This method can, however, be useful if there are no other options, and will be described.

OPERATIVE PROCEDURES

It has been our practice, whatever the chosen method of esophageal substitution, to keep all options open. A barium enema is therefore obtained on all patients to be sure that no anomalies exist that would preclude the procedure, and a standard bowel preparation is also done.

The position of the patient on the operating table differs according to the transthoracic route used. For substernal placement and for blunt esophagectomy with transposition in the esophageal bed, the patient is put in the supine position. If the retrohilar route is elected, the left thorax is elevated enough to permit a separate anterolateral left thoracotomy, which I prefer, or thoracic extension of the abdominal incision.

RIGHT COLON: RETROSTERNAL ROUTE

The abdomen is entered through a large, midline vertical incision or a bilateral subcostal incision. The right colon is mobilized and its blood supply evaluated. The right colic and midcolic vessels and the vascular arcade between the two are inspected carefully. The midcolic vessels will be used for the vascular pedicle, with the right colic and ileocolic vessels temporarily occluded by a bulldog clamp. If the color of the colon remains healthy, these vessels are divided. The terminal ileum is transected, and after an adequate length has been selected, the transverse colon is divided. Reanastomosis of the divided bowel and appendectomy are performed. Attention is then turned to the neck, where a suprasternal incision is made extending into the left side of the neck and encompassing the esophagostomy. (For purposes of discussion it is assumed that the esophageal resection in this case has been done separately, and that a cervical esophagostomy has been established.) Using a combination of blunt and sharp dissection from the neck and abdomen, a wide tunnel is made behind the sternum. This must be large enough to accommodate the colon segment and its vascular supply without compromise. The esophagostomy is dissected free for a sufficient length to permit anastomosis. Attention is then returned to the abdomen, where the colon segment and its vascular pedicle are drawn behind the stomach and through an opening made in the gastrohepatic omentum. The colon segment and pedicle are then drawn through the substernal tunnel into the suprasternal wound, bringing the cecum up to the neck. A two-layer anastomosis is performed between the transverse colon and the stomach, at a fairly low level on the anterior gastric wall, using absorbable suture for the mucosal layer and silk for the seromuscular layer. A similar anastomosis is performed between the esophagus and the cecum. The sternomastoid muscle is resutured anterior to the anastomosis. In an attempt to avoid reflux into the transposed colon, pyloroplasty or pyloromyotomy is performed.

LEFT COLON: RETROHILAR ROUTE

Again, for purposes of discussion, the damaged esophagus is presumed to have been removed.

The approach is similar to that described for use of the right colon, except that the patient will be positioned for a separate left thoracotomy or thoracic extension of the abdominal incision. The vascular arcade of interest is between the midcolic and left colic vessels. For substernal placement, the pedicle will be based on the midcolic artery. For transthoracic placement the pedicle will be the left colic vessels. If temporary occlusion of the midcolic artery leaves an adequate vascular supply, the artery is divided. A length of transverse and left colon is selected to reach easily into the neck, and the colon is divided. Re-anastomosis of the colon is performed. The chest is opened in the seventh intercostal space, and a left-sided cervical incision is also made, including the esophagostomy. Dissection is continued toward the thoracic inlet, dividing the sternomastoid muscle. Once the thoracic inlet is reached, a hand is placed into the chest and the subclavian vessels are carefully located. There is usually a difference in the sizes of the spaces anterior and posterior to these vessels. Choosing the larger space, an opening is made sharply and is enlarged bluntly to a size sufficient to accommodate the colon segment and its blood supply. A tunnel is then made posterior to the pancreas and the stomach, and the colon segment is drawn through this space. An opening in the left diaphragm is made lateral to the native esophageal hiatus and the colon is brought through this opening, placed behind the hilum of the lung, and drawn into the neck. The two anastomoses are performed as described; the one to the stomach may be on the posterior wall of the stomach, according to preference. Pyloromyotomy or pyloroplasty is also done.

GASTRIC TUBE: SIMULTANEOUS ESOPHAGECTOMY WITHOUT THORACOTOMY

The gastric tube can be placed in the substernal or retrohilar position, but the procedure to be described will involve removal of the damaged esophagus with placement of the gastric tube in the esophageal bed.

The patient is placed in the supine position on the operating table and the abdomen is opened as described in the procedure for use of the right colon. The gastrocolic omentum is opened at a distance from the greater curvature to protect the gastroepiploic vessels. A point about 2 cm proximal to the pylorus is chosen for division of the right gastroepiploic vessel, taking care that the creation of the tube at this point will not critically narrow the gastric outlet. The vessel is divided and an oblique opening made in the anterior and posterior wall of the stomach. A chest tube of appropriate size to accommodate an adequate width of gastric tube is then passed into the stomach along the greater curvature. The first part of the tube is made with a stapling device that sets two rows of staples and simultaneously cuts between them. It will be seen that the vascular arcade tends to slew onto the anterior or posterior wall of the stomach as progressive cuts are made. Care must be taken to keep the vessels out of the jaws of the stapler. I prefer to do this manually rather than by applying clamps. Three to four cuts are required for an adequate length of tube. Care must be taken not to narrow the gastric inlet. The spleen is left in place. The line of staples is reinforced with nonabsorbable seromuscular sutures. During this part of the procedure, the original chest tube is replaced with a smaller one to avoid compromise of the vascular arcade.

Next, an incision is made in the left side of the neck and the esophagus is dissected free. The dissection is continued distally, separating the esophagus from surrounding tissue as far as the aortic arch. Great care must be exercised not to injure the recurrent laryngeal nerves. The esophagus is divided above the proximal stricture and a Penrose drain sutured to the lower segment. Following this, the left triangular ligament of the liver is divided, exposing the gastroesophageal junction. Blunt dissection from below will free the rest of the thoracic esophagus. The esophagus is then drawn from the neck into the abdomen and divided at its junction with the stomach. The opening is closed in two layers. The Penrose drain attached to the native esophagus is then sutured to the gastric tube and drawn back into the neck. A two-layer anastomosis is performed between the gastric tube and upper esophagus. Pyloromyotomy is performed.

GASTRIC TRANSPOSITION

In this procedure the entire stomach is pulled up to the neck. The blood supply comes from the right gastric and right gastroepiploic vessels; the left gastric, left gastroepiploic, and short gastric vessels are all divided. The native esophagus is detached from the stomach and removed as described in the procedure for use of the gastric tube. The gastroesophageal junction is sutured closed. The duodenum is fully mobilized to allow the stomach to be pulled up, and a pyloromyotomy is performed. Stay sutures are placed at the highest point on the greater curvature of the stomach, and dissection of the cervical esophagus is done. The stay sutures are used to draw the stomach into the neck by whatever route has been selected, and the esophagus is anastomosed to the previously selected point of the stomach. The spleen remains intact and is left in the abdomen.

JEJUNUM

The portion of jejunum chosen for transposition is usually just beyond that supplied by the first artery and vein distal to the ligament of Treitz. The next two to three vessels are divided (after being temporarily obstructed by occluding them with a bulldog clamp to ensure adequacy of the distal blood supply), and the jejunum is divided at two points to provide an adequate length to reach the neck. Reanastomosis of the divided jejunum is done. Some of the vessels of the arcade may have to be divided in order to straighten the jejunum sufficiently to permit it to reach its destination. This is done by dividing vessels just proximal to the arcade and immediately adjacent to the bowel. The other details of the procedure differ little from those already described for other segments of bowel.

POSTOPERATIVE CARE

Prophylactic antibiotics are continued for 48 hours and intravenous feedings are maintained. Oral or gastrostomy feedings are delayed until a barium study (usually performed on the seventh postoperative day) shows integrity of the new esophagus without anastomotic leakage. Drains left in the neck in all procedures are removed following this study. The patient can then gradually resume oral feedings and be discharged for careful long-term follow-up.

COMPLICATIONS

The major complication of loss of the entire transposed bowel is rare, especially when meticulous attention has been paid to its vascularity at the time of surgery. A minor complication of vascular compromise is usually manifested as a cervical anastomotic leak, which usually heals spontaneously. Stricture at the cervical anastomosis may follow such a leak, especially if the cervical esophagus was scarred by the original injury. Occasional dilatation is usually successful and may be necessary at times of growth spurts in children who have undergone esophageal replacement, especially during puberty. Ulceration in the esophageal replacement is also rare, but precautions must be taken against it at all times. Long-term use of antacids may be necessary for some children. Reflux occurs with all esophageal replacement procedures and may be severe. This tends to diminish with age, but if intractable may be remediable with reported antireflux procedures for the colon and gastric tube.

SUMMARY

The large number of procedures for replacement of the esophagus attests to the lack of a single ideal substitute. In experienced hands, all of the methods described here will support adequate nutrition for the growing child, permitting regular meals to be taken with family and friends and a normal life.

BIBLIOGRAPHY

1. Buras R, Jacir N, Anderson KD: An antireflux procedure for use with the reversed gastric tube. *J Pediatr Surg* 1986; 21:545.
2. German JC, Waterson DJ: Colon interposition for the replacement of the esophagus in children. *J Pediatr Surg* 1976; 11:227.
3. Guzetta PC, Randolph JG: Antireflux cologastric anastomosis following colonic interposition for esophageal replacement. *J Pediatr Surg* 1986; 21:1137.
4. Heimlich HJ: Elective replacement of the esophagus. *Br J Surg* 1966; 53:913.
5. Malcolm JA: Occurrence of peptic ulcer in colon used for esophageal replacement. *J Thorac Cardiovasc Surg* 1968; 55:763.
6. Orringer MD, Sloan H: Esophagectomy without thoracotomy. *J Thorac Cardiovasc Surg* 1978; 76:643.
7. Saeki M, Tsuchida Y, Ogata T, et al: Long-term results of jejunal replacement of the esophagus. *J Pediatr Surg* 1988; 23:483.
8. Spitz L: Gastric transposition via the mediastinal route for infants with long gap esophageal atresia. *J Pediatr Surg* 1984; 19:149.

23

Achalasia of the Esophagus

Richard G. Azizkhan, M.D.

A 15-year-old girl complained of swallowing difficulty and mid-chest pain. Her breath was malodorous. The symptoms were worse after meals and the patient described food "getting stuck" at the sternal level. Her course was complicated by coughing episodes at night. She had had two episodes of pneumonia during the previous 2 months. A barium swallow demonstrated a dilated esophagus ending at a narrow "bird's beak" appearance at the esophagogastric junction.

This superb case scenario provides an excellent springboard for a review of esophageal achalasia in childhood. The discussion in this chapter will focus on the diagnostic evaluation for this condition as well as on current concepts and controversies in the treatment of achalasia in children. In addition, significant complications related to both the disorder and its management will be highlighted.

Esophageal achalasia is an uncommon cause of functional obstruction of the esophagus in children. Less than 4% to 5% of all affected patients are symptomatic prior to age 15.[1] The disorder is characterized by the absence of normal esophageal peristalsis; a high resting pressure of the lower esophageal sphincter (LES); and failure of the LES to relax in response to swallowing.[5–7] The achalasia is thought to be a neuromuscular disorder of unknown etiology. However, degenerative abnormalities have been described in the dorsal vagal nuclei, vagus nerves, and Auerbach's plexus of the esophagus.[5]

Almost all patients with achalasia present with dysphagia as well as retention and regurgitation of undigested food. Vomiting may occur long after meals, and in the case of some children, regurgitated food particles may be found on their pillows in the morning. Nocturnal coughing, asthma, and pneumonia from presumed aspiration complicates at least 25% of reported pediatric cases of the condition.[1] Children with achalasia may also exhibit profound weight loss or significant retardation of growth and development. Unremitting halitosis is often reported by the family as a problem.

DIAGNOSTIC EVALUATION

Esophageal achalasia can be suspected on the basis of the history alone. However, physical examination is often unrevealing in these patients. The diagnosis may be strongly supported by visualizing an air–fluid level in a dilated esophagus in conjunction with acute or chronic pulmonary changes on an upright chest roentgenogram.[1] Radiographic contrast studies typically demonstrate aberrant motility, a megaesophagus, and a severely tapered "bird's beak" distal esophagus (Fig 23–1,A).

Esophageal manometry is one of the most useful tools for confirming the diagnosis of achalasia. Typical manometric features include: (1) absence of peristalsis in the esophageal body, (2) a markedly elevated resting LES pressure (often greater than 30 mm Hg), and (3) incomplete relaxation of the LES in response to swallowing. Early in the course of achalasia, spontaneous but ineffective low-amplitude, nonperistaltic waves may be seen.

In difficult cases, esophagoscopy may be crucial for differentiating achalasia from other obstructing esophageal lesions such as benign or malignant strictures.[16] The esophagoscope readily passes through the gastroesophageal junction in patients with achalasia, confirming the functional nature of the esophageal obstruction. Although not routinely performed in children, esophagoscopy and cytologic examination to screen for malignancy play an important role in the long-term followup of adult patients with achalasia. Esophageal cancer occurs with a much higher incidence and at a younger age in patients with achalasia than in those without it.[7]

DIFFERENTIAL DIAGNOSIS

Achalasia and severe gastroesophageal reflux may be confused in small children because of similar symptoms, including frequent regurgitation, choking, apnea, pneumonia, and failure to thrive.[14] Although barium studies usually differentiate these two pathologic entities, stricture of the esophagus due to chronic reflux esophagitis may be associated with esophageal dilatation and retention of food material. The radiographic picture in the two conditions may be quite similar, but there are several features that distinguish achalasia from reflux strictures. Esophageal shortening and mucosal asymmetry and irregularity are common in strictures associated with reflux, in contrast to the smooth, tapered appearance of the intact mucosa seen in patients with achalasia. If radio-

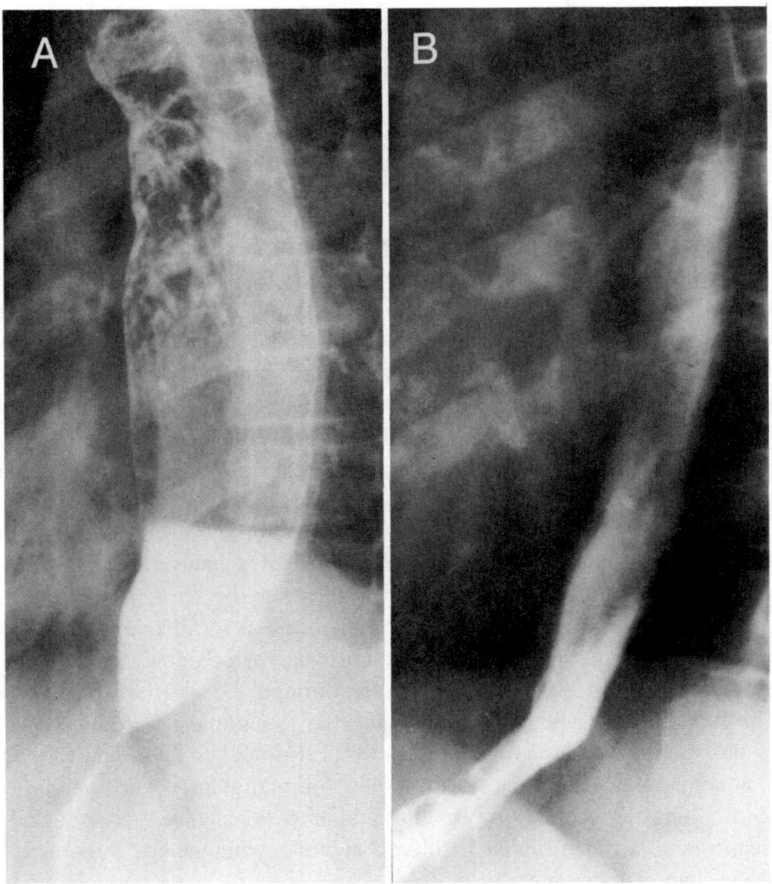

FIG 23–1.
A, barium esophagogram in a 15-year-old girl with achalasia, demonstrating a severely dilated esophagus with a characteristic "bird's beak" narrowing just proximal to the gastroesophageal junction. **B,** the same patient several months after a modified Heller esophagomyotomy. The esophagus empties promptly and has returned to a normal caliber.

graphic studies are inconclusive, the definitive diagnosis can be established by esophageal manometry or esophagoscopy.

The disordered motility and the appearance of the esophagus in scleroderma can also resemble that in achalasia. Evidence of scleroderma in other regions of the body is almost always present, thus aiding the clinician in differentiating these two diseases. In scleroderma, ingested barium may be retained when the patient is in the supine position, but empties rapidly from the esophagus when the patient assumes an erect posture. This finding reflects absent or diminished esophageal peristasic activity and usually very low LES pressures.[6]

Furthermore, distal esophageal narrowing in patients with scleroderma is very uncommon unless a concomitant reflux-induced stricture exists.

Diffuse esophageal spasm may also present with a radiographic picture resembling that in the early stages of achalasia. The observation of aberrant peristaltic activity and the presence of pulsion diverticulae provide presumptive evidence for the diagnosis of diffuse esophageal spasm. Esophageal manometry is the most reliable method for differentiating these lesions and establishing the correct diagnosis.

THERAPEUTIC OPTIONS AND OUTCOME

Since Thomas Willis first described achalasia in 1674, a variety of pharmacologic agents, along with forceful dilatation and an array of surgical approaches, have been used to treat patients with achalasia.[8, 12, 16] Recently, calcium-channel blockers such as nifedipine have been shown to reduce LES pressure with symptomatic relief.[3] Unfortunately, the effect is very short lived and its clinical usefulness is limited by significant side effects. The use of parasympathomimetic agents to stimulate esophageal peristasis in these patients has proven ineffective.[7, 16]

In patients with achalasia, disruption of the LES spasm is the goal of therapy. Forceful esophageal dilatation has been widely advocated for three centuries as a form of therapy for achalasia. However, simple bougienage alone is clearly ineffective and has been abandoned in favor of pneumatic dilatation.[1, 11, 13, 14] Pneumatic dilatation is performed under fluoroscopic control using Mosher or Brown-Hardy balloon catheters. Approximately 65% to 80% of adults with achalasia are significantly improved with pneumatic dilatation, in which there is a 4% to 5% incidence of esophageal perforation.[6, 9, 15, 16] In contrast, the results of pneumatic dilatation in children have been generally disappointing, although significant controversy surrounds this issue. Some studies advocating the use of pneumatic dilatation in children report impressive symptomatic improvement in 70% to 80% of cases.[4] Unfortunately, these studies have had an insufficient follow-up and have not considered delayed recurrence of symptoms requiring repeated dilatation and the risk of perforation. In other studies the majority of children have derived only transient benefit from pneumatic dilatation and have subsequently required a modified Heller esophagomyotomy for relief of symptoms.[1, 14] Pneumatic dilatation has had an especially poor track record in younger children less than 9 to 10 years of age.[1] For this reason the modified Heller esophagomyotomy has become the initial procedure of choice in younger children (Fig 23–1,B).[1, 2, 10, 11, 13, 14]

In older children, pneumatic dilatation may be an appropriate initial therapeutic procedure. Recently, Nakayama and associates reported that 47% of children with achalasia who were older than 9 years of age had prolonged relief of symptoms (average follow-up: 18 months), with one pneumatic dilatation.[11] Furthermore, an additional 26% had lasting improvement following two to four dilatations. In this study, there were minimal morbidity and no documented esophageal perforations attributed to pneumatic dilatation. Pneumatic dilatation is clearly less effective than a modified Heller esophagomyotomy, but by avoiding the need for a surgical procedure it becomes an acceptable initial therapy in older children. Rapid recurrence of symptoms or the need for two or more pneumatic dilatations within a year are clear indications for a modified Heller esophagomyotomy. The modified Heller operation is reported to be even more effective in children than adults, with a success rate in the range of 85% to 95%.[1, 2, 10, 11, 13, 14]

Since Heller's original description of it in 1913, the double esophagomyotomy technique has been modified, and currently only an anterior myotomy is performed, through either the chest or abdomen.[1, 2, 10, 12] The thoracic approach may be superior, however, particularly in those patients who have a long segment of esophageal involvement and may require a longer esophagomyotomy. Amid significant controversy, several authors have advocated routine concomitant antireflux procedures. When a concomitant antireflux operation is anticipated, some surgeons prefer the transabdominal approach.[2] Others prefer to combine a transthoracic esophagomyotomy with the Belsey procedure.[10] However, clinically significant gastroesophageal reflux is reported to occur in only 15% to 20% of children following a modified Heller esophagomyotomy.[1, 11] The addition of an antireflux procedure in all patients has at least theoretical disadvantages, including the creation of a relative esophageal obstruction from the fundus wrap in the face of significantly impaired esophageal motility. In this regard, a moderate approach is personally more appealing, with antireflux procedures reserved only for patients with evidence of symptomatic gastroesophageal reflux following esophagomyotomy. Ellis made an important point in emphasizing that limiting the distal aspect of the myotomy to 1 cm beyond the gastroesophageal junction reduces the complications of reflux and esophagitis.[8] Furthermore, pathologic gastroesophageal reflux is not limited to those patients who have undergone an esophagomyotomy, and has been documented in both children and adults who have had pneumatic dilatation alone.[1, 16]

Failure of the modified Heller operation, necessitating postoperative dilatation or reoperation, is very uncommon. Recurrence of symptoms may be caused by an inadequate myotomy, particularly when the mucosa has not been sufficiently separated from either side of the lateral esophageal muscle. At least half of the esophageal mucosa should be freed to permit mucosal protrusion

through the incision in the muscularis, thereby preventing the two ends of the esophageal wall to coapt with the formation of scar tissue.

Long-term follow-up is essential for patients with achalasia. Although the treatment of achalasia may relieve the symptoms of esophageal obstruction, the basic pathophysiology characterized by abnormal esophageal motility remains throughout life. Nearly 5% to 15% of adults with achalasia will develop squamous cell carcinoma of the esophagus.[7, 16] The average interval from the onset of initial symptoms to the development of esophageal cancer is approximately three decades. Adults require periodic endoscopy and cytologic studies to detect early neoplastic changes.

SUMMARY

In conclusion, achalasia of the esophagus in childhood is very rare. Older children frequently present with dysphagia and regurgitation, but in the younger child the symptoms of this condition can be confused with those of gastroesophageal reflux. Bougienage has an unacceptable rate of symptom recurrence, and the results of pneumatic dilatation in general have been disappointing, particularly in small children. Pneumatic dilatation may be appropriate as an initial therapy in the older child. However, if symptoms rapidly recur following dilatation, or more than two dilatations are required within a year, a modified Heller operation is the treatment of choice. Although the need to perform a concomitant antireflux procedure is controversial, I believe that the procedure should be reserved for patients with evidence of symptomatic gastroesophageal reflux following a modified Heller procedure. Since esophageal neoplasia is more common in these patients, long-term follow-up is essential.

REFERENCES

1. Azizkhan RG, Tapper D, Eraklis A: Achalasia in childhood: A 20-year experience. *J Pediatr Surg* 1980; 15:452–456.
2. Ballantine TV, Fitzgerald JF, Grosfeld JL: Transabdominal esophagomyotomy for achalasia in children. *J Pediatr Surg* 1980; 15:457–461.
3. Berger K, McCallum RW: Nifedipine in the treatment of achalasia. *Ann Intern Med* 1982: 96:61–62.
4. Boyle JT, Cohen S, Watkins JB: Successful treatment of achalasia in childhood by pneumatic dilatation. *J Pediatr* 1981; 99:35–40.
5. Cassella RR, Brown AL, Sayre GP, et al: Achalasia of the esophagus. *Ann Surg* 1964; 160:474–487.
6. Castell DO: Lower esophageal sphincter; physiologic and clinical aspects. *Ann Intern Med* 1975; 83:390–401.

7. Cohen SE: Motor disorders of the esophagus. *N Engl J Med* 1979; 301:184–192.
8. Ellis FH: Surgical management of esophageal motility disturbances. *Am J Surg* 1980; 139:752–759.
9. Jacobs JB, Cohen NL, Mattel S: Pneumatic dilatation as the primary treatment for achalasia. *Ann Otol Rhinol Laryngol* 1983; 92:353–356.
10. Lemmer JH, Coran AG, Wesley JR, et al: Achalasia in children: Treatment by anterior esophageal myotomy (modified Heller operation). *J Pediatr Surg* 1985; 20:333–338.
11. Nakayama DK, Shorter NA, Boyle JT, et al: Pneumatic dilatation and operative treatment of achalasia in children. *J Pediatr Surg* 1987; 22:619–622.
12. Steichen FM, Heller E, Ravitch MM: Achalasia of the esophagus. *Surgery* 1960; 47:846–876.
13. Tachovsky TJ, Lynn HB, Ellis FH Jr: The surgical approach to esophageal achalasia in children. *J Pediatr Surg* 1968; 3:226–231.
14. Vane DW, Cosby K, West K, et al: Late results following esophagomyotomy in children with achalasia. *J Pediatr Surg* 1988; 23:515–519.
15. VanTrappen G, Hellemans J, DeLoof W, et al: Treatment of achalasia with pneumatic dilatation. *Gut* 1971; 12:268–275.
16. Yon J, Christensen J: An uncontrolled comparison of treatments for achalasia. *Ann Surg* 1975; 186:672–676.

24

Gastroesophageal Reflux

Dale G. Johnson, M.D.

A 14-month-old girl was referred because of failure to thrive and nonbilious vomiting. The vomiting began shortly after birth and has continued despite treatment with metoclopramide and upright feedings of thickened formula. The child frequently coughs while sleeping, and has had recurring respiratory infections. She is currently below the 5th percentile for both height and weight on the growth grid. A gastric scintiscan showed gastroesophageal reflux to the level of the thoracic inlet, and delayed gastric emptying.

The case presentation describes a 14-month-old infant with a prolonged (lifelong) history of vomiting. Her growth appears to be significantly retarded, with a height and weight below the 5th percentile on the growth grid, and she suffers from recurrent respiratory infections and frequent coughing during sleep. Since a gastric scintiscan has demonstrated gastroesophageal reflux to the thoracic inlet plus a delay in gastric emptying, the vomiting, growth retardation, and respiratory symptoms may all be related to the uncontrolled reflux of gastric content. Standard medical treatment for reflux (upright positioning, thickened feedings, metoclopramide medication) has not provided control of the vomiting or its presumed side-effects on the infant's growth and respiratory function. What is the next step in management?

DISCUSSION

This infant appears to have at least three indications for surgical control of gastroesophageal reflux (GER). The presence of reflux, in itself, is not an indication for surgery, but specific complications of reflux that have not responded to nonoperative treatment are indications for operation. This infant's intractable vomiting, recurrent respiratory infections, and failure to thrive are all common complications of reflux in children. Each of these problems can, however, have a cause other than reflux. Before proceeding with an antireflux procedure, we need to be reasonably certain that the symptoms are caused by and not merely coexistent with the reflux. It is frustrating to cure the reflux but not the patient.

DIAGNOSTIC STUDIES

Barium Swallow

A barium study of the stomach and esophagus is my own preference for a first approach to the evaluation of persistent vomiting. Good anatomic imaging with barium is important to rule out possible distal obstruction or pathologic anatomy of the stomach or esophagus. Estimates concerning the degree of reflux or the presence of delayed gastric emptying of barium are also useful when the abnormality is gross, even though the quantitative accuracy of the procedure is very limited for most cases. Early stages of esophagitis are not detectable by barium study, but advanced esophagitis and stricture are, and their presence is a clear indication for antireflux surgery.

Gastric Scintiscan

The patient in question had reflux demonstrated by gastric scintiscan rather than barium swallow. Delay in gastric emptying was also demonstrated by this study. These data require experienced interpretation. Published normal values of gastric emptying for children are tentative, because normal children are not given radionuclides. Because esophageal pH monitoring has shown that normal children may reflux for the first 1 to 2 hours after a liquid feeding, data that identify the range between normal and abnormal are important. Our own experience with scintiscanning compared with pH monitoring for the demonstration of reflux outside the normal range suggests that scintiscanning has a higher false-positive error. The hope that scintiscanning might be the answer for proving a cause-and-effect relationship between reflux and respiratory complications also has been disappointing. Scintiscanning infrequently demonstrates the aspiration of gastric content into the lungs, even though the relief of recurrent pneumonias in a large number of refluxing infants is clinically well-established. Finally, quantitation of gastric emptying is the most useful aspect of the scintiscan study, but even here there are pitfalls. The study depends on the medium that is mixed with the radionuclide, the emptying of liquids giving different values than that of semisolids. Moreover, the presence of reflux requires some sort of correction factor because of recycling through the stomach. The separation between normal and abnormal is therefore dependent upon technique, institutional experience, and a fairly wide standard deviation.

Endoscopy

Esophagoscopy with mucosal biopsy is the only direct way to evaluate esophagitis. By itself, esophagoscopy is highly subjective for diagnosing esophagitis in its early stages of grades I and II. Mucosal biopsy is essential for any objective comparisons. Advanced stages of esophagitis, however, are easily recognized, and the diagnosis is consistent between observers. We do not know whether our discussion case does or does not have esophagitis, since esophagoscopy was not done. The long history of vomiting makes some degree of esophagitis a likely possibility. Not infrequently, esophagitis may contribute to growth retardation by causing pain on swallowing and secondary refusal of feedings. Knowing the presence or absence of esophagitis is not essential to the decision for operation in this child, however, since there are three other reasons for surgical treatment.

If I were beginning the work-up in this case, I would have requested a barium study initially, to rule out distal obstruction, esophageal stricture, or gross intrathoracic herniation of the stomach. I would then have added further studies only if I did not have sufficient reason to proceed with surgical operation on the basis of the barium study, the history of unrelieved vomiting, and the type of secondary complications thought to be related to the vomiting.

If the focus were on control of respiratory complications, I would proceed with a 24-hour pH study. The pH monitoring gives the most accurate quantitation of reflux, and the correlations between respiratory complications and a prolonged duration of reflux during sleep, while not perfect, are better than other studies can provide. The gastric scintiscan showed reflux to the thoracic inlet, and this is suggestive but not diagnostic of a cause-and-effect relationship between this and the patient's respiratory complications.

If failure to thrive were the major reason for considering antireflux surgery, I would require careful evaluation of the patient for other possible causes of growth retardation, including cardiac, neurologic, metabolic, and renal evaluations. A cause-and-effect relationship between the vomiting and growth retardation is often difficult to establish with certainty. If reflux is the cause of failure to thrive, one should be able to show a significant deficit in caloric intake even though the infant may be refed after vomiting. A period of observation in the hospital for careful calorie counts of retained feedings is often useful in trying to identify which infants who fail to thrive will benefit from antireflux surgery. The desirability of reversing growth retardation, particularly in the critical first 2 years of life, is unquestioned. Unfortunately, the elimination of reflux does not always reverse the slow growth trend. Screening for other causes of failure to thrive is therefore important. In cases in which caloric retention is clearly deficient because of constant vomiting, the benefits of an antireflux operation for improved growth are more predictable.

MEDICAL MANAGEMENT

Nonsurgical treatment of reflux is designed to control its symptoms, in the hope that time, anatomic growth, and physiologic maturation will allow spontaneous resolution of its underlying cause.

Spontaneous resolution of reflux in infants is a common phenomenon, thus justifying an initial, rigorous medical effort to control its symptoms in virtually all refluxing infants. In our experience, however, spontaneous resolution of reflux in symptomatic infants usually occurs within the first 10 months of age. Medical treatment beyond 1 year of age may produce temporary control of symptoms, but seldom results in a cure that obviates the need for further treatment.

Before embarking on a course of treatment, either medical or surgical, one should ask if the symptoms are sufficiently significant to justify or require treatment. It is often stated that "all babies reflux," and that "spitting up" of feedings is a normal phenomenon. While this may be true, it is obviously a matter of degree. We are not told how much or how often the infant in the case described here vomited, but 14 months of vomiting since early infancy is highly abnormal. Other side effects of reflux in infants may have more damaging effects, but the persistence of repeated vomiting alone may occasionally be justification for surgical control when other measures have failed. An antireflux operation after months of ineffective treatment with diet changes and medication may be a godsend for the parents of an infant continually soiled and smelling from vomitus.

Positioning

Upright or prone positioning for infants is perhaps the most effective component of a nonsurgical program for the management of reflux. This becomes difficult to achieve after 6 to 8 months of age, however. The objectives are to position the gastroesophageal junction in the gastric air bubble, rather than below the gastric fluid level, and to utilize gravity for increased resistance against esophageal reflux. The effect of positioning is often unpredictable, however, and some infants reflux more often when erect than when supine.

Feedings

Thickening of feedings is a time-honored approach in the management of reflux and probably helps to some degree in most refluxing infants.

Medication

Pharmacologic manipulation of lower esophageal sphincter pressures and gastric emptying also has its enthusiasts, and is attempted in most infants. Bethanechol and metoclopramide are the agents most commonly used in the United States. Cisapride, a "prokinetic" agent said to have enhanced peripheral effectiveness at the myenteric nerve ending, without central side effects, has been used in European and South African trials, but is not yet approved for use in the United States. Cimetidine and ranitidine have been used to block acid secretion in cases in which symptoms of esophagitis are manifest. The reduction of acid secretion is clearly useful in treating reflux esophagitis, but is directed at the symptoms and not the cause of the esophagitis. Attempts to increase lower esophageal sphincter pressures and to increase gastric emptying seem to have a less predictable benefit, and are occasionally associated with unpleasant side effects.

Surgical Management of Reflux

The infant presented for discussion has persisting reflux symptoms at 14 months of age. Spontaneous resolution of the condition is unlikely, and medical treatment has been ineffective. The growth retardation is severe enough to demand urgent treatment, since the critical period for growth of the brain and nervous system is within the first 2 years of life. If, however, we assume for the sake of argument that careful calorie counts have documented an adequate caloric intake for growth, and that the growth response to the control of reflux will be questionable, we still have the repeated pulmonary infections and the vomiting. After 24-hour pH monitoring and our best efforts to relate the respiratory problems to the reflux, we may still be left with the option of surgical elimination of the reflux to see what happens to the lungs. The result is usually favorable. Even if the respiratory symptoms are not completely eliminated the elimination of repeated vomiting of feedings, after 14 months, will still justify the antireflux operation.

Choice of Operation

My own preferred procedure for the surgical treatment of gastroesophageal reflux is the Nissen fundoplication. I like a short wrap (1.5 to 2.0 cm) performed loosely over a large intraesophageal bougie (34 to 38 F for a 14-month-old infant). The short gastric vessels are usually divided to provide adequate mobility of the fundus. The crura are closed behind the esophagus with two mattress sutures over Teflon pledgets. The fundoplication is then performed by wrapping the posterior fundus behind the esophagus and the anterior fundus in front. The first layer of sutures passes from the anterior fundus through the right margin of the esophagus and to the posterior fundus. A second layer of sutures between the anterior and the posterior fundus is added for security. Additional sutures fix the left side of the wrap to the diaphragm.

Surgical alteration of the gastric outlet remains controversial in my mind. I am not convinced that preoperative studies demonstrating a delay in gastric emptying necessarily mean that postoperative gastric emptying will be delayed in the same patient. In fact, our own data document that some patients have delayed emptying preoperatively and some have delayed emptying postoperatively, but in most cases they are not the same patients. Our experience confirms published data[1, 2] suggesting that the antireflux procedure may significantly increase gastric emptying postoperatively. Although a postoperative delay in gastric emptying clearly causes symptoms, and may contribute to breakdown of the repair, we find it difficult to predict from preoperative studies which patients will have problems. Fortunately, the delayed emptying is self-limited in most patients, and improves with time. Furthermore, other centers have sent us patients who have had pyloroplasties and who have symptoms consistent with dumping and gastric pain typical of alkaline reflux. Data on the incidence of these complications are inconclusive, but for all of the above reasons I am not convinced that a pyloroplasty should be added to an antireflux procedure on the basis of a preoperative delay in gastric emptying.

SUMMARY

This infant has a long history of reflux and reflux-associated symptoms and side effects. Nonsurgical treatment has been ineffective, and I believe that a short, loose, 360-degree fundoplication will eliminate the long-term vomiting, probably diminish the repeated respiratory infections, and improve the infant's growth.

REFERENCES

1. Jolley SC, Leonard JC, Tunnel WP: Gastric emptying in children with gastroesophageal reflux: I. An estimate of effective gastric emptying. *J Pediatr Surg* 1987; 22:923–926.
2. Maddern GJ, Jamieson GG: Fundoplication enhances gastric emptying. *Ann Surg* 1985; 201:296–299.

25

Caustic Stricture of the Esophagus

Hernan M. Reyes, M.D.

A 30-month-old boy is found crying on the kitchen floor next to a half-empty, open bottle of liquid alkali. He has burns on his lips. He is taken to an emergency room and oropharyngeal examination shows alkaline burns in the buccal mucosa and pharynx. The child's temperature is 37.7° C and the WBC count is 21,000/mm^3. Chest x-ray shows no evidence of mediastinal air.

The foregoing case illustrates the typical presentation of a toddler or preschool child who has ingested liquid lye, the most common brand of which is "Drano," a potent alkali made up of 36.5% sodium hydroxide or potassium hydroxide and commonly used as a drain cleaner. The cases we currently encounter are accidental ingestions of such highly concentrated drain cleaners whose safety caps have been inadvertently left off. In some Third World countries, these liquid drain cleaners are divided into small volumes, packaged into empty soft-drink bottles, and mistakenly ingested by toddlers and older children who are unaware of the contents of the bottle.

On presentation in the emergency room, the patient should not be given any medication, liquids, or food orally, in order to prevent vomiting. Liquid lye, being a strong alkali, produces liquefaction necrosis of the esophagus and penetrates its wall, so that vomiting precipitated by oral intake will further aggravate the extent and depth of the injury, thereby converting a superficial mucosal and submucosal injury into a deeper burn or a full-thickness lesion that is likely to result in acute necrosis and perforation or late esophageal stricture.

Intravenous fluids with 5% dextrose and 0.2% sodium chloride should be started at maintenance dose. The initial blood analysis should consist of a complete blood count (CBC) and measurements of electrolytes, blood urea nitrogen

(BUN), and blood glucose. A second-generation cephalosporin should be started. Although steroids were given in our original protocol, we no longer consider this essential in the management of these patients.

A supine and an upright chest x-ray, in both the lateral and posteroanterior (PA) projections, should be obtained in the emergency room to rule out the presence of posterior mediastinal air indicating esophageal perforation. This complication will require aggressive surgical treatment on an emergency basis. Fever and leukocytosis may simply indicate the presence of an inflammatory process, which occurs almost immediately after a chemical burn of the esophagus. A high fever developing within a few hours after ingestion of a strong alkali should alert the clinician to the possibility of esophageal perforation and acute mediastinitis, and must be managed accordingly.

Direct laryngoscopy and esophagoscopy under general anesthesia should be performed within 12 hours of the patient's admission, and certainly no longer than 24 hours after admission. It is essential that the entire length of the esophagus be visualized in order to ascertain the extent and depth of the injury. In some instances, the oropharynx and proximal esophagus may be completely spared from a severe injury that may affect the middle or distal esophageal segments. This finding is especially true in the case of ingestion of granular Drano or Clinitest tablets. Endoscopic examination further determines the type of treatment that will be provided to these patients.

If the endoscopic findings consist of burns involving the mouth, tongue, and oropharynx, with or without esophageal injury, and provided that the esophageal burn is superficial as evidenced by hyperemia, mucosal friability, and edema without ulcerations, no further treatment is necessary. The patient is simply given nothing by mouth for another 24 hours, after which the diet progresses from clear liquids to a soft diet. Antibiotics are discontinued and the child is discharged after solid foods are tolerated. No follow-up radiographic study is necessary, provided the patient is totally asymptomatic 12 weeks after the initial injury. The onset of dysphagia within this period is suggestive of a deeper esophageal burn that was misdiagnosed at the original examination, with underestimation of the gross findings at the time of initial esophagoscopy. An esophagogram followed by immediate esophagoscopy is mandatory in this instance.

If deep ulcerations, eschar formation, or sloughing of the esophageal mucosa is noted, especially when these lesions are circumferential, we advocate the insertion of a full-length, intraluminal esophageal stent with a silicone-coated tube, as we described in 1976.[1] With the patient under general endotracheal anesthesia, a hollow, 28 F, silicone-coated tube is inserted under direct vision throughout the entire length of the esophagus. This is made possible by sheathing the stent over either a 3.5 × 20-mm rigid bronchoscope with a Storz telescope or a flexible pediatric gastroscope. The esophageal stent is in most cases approximately 20 cm long, spanning the length of the esophagus from slightly above the cricopharyngeus to below the gastroesophageal junction. The distance between the cricothyroid cartilage proximally and the xiphoid process distally provides a guide to the approximate length of the stent to be used. A medium-size Penrose drain, divided in half, is sheathed over the distal end of the stent prior to insertion. This drain is anchored with two separate transfixing sutures of 0 silk, and will serve to prevent reflux of gastric contents through the hollow lumen of the stent. The proximal end of the esophageal stent is anchored to the distal end of a 10 F Replogle sump tube previously passed through the nasopharynx. This will serve as a suspension mechanism for the stent, and provides a means for aspirating oropharyngeal secretions, which almost invariably pool in the posterior pharyngeal space. It is essential that the proximal end of the stent be at least 1 cm above the cricopharyngeal opening, while the distal end should be below the gastroesophageal junction without pressure on the gastric wall. An x-ray of the chest that includes parts of the neck and abdomen is obtained in the operating room to ascertain the position of the intraluminal splint (Fig 25–1).

If the burns are so severe that the larynx is also injured, it is prudent to place a standard tracheostomy tube before terminating general anesthesia. A separate 8 F feeding tube may likewise be inserted through the opposite nostril, down the lumen of the stent, and into the stomach to be used for future enteral feedings. The nasogastric suspension tube should be anchored to the nose with a Logan bow (Fig 25–2). This stent should stay in place for a minimum of 3 weeks.

Care of the patient following insertion of an intraluminal esophageal stent consists of the following measures:

1. The nasogastric tube should be connected to low intermittent suction.
2. The patient should be kept in a semisitting position at all times.
3. Oropharyngeal secretions should be aspirated frequently.
4. Mittens must be placed on both of the child's hands to prevent him from grabbing the nasogastric tube.
5. Antibiotics should be continued for a total of 5 days unless the patient remains septic or develops aspiration pneumonia. Appropriate antibiotics should then be started, on the basis of cultures of the tracheal aspirate.
6. Enteral feedings can be started within 24 hours after the stent placement, and an accurate calorie count should be kept on a daily basis.
7. Chest x-rays in both the PA and lateral projections should be obtained daily for 3 days and once a week therafter unless otherwise indicated.
8. A CBC and measurements of blood electrolytes, fasting blood glucose, BUN, and total proteins are obtained weekly.

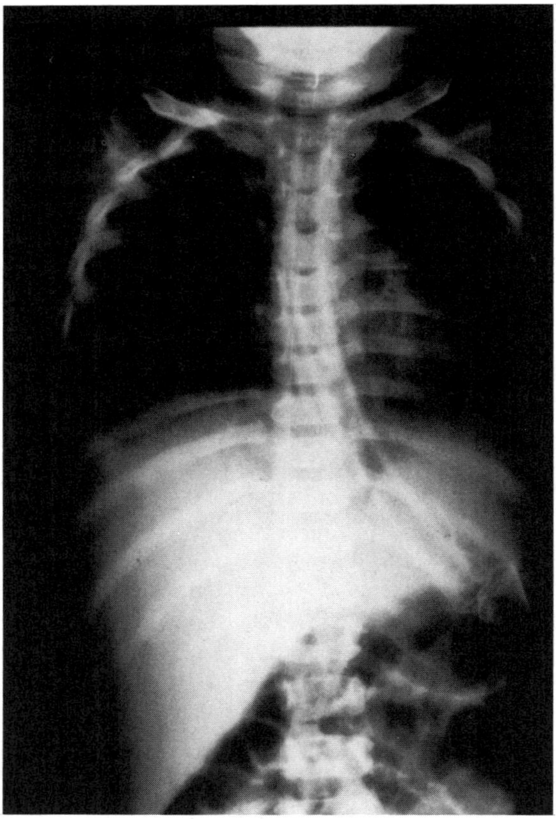

FIG 25–1.
Radiologic appearance of esophageal intraluminal stent.

After 21 days, the stent is removed under general anesthesia and the entire esophagus is visualized using either a flexible or a rigid endoscope. The presence of unhealed burns in the form of deep ulcers, especially when circumferential, is an indication to replace the stent. The procedure of stent removal and repeat endoscopy is performed a week later and weekly thereafter until all lesions have completely healed. Whenever reinsertion of the stent is difficult, no further attempts should be made, lest perforation of the esophagus occur. In our series, two patients with unhealed esophageal ulcers 3 weeks after injury and intraluminal splinting did not develop esophageal strictures despite our failure to restent the esophagus.

The initial procedure following stent removal is an esophagogram, done 24 hours later. Demonstration of a patent esophageal lumen, despite a slight narrowing or extreme dilatation, should not be a reason to delay oral feedings,

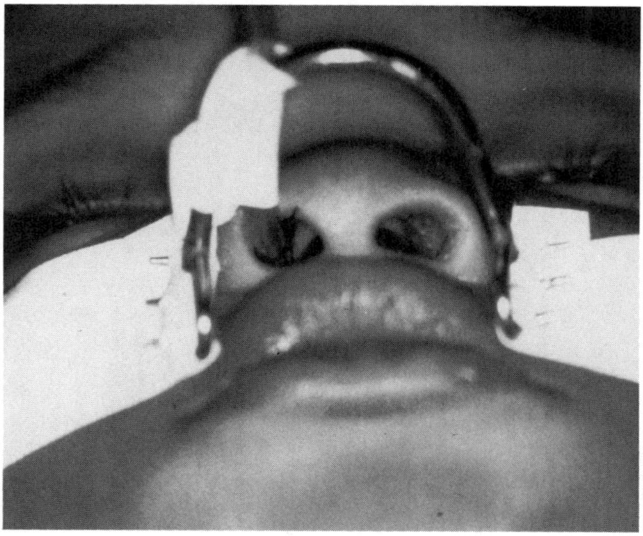

FIG 25–2.
Intraluminal stent suspension mechanism anchored with a Logan bow.

which should start with a liquid diet and gradually progress to solids (Fig 25–3). Unless the patient is symptomatic, an esophagogram, manometry, and 24-hour intraluminal pH study of the lower esophagus is obtained 12 weeks after removal of the intraluminal esophageal stent, and should be repeated at 24 weeks. The occurrence of dysphagia is an indication for prompt esophagography and endoscopy. In the absence of any swallowing problems, the best method of ascertaining normal esophageal function is the nutritional status of the patient, regardless of the radiographic appearance of the esophagus.

The presence of esophageal perforation at the time of admission or a few hours thereafter, as demonstrated either radiographically or by clinical evidence of acute mediastinitis, is an indication for emergent, aggressive surgical intervention. At surgery, the patient's neck, chest, and abdomen are fully prepped and draped. A limited laparotomy should be performed initially to identify the extent of the necrosis and involvement of the distal esophagus and stomach. Thereafter, a right posterolateral thoracotomy is performed through the fifth intercostal space, preferably using an extrapleural approach. A limited perforation and necrosis can be treated by limited resection and primary repair in conjunction with posterior mediastinal drainage, cervical esophagostomy, and gastrostomy. Diffuse necrosis of the intrathoracic esophagus will require an end-cervical esophagostomy, esophagectomy, closure by stapling of the distal esophagus or proximal segment of the stomach beyond the level of full-thickness necrosis, and a Stamm gastrostomy. This aggressive approach is a lifesav-

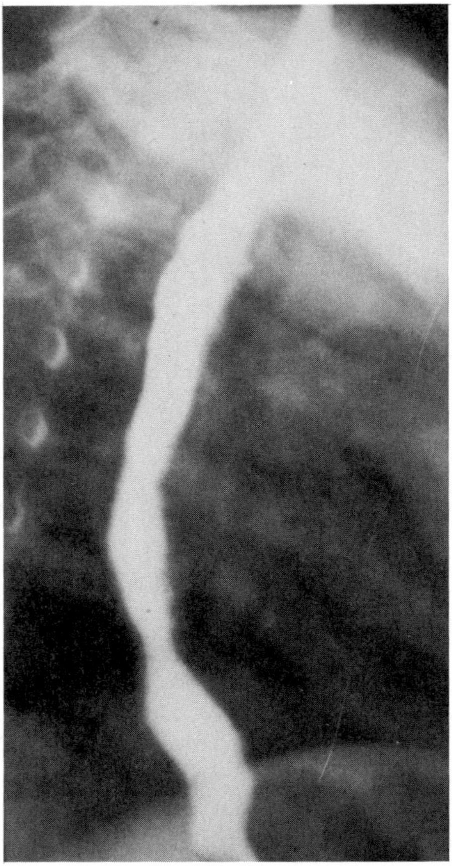

FIG 25–3.
Esophagogram 12 weeks after removal of a stent, showing a deformed esophageal wall with areas of narrowing. The patient is, however, asymptomatic and tolerating all feedings 8 months after an esophageal lye burn.

ing procedure in an infant or child with extremely severe chemical burns of the esophagus. Broad-spectrum antibiotics should be started and enteral nutrition initiated as soon as it becomes feasible. Esophageal replacement by colon or small-bowel transplantation can be accomplished within 6 months to a year after the initial injury.

Since our first attempt, in 1976,[2] to treat severe nonperforated esophageal burns with a full-length intraluminal esophageal stent, incorporating our observations in an experimental study[3] completed and published two years previously, we have treated seven children and one adult in this way. All of these patients were treated with an intraluminal esophageal stent, on the basis of our initial assessment of the gross burn injury. These patients represent a small percentage of the number of infants and children admitted to our institution for accidental lye ingestion, which approximates 10 a year. The longest follow-up in such cases has been 10 years, in three of our patients, and the shortest has been for a patient we treated in December 1989. All have remained asymptomatic, with no evidence of stricture formation. Two patients with narrowed esophagi on radiographic studies are tolerating solid foods well without the need for bouginage. No patient has required dilatation or esophageal replacement. Two patients have required tracheostomy because of respiratory obstruction from a burned larynx. In both patients symptoms became evident after endotracheal extubation. Both patients currently have normal respiratory status, both functionally and by endoscopy, and their tracheostomies have since been removed.

A 2-year-old girl who was treated with an intraluminal stent in July 1988 showed what appeared to be a distal esophageal narrowing 6 weeks after removal of the stent. A gastrostomy tube had to be placed for feeding. A repeat esophagogram 2 weeks later showed an abnormal esophagus with markedly decreased peristalisis, including a deformity of the esophageal wall with some degree of narrowing of the entire lumen of the esophagus. The child was gradually given oral feedings, and 3 months after removal of the stent was tolerating solid foods without any problems whatsoever. The gastrostomy tube has since been removed. Eight months after the initial injury, she remains completely asymptomatic, tolerating liquid and solid foods well and maintaining a normal nutritional status.

Discussion

Numerous investigators have now reported their results in the treatment by intraluminal esophageal stenting of severe burns of the esophagus caused by the ingestion of caustic drain cleaner.[4–7] As shown in Table 25–1, a number of patients subsequently developed strictures even after intraluminal splinting of the esophagus for a period of 3 weeks. These patients, however, have been adequately managed with dilatation, and have not undergone esophageal replacement. Granting that in some patients with severe esophageal burns, stricture will develop after intraluminal esophageal stenting for 3 weeks, the overall stricture incidence of 21% (8/38) in this highly selective group of patients with severe esophageal burns (see Table 25–1) is certainly very low, considering the alternative results without intraluminal stent treatment, in which the expected stricture rate would be greater than 90% based on our experimental data.[3] Endoscopy should be performed after the initial removal of the intraluminal stent 3 weeks after its placement. If at that time unhealed lesions are still present, the intraluminal stent should be reinserted and the patient re-endo-

TABLE 25–1.
Experience With Intraluminal Esophageal Stenting in the Treatment of Caustic Esophageal Burns: 1976–1989

AUTHOR (YR)	NO. OF PATIENTS	EXTENT OF BURNS	DURATION OF INTRALUMINAL STENT (WK)	NO. OF PATIENTS WITH STRICTURE (TREATMENT)	ESOPHAGEAL REPLACEMENT	LENGTH OF FOLLOW-UP
Reyes et al. (1976–present)	8	Severe, nonperforated	3	0	0	2 mo–13 yr.
Mills et al. (1978)	4	Severe, nonperforated	3	0	0	6 mo–$2\frac{1}{2}$ yr
Coln et al. (1986)	7	Severe, nonperforated	3	3 (Dilatation)	0	2–7 yr
Pawlik et al. (1989)	8	Severe, nonperforated	3	4 (Dilatation)	0	5–21 mo
Wijburg et al. (1989)	11	Severe, nonperforated	5–6	1 (Dilatation)	0	5–19 yr
Total	38			8 (21%)		2 mo–19 yr

scoped on a regular weekly basis thereafter, with reinsertion of the stent until complete healing has taken place. One source has suggested that steroids are not an important factor in preventing strictures in patients treated with an intraluminal splint.[7] We have not used steroids in our last two patients, and are confident that these drugs are no longer an important adjunct in the management of the patient with severe caustic burns of the esophagus who is being treated with an intraluminal esophageal stent.

We still subscribe to the conclusion stated in our experimental studies reported in 1974,[3] that the intraluminal esophageal stent prevents cross-fusion of mural ulcers and obliteration of the esophageal lumen by exuberant granulation tissue. Esophageal intubation for a 3-week period was associated with a lesser degree of inflammation, reduced amount of granulation tissue, and minimal formation of scar tissue. It also compresses the granulation tissue, thereby leaving a clean base for complete epithelialization of the esophagus, and establishes a patent esophageal lumen.

The clinical studies that have now been reported, however, strongly suggest that the presence of unhealed lesions 3 weeks after the initial splinting requires additional esophageal intubation until the lesions are healed, in order to prevent late stricture formation. Despite the alteration of esophageal motility that follows stenting of a severely burned esophagus, the procedure provides an adequate conduit for the passage of food and fluid to the stomach, and one that is functionally as good as or better than the colon, stomach, or small-bowel segment needed to replace this organ. On the basis of our experience and that of others, we fail to see the rationale for early esophagectomy and esophageal replacement for deep esophageal burns in the absence of diffuse necrosis and perforation, as some sources have advocated.[8, 9] Treatment of deep, severe, nonperforated caustic burns of the esophagus by intraluminal splinting as originally advocated by Fell and co-workers[10] is, in my opinion, the best method currently available for preventing late esophageal stricture in the majority of patients.

REFERENCES

1. Reyes HM, Hill JL: Modification of the experimental stent technique for esophageal burns. *J Surg Res* 1976; 20:65.
2. Hill JL, Norbert HP, Smith MD, et al: Clinical technique and success of the esophageal stent to prevent corrosive strictures. *J Pediatr Surg* 1976; 11(3):443.
3. Reyes HM, Lin CY, Schlunk FF, et al: Experimental treatment of corrosive esophageal burns. *J Pediatr Surg* 1974; 9(3):317.
4. Mills LJ, Estrera AS, Platt MR: Avoidance of esophageal stricture following severe caustic burns by the use of an intraluminal stent. *Ann Thorac Surg* 1979; 28:60.
5. Coln D, Chang JHT: Experience with esophageal stenting for caustic burns in children. *J Pediatr Surg* 1986; 21(7):588.
6. Annual Meeting Poster Session, American Pediatric Surgical Association, May 28-31, 1989, Baltimore, Maryland.
7. Wijburg FA, Heymans HSA, Urbanus NAM: Caustic esophageal lesions in childhood: Prevention of stricture formation. *J Pediatr Surg* 1989; 24(2):171.
8. Meridith JW, Kon ND, Thompson JN: Management of injuries from liquid lye ingestion. *J Trauma* 1988; 28(8):1173.
9. Moazam F, Talbert JL, Miller D, et al: Caustic ingestion and its sequelae in children. *South Med J* 1987; 80(2):187.
10. Fell SC, Denize A, Becker NH, et al: The effect of intraluminal splinting in the prevention of caustic stricture of the esophagus. *J Thorac Cardiovasc Surg* 1966; 52:675.

26

Hypertrophic Pyloric Stenosis

Marshall Z. Schwartz, M.D.
Donald B. Shaul, M.D.

A 3-week-old boy developed nonbilious vomiting following feedings. Although he experienced weight gain in the first 2 weeks of life, his weight remained the same throughout the third week. His mother noted a decrease in the amount of urine produced and a reduction in the number of bowel movements. The vomiting became projectile. Scleral icterus was observed in association with an elevated indirect bilirubin fraction. Serum electrolytes were obtained and showed Na^+, 135 mEq/L; Cl^-, 84 mEq/L; K^+, 2.9 mEq/L; and CO_2-combining power, 36 mEq/L.

A 3-week-old infant is described as having projectile vomiting. The infant has biochemical evidence of hypochloremic, hypokalemic metabolic alkalosis. Although this is the classical presentation for hypertrophic pyloric stenosis (HPS), other entities, including pylorospasm and gastroesophageal reflux, may present in a similar fashion. All too often in this era of advanced technology, the desire is to request an imaging procedure to obtain a definitive diagnosis. That at least 75% of infants with HPS can be identified by a careful and patient physical examination is frequently ignored. To be successful in this endeavor, it is appropriate to create the best circumstances for it. Although the method of accomplishing this may vary from one examiner to the next, the infant must be calm to allow cooperation during careful palpation of the epigastrium. The use of a pacifier, or even feeding with a small amount of 5% dextrose in water, is frequently helpful. It will be much easier to palpate the hypertrophied pylorus or "olive" if the infant's stomach is empty. It may be necessary to aspirate the stomach with a nasogastric tube if the infant has recently been fed and not had an emesis. Covering the abdomen and legs with a blanket will prevent the infant from getting cold and being less cooperative. With the infant supine, the examining hand (underneath the blanket) should be placed in the epigastrium. After the edge of the liver has been identified with the fingertips, gentle pressure applied posteriorly, deep to the liver and progressing caudally, should reveal a palpable pylorus against the spine or posterior abdominal wall in infants with HPS. It is important to note that gentle pressure will allow a better examination and provoke less resistance from the infant. One should be able to "roll" the hypertrophied pylorus under the fingertips on at least two occasions to be convinced of the diagnosis. Patience in securing the optimum circumstances for palpation of the hypertrophied pylorus is critical. It may take 5 to 15 minutes to be successful, and the examiner should be willing to commit this amount of uninterrupted time if necessary. If a hypertrophied pylorus is not palpable, then further work-up is indicated. In the recent past, ultrasound has become a frequently used imaging technique for diagnosing HPS. Under optimum circumstances, this technique can be very reliable. However, it is greatly dependent on the level of experience and expertise of the ultrasonographer. Also, criteria for a positive diagnosis vary between different institutions. A barium upper gastrointestinal (UGI) study has generally been the definitive way of evaluating suspected HPS in infants when the hypertrophied pylorus is not palpable. Oral or nasogastric administration of thin barium to infants with HPS usually reveals a narrowed and elongated pyloric channel, referred to as either the "railroad track" sign (two narrow channels) or the "string" sign (one narrow channel). These findings are associated with indentation on the antral outline produced by the hypertrophied pyloric mass. In the absence of radiographic signs of HPS, the UGI study may reveal pylorospasm or gastroesophageal reflux. Although the UGI study is a reliable method of diagnosing HPS, it has the disadvantage of filling the stomach with barium, which can subsequently be aspirated either preoperatively or intraoperatively. Therefore, it is advisable for the radiologist to aspirate residual barium from the stomach after termination of the radiographic procedure.

Once the diagnosis of HPS is made, either by physical examination or imaging techniques, the appropriate next step is to optimally prepare the infant for surgical correction of the condition. It is important to remember that HPS is not a surgical emergency. In the case synopsis given here, it is suggested that the infant is hypovolemic, on the basis of a decreased urine output. In addition, the serum chloride and potassium levels are low and the bicarbonate level is markedly elevated, which are collectively indicative of hypochloremic/hypokalemic metabolic alkalosis. Unless there is significant hypovolemia (>10% dehydration), there is no urgency to correct hypovolemia. In infants with moderate to severe fluid, electrolyte, and metabolic imbalances, it is appropriate to take 24 to 48 hours to correct them. Intravenous fluid resuscitation with 5% dextrose in

0.45N saline containing 20 to 40 mEq KCl/L is frequently the optimum solution for fluid and electrolyte replacement. As in the case described above, potassium-, chloride-, and hydrogen-ion depletion are the most common findings in patients with HPS. Because hyponatremia is generally not a significant problem, excessive sodium chloride replacement with normal saline is usually not indicated. The rate of intravenous infusion should be correlated with the level of dehydration, and can range from 1.25 to 1.5 times the normal maintenance rate until adequate fluid replacement is achieved. In severe cases, initial bolus intravenous therapy may be warranted. The concentration of KCl in the intravenous fluid should be based on the level of hypokalemia, remembering that a KCl concentration exceeding 30 to 40 mEq/L is rarely indicated. There is little justification in attempting to correct the hypokalemia over a short period. It is appropriate to monitor urine output and to diminish the intravenous infusion rate when an adequate urine output is obtained (>1 cc/kg/hr). Serum electrolytes (Na^+, K^+, Cl^+, and CO_2) should be monitored every 6 to 12 hours as a guide for the adequacy of electrolyte repletion. In instances of moderate to severe metabolic alkalosis, there may be a delay in obtaining a normal serum bicarbonate level despite normalization of fluid volume and electrolyte status. Continued fluid and electrolyte resuscitation is usually sufficient to correct the persistent metabolic alkalosis. Administration of ammonium chloride or dilute hydrochloric acid is rarely necessary.

In the case presented, indirect hyperbilirubinemia was identified. This should not lead to an extensive work-up for liver disease. Of importance is that 5% to 10% of infants with HPS present with indirect hyperbilirubinemia that may exceed 15 mg%. The etiology of this finding is not completely known, but it appears to be partly related to the glucuronyl transferase deficiency commonly seen in neonates.[1] It has been routinely observed that the jaundice rapidly disappears after correction of the HPS and the resumption of oral feedings.

Following normalization of the patient's fluid, electrolyte, and acid–base status, it is safe to proceed with the surgical correction of HPS. Pyloromyotomy is the surgical procedure of choice because it is straightforward, curative, and associated with a remarkably low morbidity. A transverse incision, approximately 3 cm long, is made over the right rectus muscle in the right upper quadrant. It is not necessary to divide the rectus muscle to enter the peritoneal cavity; it may be retracted or split longitudinally in the middle. The pylorus should be delivered by initially grasping the greater curvature of the stomach and pulling it out through the incision. Using traction in an inferior and lateral direction, the pylorus can be brought out through the incision. Grasping the duodenum or pylorus directly with a forceps can result in injury to or perforation of these structures. Following delivery of the pylorus from the peritoneal cavity, the serosa on the anterior wall of the hypertrophied pylorus is incised from the duodenal junction proximally to a point proximal to the area of hypertrophied muscle. We prefer to use the back of a scalpel handle to bluntly split the hypertrophied muscle down to the submucosa. At this juncture, a careful check for entrance into the lumen of the stomach should be made before returning the pylorus to the peritoneal cavity. It is important to be sure that bleeding from the muscle edges has stopped before closing the abdominal-wall incision. Usually, the bleeding will stop spontaneously. We routinely avoid the use of cautery on the submucosa, to prevent a subsequent perforation.

Entrance into the lumen during pyloromyotomy should be a rare event. If this occurs, the submucosa should be approximated with fine interrupted sutures, followed by reapproximation of the hypertrophied muscle. The pylorus can then be rotated 180 degrees and a myotomy performed on the posterior wall of the pylorus.

The majority of infants can be started on feedings at 6 to 8 hours after the surgical correction of HPS. Infants who present with hematemesis from gastritis may benefit by delaying feedings for 24 hours after surgery. Our feeding schedule is shown in Table 26–1. It has been customary to initiate feedings with 5% dextrose solution at 15 to 30 cc per feeding every 3 hours. Over the course of the next 30 to 36 hours, the concentration and volume of feeding can gradually be increased to obtain appropriate caloric and fluid inputs. In the first few days after pyloromyotomy, it is common for infants to have intermittent

TABLE 26–1.
Postpyloromyotomy Feeding Schedule*

Pedialyte, 30 cc p.o. every 3 hr × 2
Half-strength formula, 30 cc p.o. every 3 hr × 1
Full-strength formula, 30 cc p.o. every 3 hr × 1
Full-strength formula, 45 cc p.o. every 3 hr × 2
Full-strength formula, 60 cc p.o. every 3 hr × 2
Full-strength formula, 75 cc p.o. every 3 hr × 2
Full-strength formula, 90 cc p.o. every 3 hr × 2
Full-strength formula ad lib

*For very small infants, the starting feeding volume may be reduced to 15 cc and the schedule stopped at volumes of 60 to 75 cc, which would provide an adequate calorie supply.

emesis. However, this should not delay the advancement of the feeding schedule, since persistent vomiting is unusual. Intravenous hydration can usually be stopped 12 hours after the feedings are begun, and discharge generally occurs 30 to 48 hours postoperatively. Nutritional repletion rapidly occurs and infants will resume growth at a normal rate.

The postoperative course for patients with HPS treated by pyloromyotomy is an excellent one. An infrequent complication is incomplete division of the pyloric musculature. This will result in persistent gastric-outlet obstruction evidenced by persistent vomiting. Another uncommon complication is submucosal injury during the myotomy, leading to perforation. This complication can be avoided by the use of careful technique, a search for this injury prior to terminating the surgical procedure, and the avoidance of cautery.

The long-term outlook for infants with HPS treated surgically is excellent, and the parents should be assured that further gastrointestinal problems from HPS are unlikely.

It is said that the first report of HPS was made in 1788.[2] Ramstedt, in 1912, is credited with describing pyloromyotomy.[3] The incidence of HPS in North America is between 1 in 300 and 1 in 900 births, with males having a fourfold higher incidence than females. Many authors report a higher incidence in firstborn males. The most characteristic pathologic finding is an increase in the thickness of the pyloric musculature. Histologic evaluation of the pyloric muscle reveals an increased cytoplasmic-to-nuclear ratio and an absence of mitotic figures indicative of hypertrophy rather than hyperplasia.[4]

The etiology of HPS remains unknown. Persistent spasm of the pylorus has been suggested as a possible etiology. Evaluation of the innervation of the pylorus has shown the neurons to be normal in number and maturity but lacking in substance P, an important neurotransmitter responsible for enteric muscle contraction.[4] Chronic pylorospasm could lead to exhaustion of substance P as well as to muscle hypertrophy. Chronic pylorospasm could also be related to mucosal erosion or ulceration.[5]

Several gastrointestinal hormones have been investigated as possible etiologic factors in HPS. They include gastrin, secretin, enteroglucagon, and neurotensin.[5–7] However, these peptides have not been definitively associated with HPS.

In summary, the diagnosis of HPS can usually be made by careful physical examination. Ultrasound or UGI can be employed if abdominal palpation is unsuccessful. Fluid, electrolyte, and metabolic abnormalities should be completely corrected before pyloromyotomy is undertaken.

The diagnosis, preoperative preparation, and surgical treatment of infants with pyloric stenosis remain among the most rewarding endeavors for the children's surgeon. A short hospitalization and an excellent outcome should be anticipated in almost all of these infants.

REFERENCES

1. Roth B, Statz A, Heinisch HM, et al: Elimination of indocyanine green by the liver of infants with hypertrophic pyloric stenosis and the icteropyloric syndrome. *J Pediatr* 1981; 99:240–243.
2. Donovan EJ: Congenital hypertrophic stenosis of the pylorus. *Arch Pediatr* 1958; 75:359.
3. Ramstedt C: Zur operation der angeborenen pylorus-stenose. *Med Klin* 1912; 8:1702.
4. Tam PK: Observations and perspectives of the pathology and possible aetiology of infantile hypertrophic pyloric stenosis—A histological, biochemical, histochemical and immunocytochemical study. *Ann Acad Med Singapore* 1985; 14:523–529.
5. Markowitz RI, Wolfson BJ, Huff DS, et al: Infantile hypertrophic pyloric stenosis—Congenital or acquired? *J Clin Gastroenterol* 1982; 4:39–44.
6. Moazam F, Kolts BE, Rodgers BM: In pursuit of the etiology of congenital hypertrophic pyloric stenosis. *J Pediatr Gastroenterol Nutr* 1982; 1:97–99.
7. Christofides ND, Mallet E, Ghatei MA, et al: Plasma enteroglucagon and neurotensin in infantile pyloric stenosis. *Arch Dis Child* 1983; 58:52–55.

27

Acute Peptic Ulcer in Infants and Children

Stephen P. Dunn, M.D.

A premature infant of 29 weeks' gestational age, weighing 1.2 kg, developed severe respiratory distress syndrome shortly after birth. The infant required intubation and mechanical ventilation for severe hypoxia. A prolonged ventilator run resulted in bronchopulmonary dysplasia with reactive airway disease. The infant was put on steroid therapy. One week later, the stools became positive for blood in a stool guaiac test. Antacid therapy was begun when gastric residuals demonstrated the presence of coffee-ground material. The infant suddenly deteriorated and abdominal distension was noted. An abdominal roentgenogram showed free air in the peritoneal cavity.

This infant has clearly suffered an intra-abdominal catastrophe that will require urgent resuscitation and surgical operation. Although there are several possible causes of free air in this child, we will be discussing the management of acute peptic ulcer disease in infants and children, which is the most probable cause of this child's acute perforation and deterioration. A knowledge of peptic ulcer disease in infants and children will allow us to better select the surgical approach to this infant and better predict the infant's response to treatment and long term prognosis. We will begin by discussing peptic ulcer disease in children in general.[1, 2]

Peptic ulcer disease occurs in children of all ages beyond the newborn period. The newborn does not make gastric acid, which is the common ingredient in all peptic ulcer disease in children.

The disease can be divided into two patient groups. Acute peptic ulcers can occur in any stressed infant or child at any age beyond the newborn period. Generally, these children have an underlying illness that has resulted in significant physiologic stress. Poor systemic perfusion or oxygenation, or inadequate nutrition are often present. The underlying illness may require treatment with an ulcerogenic medication such as aspirin, nonsteroidal anti-inflammatory drugs, or steroids. These infants and children present acutely with symptoms of hematemesis, melena, or perforation. The ulcerogenic process in these patients seems to be related to their physiologic stress or to the ulcerogenic medication they are receiving, and the incidence of later recurrence is uncommon, as are chronic symptoms. The prognosis in these cases is most affected by the underlying illness that has created the physiologic stress leading to the acute ulcer.

The second group of children with peptic ulcer disease present later in life with symptoms of abdominal pain. They frequently do not have identifiable risk factors except a positive family history of ulcerative disease. Diagnostic investigation will reveal the etiology of the abdominal pain as a gastric or duodenal ulcer. Recurrence of symptoms after completion of treatment is not uncommon, and many of these children go on to suffer lifelong symptoms of chronic ulcer disease. Many methods have been used to diagnose peptic ulcer disease in infants and children who manifest its signs or symptoms. The diagnosis can usually be made by a barium or double-contrast upper gastrointestinal (GI) study or upper GI endoscopy. Symptoms of gastrointestinal hemorrhage are best diagnosed by endoscopy, although an occasionally stable patient with bleeding may benefit from arteriography for diagnosis of the condition and its treatment with embolization. Rapid control of bleeding from a single point can be achieved transendoscopically. Neither of these methods should, however, prevent the unstable patient from being moved rapidly to definitive surgery.

Once a diagnosis of peptic ulcer disease has been made, most patients will respond to medical treatment for it. This includes a regimen of antacids, H-2 blockers, or sucralfate. In patients with active hemorrhage, transendoscopic application of cautery to exposed vessels may be successful. Surgical treatment is indicated for patients whose estimated blood loss is greater than 60% of their estimated blood volume. The surgical goal is to control bleeding with the most limited operative procedure required. Usually this will include gastrotomy with direct suture of the bleeding vessel. Acid-reducing operations are reserved for those patients with the chronic symptoms of a nonhealing ulcer and pain, recurrent bleeding, or obstruction. These operations include vagotomy with pyloroplasty, vagotomy with antrectomy, or highly selective vagotomy. The operation selected for treating the symptoms of chronic ulcer may partly be dictated by the problem. As an example, gastric outlet obstruction may be best treated by antrectomy and vagotomy. Patients with perforation do not need further testing, but should undergo surgery after proper resuscitation. The patient presented in this case offers many areas for comment in the care and management of a very small and very sick infant. The surgical management of the operative findings is only one of these areas. We will begin by discussing the resuscitation of this infant in a step-by-step approach.

This infant has a perforated viscus from peptic ulcer disease. There will be a rapid onset of diffuse chemical peritonitis resulting in massive fluid shifts and systemic hypotension. Adequate resuscitation will require a supportive approach to the whole patient. This patient is known to have bronchopulmonary dysplasia and to have required long-term endotracheal intubation. The status of the patient's ventilation should be evaluated. This would involve an examination of the chest to verify that adequate breath sounds are heard on both sides and that the endotracheal tube is adequately secured. The infant's arterial blood gases should be measured, and any ventilator or respiratory therapy changes should be made to optimize oxygenation and correct respiratory acid-base abnormalities. Intravenous therapy should be begun with a balanced salt solution. A Foley catheter should be inserted and the urine output should be monitored hourly. With appropriate resuscitation, this infant should excrete 1 to 2 cc/kg/hr of urine. Until good urine output has been established, fluid should be given in aliquots of 10 to 20 cc/kg over short intervals. Laboratory studies should be done for blood type and crossmatch characteristics, hemoglobin, platelet count, and clotting. Fresh-frozen plasma and platelets should be available for surgery. The appropriate intravenous infusion lines will have to be established prior to laparotomy. At least one relatively short, large-bore "volume" line will usually be required for a laparotomy of this nature. Antibiotics should be administered. Ampicillin and an aminoglycoside will appropriately cover the oral flora and any unusual organisms that may have colonized the infant in the hospital. Stress-reducing steroids should be administered prior to the induction of anesthesia. These may be rapidly tapered in the postoperative period. An adequate approach before surgery consists of 20 to 40 mg/m^2 of methylprednisolone given intravenously over 30 minutes. Resuscitation of this infant can be accomplished safely in 1 to 2 hours, while the operating room is being prepared for emergent surgery.

The infant should be moved to the operating room under the careful supervision of experienced personnel. After it has been positioned on the operating table and the anesthesiologist has completed a review of the airway and the intravenous lines, anesthesia should be induced. The operation will involve exposure of the abdominal viscera, and nitrous oxide should be avoided. An electrocautery grounding pad is attached to a dry, clear area of skin. Everything except the operative field is covered with a plastic material that will ensure dryness of the patient during the course of the surgical procedure. The infant is positioned on a warming blanket on the operating table, and temperature monitoring is maintained throughout the course of the procedure. The abdomen is prepared for operation with a povidone/iodine (Betadine) scrub and followed by a warm Betadine preparative solution. The surgical draping should include the entire abdomen.

The surgery is begun with a left transverse upper abdominal incision.

When the abdomen is entered, culture specimens should be obtained. A thorough examination of the abdomen should be undertaken and the site of the perforation identified. Perforations can be detected by direct observation of both surfaces of the stomach and careful inspection of the duodenum. Once the perforation has been identified, its management must be selected. Small perforations can be best managed by freshening of the edge and simple suture closure reinforced by an omental patch. This treatment is quite adequate, since these ulcers do not have a high propensity for recurrence, and a definitive ulcer operation is not required. In some rare cases, gastric perforations can be quite large and present difficult technical problems for closure. If possible, simple plication of the defect in such cases is still preferable to gastric resection. Difficult duodenal perforation may require a more extensive procedure. This includes the diverticularization of the duodenum by oversewing of the pyloric outlet to the stomach and creation of a gastrojejunostomy. After closure of the duodenal perforation, the area should be drained laterally. In most cases, simple plication will be adequate for managing a perforation. Once the perforation has been appropriately managed, the abdomen should be copiously irrigated with warm saline. A nasogastric tube should be positioned, under direct vision, in the most advantageous portion of the stomach, without pressure being applied to the suture line.

The principles of postoperative management for this patient are straightforward. Good perfusion should be maintained by the adequate administration of fluids. There will be third-space losses into the peritoneum, related to the ongoing peritoneal inflammation, which will require one-and-a-half to two times the usual volume of fluid for maintenance during the first 24 hours after surgery. The infant's urine output should be monitored with an indwelling bladder catheter. The dosage of stress-reducing steroids given at the time of surgery should be tapered in the postoperative period. A normal schedule would involve tapering the dose of methylprednisolone over a 2-week period. After surgery, the patient should receive an H-2 blocker intravenously. The pH of the nasogastric aspirate should be determined frequently. A pH below 5 should be treated with antacid therapy. This can be done with 5 cc of an antacid administered by nasogastric tube every 2 hours until the pH is consistently greater than 5. After 24 hours, parenteral nutrition should be started. This child will require 100 to 120 calories per kilogram for adequate nutrition. Because of the child's bronchopulmonary dysplasia, 30% to 40% of these calories should be given as fat, to decrease the respiratory quotient and excess CO_2 production. Antibiotic therapy should be continued for 7 to 10 days.

This infant, suffering from bronchopulmonary dysplasia, has been further compromised by the complication of acute peptic ulcer disease. If, however, it is appropriately managed, its prognosis is good, and recurrent ulcerations should not be expected. Physicians caring for children with stressful illnesses need to be alert to the possible complication of acute peptic ulcer secondary to stress, medication, or both. The long-term outlook for these patients is good if their acute management is prompt and judicious.

REFERENCES

1. Dunn SP, Weber TR, Grosfeld JL: Acute peptic ulcer in childhood: Emergency surgical therapy in 39 cases. *Arch Surg* 1983; 118:656–660.
2. Drum B, Rhoads JM, Stringer DA, et al: Peptic ulcer disease in children: Etiology, clinical findings and clinical course. *Pediatrics* 1988; 82:410–414.

PART FOUR

Hepatobiliary and Pancreatic Disorders

28

Biliary Atresia

F. M. Karrer, M.D.
John R. Lilly, M.D.

A 6-week-old infant presents with scleral icterus, hepatomegaly, and light-colored stools. The infant was full-term and had an uneventful vaginal delivery. On physical examination, the abdomen was slightly protuberant and an enlarged, firm liver edge was palpable 2.0 cm below the right costal margin in the midclavicular line. The tip of the spleen was palpable. There was no cardiac murmur. Fasting abdominal ultrasound examination showed a small gallbladder that did not contract with feeding. The total serum bilirubin was 10 mg/dL, with a 6.2 mg/dL direct fraction. A hepatobiliary iminodiacetic acid (IDA) scan was consistent with biliary obstruction. The α_1-antitrypsin level was normal.

In infancy, jaundice that persists beyond 2 weeks should no longer be considered physiologic, particularly when the bilirubin elevation is primarily of the direct type (conjugated fraction). A host of conditions may be responsible for jaundice in infancy, including infectious, metabolic, hematologic, cholestatic, and obstructive disorders. The diagnostic evaluation for all possible etiologies would take weeks, time that is critical to successful relief of the most common obstructive cause of jaundice, biliary atresia.

DIAGNOSTIC EVALUATION

The clinical features of infants with neonatal cholestasis provide little indication as to the etiology. Most infants have icterus, light-colored (rarely acholic) stools, dark urine, and hepatomegaly. Often, infants with biliary atresia appear healthy and do not have marked jaundice at birth. Infants with hepatocellular jaundice frequently appear sick and more commonly are icteric from birth.

We employ ultrasonography and technetium-99m iminodiacetic acid (IDA)

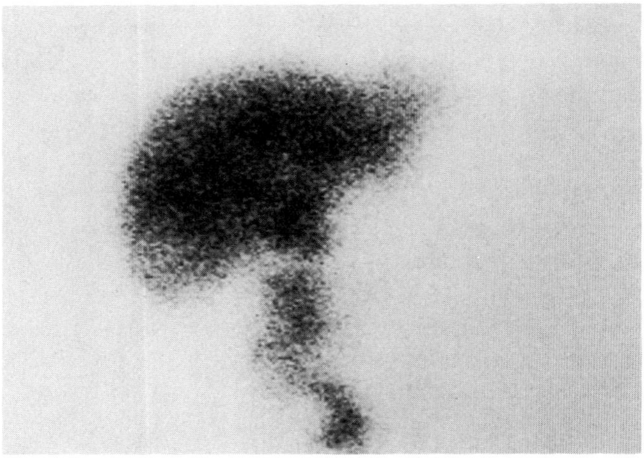

FIG 28–1.
In addition to preoperative diagnostic imaging, 99m-technetium-iminodiacetic acid (IDA) imaging is also useful for postoperative follow-up studies in patients with biliary atresia. This IDA scan of a 4-month-old infant, done after a successful portoenterostomy, shows good hepatocyte uptake and prompt excretion into the Roux-en-Y limb.

imaging early in the work-up. In biliary atresia, abdominal ultrasound examination typically shows increased echogenicity of the liver, with a small, shrunken gallbladder that does not contract with feeding. Hepatobiliary IDA scintigraphy demonstrates adequacy of hepatocyte uptake which, particularly early in the course of biliary atresia, is rapid. However, excretion into the bowel is absent, even on delayed images. In contrast, hepatocellular causes of jaundice are characterized by delayed isotope uptake due to parenchymal disease, but excretion into the intestine usually eventually ensues (Fig 28–1). Percutaneous liver biopsy may also be helpful, and is safe, provided that the patient's coagulation status is normal. However, the characteristic diagnostic features of biliary atresia (i.e., bile-duct proliferation, canalicular bile stasis, and fibrosis) tend to occur later in the course of the disease; earlier there may be histologic overlap with the features of neonatal hepatitis. Alpha-1-antitrypsin deficiency should be specifically ruled out, since the PiZZ phenotype causes a cholestatic jaundice easily confused with biliary atresia.

PATHOLOGY

About 10% to 15% of infants with biliary atresia have a peculiar constellation of associated anomalies (i.e., polysplenia, a bilobed liver, situs inversus, an

absent inferior vena cava, a preduodenal portal vein, and intestinal malrotation). This association suggests an early embryologic etiology.

Biliary obstruction is not static, but rather a dynamic, sclerosing, obliterative process. Serial sectioning of the extrahepatic bile ducts in infants with biliary atresia reveals patent, tiny biliary channels in the bile-duct tissue at the porta hepatis.[1] These structures communicate through an arborizing network with the intrahepatic bile ducts. We have demonstrated this histologic picture in a patient shortly after birth.[2] Patency of this arborizing biliary network is lost in time, and by 4 months these structures are completely replaced by fibrous tissue.

In the majority of patients (80% to 85%), the entire extrahepatic biliary tree is obliterated (Fig 28–2). In 10% to 15% of infants, however, the distal ducts are spared (i.e., the patency of the gallbladder, cystic duct, and common bile duct is retained). A third group of patients (5% to 10%) are found to have dilated proximal bile ducts. These most often represent bile pseudocysts in the liver hilum, not true ducts. They have no epithelial lining and the wall is composed only of fibrous tissue. Communication with the intrahepatic ducts, if it exists at all, is by minute biliary radicles.

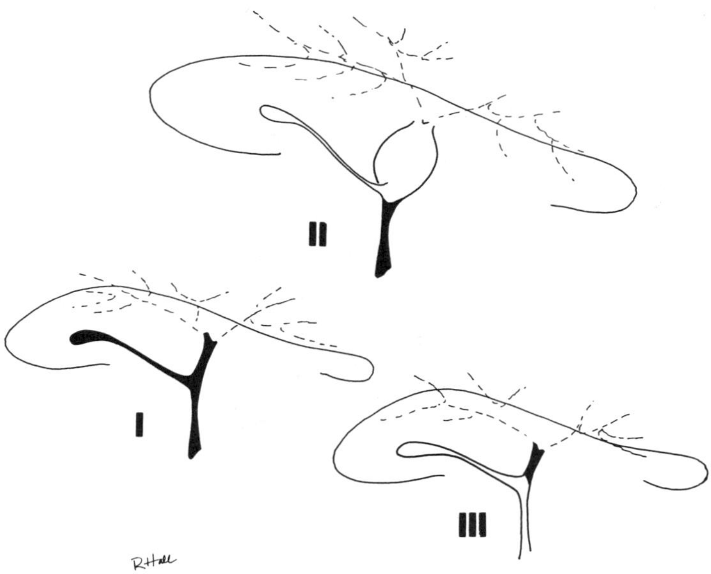

FIG 28–2.
The different types of extrahepatic anatomy in biliary atresia. Complete obliteration of the extrahepatic ducts *(I)*. Proximal "patency" with dilated hilar bile cysts, usually devoid of epithelial lining and communicating with the intrahepatic ducts only by minute biliary channels *(II)*. Distal patency of the gallbladder, cystic duct, and common bile duct *(III)*.

SURGICAL MANAGEMENT

Exploratory laparotomy and cholangiography should be done if the diagnostic evaluation suggests biliary atresia. Through a limited right-upper-quadrant incision, surgical cholangiography can be attempted via the gallbladder, and the liver can be biopsied. In most instances the liver is firm and nodular, with a green-brown color, while the small atretic gallbladder makes cholangiography impossible. If the gallbladder is patent, cholangiography is performed, and if the biliary ducts are visualized from the intrahepatic ducts to the duodenum, the diagnosis of biliary atresia is excluded.

In biliary atresia, the incision is extended and full exploration of the extrahepatic biliary tree is required. In those patients with only distal patency of the bile ducts, the gallbladder and distal common bile duct are preserved for subsequent reconstruction (see below). Otherwise, the common bile duct is dissected to the liver hilus (at the bifurcation of the portal vein). Here the duct broadens to form a cone of fibrous tissue. Sutures are placed at the lateral edges of the fibrous cone and also posteriorly, behind the crotch of the portal vein, and the cone is then transected flush with the liver surface (Fig 28–3). The

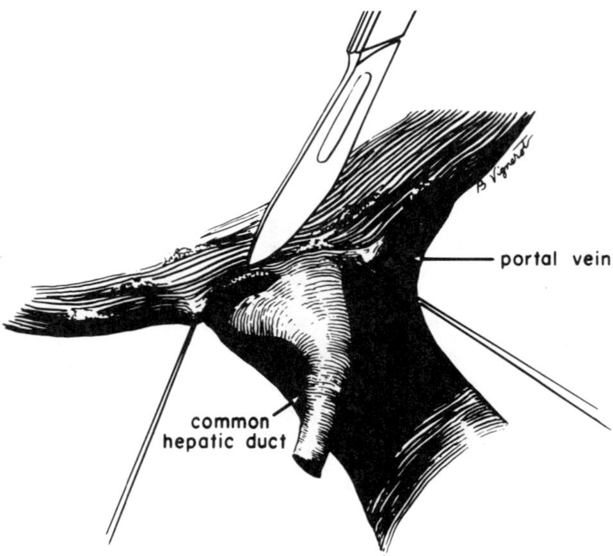

FIG 28–3.
The hilar dissection is critical to the success of the Kasai procedure. The extrahepatic-duct remnants are dissected out to the bifurcation of the portal vein. The fibrous cone is then transected flush with the liver. (From Lilly JR: Biliary atresia: The jaundiced infant, in Welch K, Randolph J, Ravitch M, O'Neill, J, et al (eds): *Pediatric Surgery,* ed 4. Chicago, Year Book Medical Publishers, Inc., 1986, pp 1047–1056. Used by permission.)

presence of minute biliary structures is confirmed by frozen-section examination. If no such structures are found, the porta hepatis should be re-excised, since bile drainage does not occur if these structures are not breached. Bilioenteric continuity is re-established by anastomosis of the transected liver hilus to a Roux-en-Y jejunal loop.

A variety of modifications have been advanced to reduce the incidence of cholangitis. We prefer to temporarily exteriorize the jejunal conduit as a double-barreled enterostomy during the critical early period of bile drainage, which lasts for the first 6 to 12 postoperative weeks. In addition, we incorporate an intussusception "valve" into the distal intestinal conduit (Fig 28–4). The valve modifications are thought to decrease colonization of the conduit with enteric flora, and thereby reduce the incidence of cholangitis. The biliary stoma is closed intraperitoneally when the infant is 3 to 4 months old.

An identical operation is performed when proximal patency is demonstrated. The dilated proximal duct communicates with the intrahepatic ducts only by minute radicles. Simple intestinal anastomosis to the hilar cyst is usually not followed by sustained bile drainage. We therefore recommend excision of the cystic structures at the liver hilus, followed by portoenterostomy.

In those infants in whom the gallbladder, cystic duct, and common bile duct are patent to the duodenum, the gallbladder is carefully shelled out of the hepatic bed while preserving the cystic arterial blood supply. The proximal hilar transection is identical to that described above. The gallbladder is opened and anastomosed to the liver hilus to re-establish biliary continuity. Because the small, unused common duct may be inadequate to accommodate all of the bile drainage, temporary tube decompression of the gallbladder is employed.[3] Use of the portocholecystostomy has the advantage of almost eliminating postoperative cholangitis.

With timely referral for surgical operation (age <10 weeks), successful bile drainage can be achieved in more than 80% of infants with biliary atresia. Because bile flow in the first few postoperative weeks may be tenuous, careful monitoring of bile volume and bile bilirubin is essential. Intravenous antibiotic or corticosteroid therapy or both should be instituted early if cholangitis or bile shutdown is threatened. The collected bile is refed through the distal stoma to avoid dehydration and electrolyte abnormalities, and to improve the absorption of fats and fat-soluble vitamins.

POSTOPERATIVE COMPLICATIONS

Cholangitis

Because the intrahepatic ducts are hypoplastic and incompletely drained in patients with biliary atresia, bile stasis persists for months, even after "success-

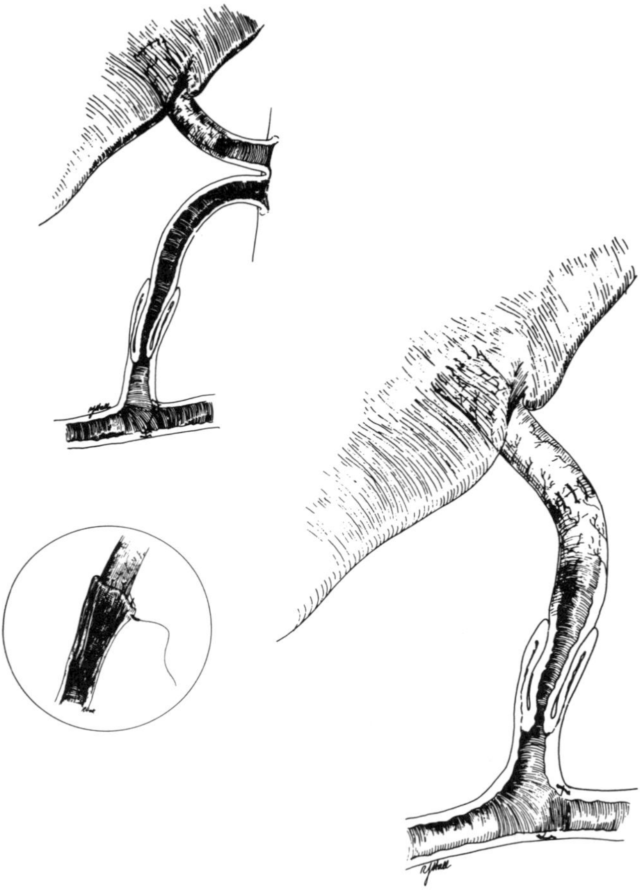

FIG 28–4.
The reconstruction currently used at the University of Colorado-Children's Hospital in Denver. The Roux-en-Y loop is anastomosed to the porta hepatis and then immediately exteriorized as a double-barreled stoma. An intussusception valve is created in the distal limb to prevent reflux and decrease bacterial colonization by enteric flora. (Lilly JR, Karrer FM, Hall RJ, et al: *Ann Surg* 1989; 210:289. Used by permission.)

ful" portoenterostomy. In combination with the bacterial flora present in the intestinal conduit, this constitutes the prerequisite for the development of cholangitis. Most children suffer one or more episodes of cholangitis within the first year after Kasai's operation. Thereafter, the liability of cholangitis wanes. Typically, cholangitis presents with fever, leukocytosis, and elevations in the serum bilirubin level and hepatic enzyme activity. The responsible bacteria are almost always enteric pathogens, but can rarely be isolated by blood culture. Prompt institution of broad-spectrum antibiotics [we are currently using imipenem-cilastatin sodium (Primaxin) with or without aminoglycosides] will control most episodes. For refractory cholangitis, corticosteroids are effective in increasing bile flow and decreasing periductular inflammation.[4] In some instances of recurrent cholangitis, long-term "prophylactic" antibiotics may be needed.

Fat Malabsorption

Because many patients have insufficient bile flow or poor quality bile for months after the surgical treatment of biliary atresia, their fat absorption is impaired. We routinely use formulas with fats provided as medium-chain triglycerides (MCT). These triglycerides are absorbed directly through the intestinal mucosa, without the need for micelle formation, emulsification, and hydrolysis. Fat-soluble vitamins also depend on micelle formation for absorption. The risk of deficiency diseases such as rickets (vitamin D) and ataxic neuromyopathy (vitamin E) can be minimized by careful monitoring of serum vitamin levels, with appropriate supplementation.

Portal Hypertension

Despite successful bile drainage, intrahepatic disease progresses in many patients, with the development of portal hypertension. Clinical manifestations of portal hypertension include esophageal variceal hemorrhage, hypersplenism, and ascites. Bleeding from esophageal varices can be controlled and prevented by repeated sessions of esophageal endosclerosis, or by the more recent procedure of endoscopic variceal banding.[5] Since some patients will eventually be considered for hepatic transplantation, portacaval shunt procedures should be avoided. Hypersplenism, manifested by thrombocytopenia and leukopenia, is effectively treated by partial splenic embolization, which also appears to reduce the incidence of esophageal variceal hemorrhage. Ascites, rarely a significant clinical problem, can be easily treated with spironolactone and salt restriction, and, if necessary, with furosemide. In some patients, complications of portal hypertension subside over time, either because of improvement in hepatic histology (less fibrosis) or the spontaneous development of portosystemic shunts. When hepatic function is preserved (as manifested by an anicteric, normal coagulation status and normal serum albumin), continued nonsurgical efforts at preventing portal hypertensive complications are justified. In the presence of deteriorating hepatic reserve, the patient should be referred for liver transplantation.

PROGNOSIS

Hepatic portoenterostomy has positively altered the natural history for infants with biliary atresia. Bile drainage is achieved in 80% to 90% of patients. However, the long-term survival (>10 years) is at best only 50%.[6] The major determinant of survival is the patient's age at the time of corrective surgery; the survival is over 60% if the surgery is done before 60 days of age, as opposed to 30% if done after this.[7] Furthermore, the technical details of the hilar dissection are crucial to subsequent bile drainage.

Unfortunately, establishment of bile flow does not guarantee long-term survival. Cirrhosis, portal hypertension, and ascending cholangitis complicate the postoperative course of many children. Cholangitis has a pronounced adverse effect on long-term outcome; in a series from the Netherlands, the survival among patients with cholangitis was only 51%, as compared to 91% in the group without cholangitis.[8] We have also found that the quantity and quality of bile excreted is predictive of outcome. At 1 month after surgery, a daily bilirubin excretion (the product of bile volume and bile bilirubin) of more than 6 mg/day is associated with a greater than 90% survival, as compared with a survival of less than 30% at 5 years if the daily bilirubin excretion is less than 6 mg/day.[9]

In our series, about one-third of patients with biliary atresia survive beyond 10 years, and most are completely asymptomatic.[10] For children in whom bile drainage is not achieved, or with late progression of liver disease despite relief of biliary obstruction, liver transplantation now offers the possibility of extended survival. In the largest series reported to date from Pittsburgh, children with biliary atresia had a 62% 5-year actuarial survival rate with cyclosporine/prednisone immunosuppression.[11] The postoperative complications and morbidity of transplantation are, however, high. In light of the scarcity of infant donors and the liabilities of long-term immunosuppression, we believe that Kasai's portoenterostomy should be the initial operation for infants with biliary atresia.

REFERENCES

1. Kasai M, Suzuki S: A new operation for "non-correctable" biliary atresia: Hepatic portoenterostomy. *Shujitsu* 1959; 13:733.
2. Greenholz SK, Lilly JR, Shikes RH, et al: Biliary atresia in the newborn. *J Pediatr Surg* 1986; 21:1147–1148.
3. Lilly JR, Stellin G: Catheter decompression of hepatic portocholecystostomy. *J Pediatr Surg* 1982; 17:904–905.
4. Karrer FM, Lilly JR: Corticosteroid therapy in biliary atresia. *J Pediatr Surg* 1985; 20(6):693–696.

5. Hall RJ, Lilly JR, Stiegmann GV: Endoscopic esophageal varix ligation: Technique and preliminary results in children. *J Pediatr Surg* 1988; 23:1222–1223.
6. Ohi R, Hanamatsu M, Mochizuki I: Progress in the treatment of biliary atresia. *World J Surg* 1985; 9:285–293.
7. Schweizer P: Treatment of extrahepatic bile duct atresia: Results and long-term prognosis after hepatic portoenterostomy. *Pediatr Surg Int* 1986; 1:30–36.
8. Houwen RHJ, Zwierstra RB, Severijnen RVM, et al: Prognosis of extrahepatic biliary atresia. *Arch Dis Child* 1989; 64:214–218.
9. Vazquez-Estevez JJ, Stewart BA, Shikes RH, et al: Biliary atresia: Early determination of prognosis. *J Pediatr Surg* 1989; 24:48–51.
10. Lilly JR, Karrer FM, Hall RJ, et al: The surgery of biliary atresia. *Ann Surg* 1989; 210:289–296.
11. Iwatsuki S, Starzl TE, Todo S, et al: Experience in 1000 liver transplants under cyclosporine-steroid therapy: A survival report. *Transplant Proc* 1988; 20:498–504.

29

Choledochal Cyst

Ken Kimura, M.D.

A 4-year-old girl was referred for evaluation of right-upper-quadrant pain and vomiting. On physical examination, scleral icterus was observed and a mass was palpated in the right upper quadrant. An abdominal ultrasound examination demonstrated a dilated gallbladder and a cystic mass inferior to the porta hepatis. The serum total bilirubin was 8.0 mg/dL, with a direct fraction of 5.5 mg/dL, and the alkaline phosphatase was 535 IU/L. The white blood cell count was $19{,}000/mm^3$ with a shift to the left on the differential smear. The serum amylase level was 900 IU/L.

Choledochal cyst is a rare disease of congenital origin that results in varying degrees of dilatation of the extrahepatic biliary system, and which at times involves the intrahepatic biliary radicles as well. In our experience (n=53), the incidence is three times higher in females than males.[1] More than 50% of our patients were initially diagnosed before the age of 2 years, presenting with a mass in the right upper abdomen, jaundice, abdominal pain, fever, and vomiting.

Until two decades ago, choledochal cyst was considered to represent simply a developmental anomaly of the bile duct. However, in 1969, Babbitt proposed the etiologic concept of the dilation of the biliary ducts possibly being secondary to degenerative change resulting from persistent exposure to pancreatic juice that refluxes into the biliary system through an abnormally high junction between the common bile duct and the pancreatic duct.[2] The association of this ductal anomaly was consistently demonstrated in cholangiograms of patients with choledochal cysts.[3] Later studies demonstrated an elevated amylase level in the choledochal fluid. Today, Babbitt's concept is supported by many authors.[3–8]

The clinical history of our propositus suggests that the problems in this 4-year-old girl are: (1) obstructive jaundice with elevated serum bilirubin and alkaline posphatase levels, (2) moderate pancreatitis with abdominal pain, vomiting, and an elevated serum amylase level and leukocyte count, and (3) a choledochal cyst that was detected as a palpable mass in the right upper quadrant and visualized by abdominal ultrasound examination.

This patient should be immediately admitted for further evaluation and preparation for surgery.

PREOPERATIVE EVALUATION OF THE PATIENT

Jaundice

In choledochal cyst, jaundice is intermittent and associated with hepatic enzyme elevations of various degree. The severity of the liver disorder does not always correlate with the serum bilirubin level. Therefore, an evaluation of liver function is mandatory, including tests for coagulopathy. When the liver disorder is critical, an attempt should be made to improve the defective liver functions prior to a surgical attack on the choledochal cyst. In our experience, percutaneous transhepatic cholangiodrainage (PTCD) produces effective decompression of the biliary system and rapid recovery of failed liver functions in 1 to 2 weeks.

Associated Pancreatitis

Relapsing pancreatitis is another specific association with choledochal cyst.[7] Intermittent, mild to moderate elevation of the serum amylase level is present in one third of patients.[1] Abdominal pain, vomiting, leukocytosis, and fever are frequent associated manifestations. The precise etiologic mechanism of relapsing pancreatitis is unclear, but the anomalous communication between the common and pancreatic ducts is considered the likely cause.[7]

Abdominal Mass

For diagnosing a choledochal cyst by imaging, an abdominal ultrasound examination alone can precisely demonstrate its location, size, form (cystic, cylindrical, or diverticular), and its relationship to adjacent organs. The technique clearly differentiates choledochal cyst from other masses. We prefer an additional computed tomographic (CT) scan to more precisely document the intrahepatic biliary system before and after surgery. In several institutions, endoscopic retrograde choledochopancreatography (ERCPG) is frequently used to visualize the anomalous communication between the common and pancreatic ducts[4, 6, 7]; however, we feel that this invasive study need not be part of the routine preoperative workup, since the information obtained from ERCPG does not significantly benefit the surgeon who performs the operation. Studies of bile excretion, such as by nuclear liver scanning or intravenous cholangiography, were previously used on a routine basis. Today they have been largely replaced by imaging studies.

PREPARATION FOR SURGERY

Besides routine prelaparotomy laboratory tests including a complete blood count and urinalysis, blood typing and the crossmatching of one unit of blood are mandatory. An additional unit of blood should be screened and ready before the patient is on the operating table. In our experience (n=48), the amount of blood loss during dissection of a choledochal cyst has ranged from 48 to 1,720 mL (mean 359.7 ± 392.1 mL).[1] The bowel is prepared using polyethylene glycol solution.[10]

SURGICAL OPERATION

After induction of anesthesia, the patient is placed on the operating table in the supine position, with the right upper abdomen elevated by a small pillow. Two venous routes are secured using large-bore venous catheters.

Laparotomy

A right subcostal skin incision is extended from the midline to the anterior axillary line to enter the abdomen. The proximal transverse colon is mobilized downward to expose the distal part of the choledochal cyst, the head of the pancreas, and the second portion of the duodenum. During the entire procedure, the bowel is tucked away in the abdominal cavity, using peritoneal pads.

Intraoperative Studies

Sampling of the choledochal cyst contents, cholangiography, and liver biopsy are done initially. Using a syringe with a 21-gauge needle, a small amount of choledochal cyst fluid is aspirated for culture and amylase determination. A 4-0 silk purse-string suture is placed in the fundus of the gallbladder, and an 8F feeding tube is inserted through the suture and advanced into the choledochal cyst through the dilated cystic duct. Intraoperative cholangiograms are obtained with iodinated contrast medium. When the choldedochal cyst is large, visualization of the entire biliary system is often unsatisfactory because of dilution of the contrast material. In this case, a successful cholangiogram is obtained when the choledochal cyst contents are evacuated and replaced by contrast medium.

In our experience, this technique routinely reveals the anomalous communication between the common and pancreatic ducts at a point 10 to 25 mm proximal to the papilla of Vater. The duct between this anomalous communication and the papilla is called the "common channel." A biopsy specimen is harvested from the anterior margin of the liver while the cholangiogram is being processed.

Resection of Choledochal Cyst

The gallbladder is dissected from the fundus downward, perhaps using the catheter in the gallbladder for traction. In this phase of dissection, one should look for an anomalous right hepatic artery and its relationship to the gallbladder.

A serosal incision on the choledochal cyst is extended longitudinally to reach the first portion of the duodenum (Fig 29–1,A) The anterior wall of the distal portion of a choledochal cyst is formed by layers of highly vascular fibrous tissue, and dissection in this area requires special attention to control hemorrhage. Conventional blunt dissection may invite uncontrollable massive bleeding. Electrocautery usually fails to achieve satisfactory hemostasis. Only tedious and meticulous dissection using numerous hemostats and ligatures will avoid massive blood loss. The danger of massive blood loss in this phase of the dissection cannot be overemphasized. To avoid hemorrhage, shunt operations employing choledochocystoenterostomy were previously advocated. However, recent studies report a high incidence of cancer developing in the unresected choledochal cyst, mandating its complete resection.[8, 10]

When dissection reaches the distal end of the choledochal cyst, the duodenum and pancreas are retracted downward to expose the common duct, which communicates with the choledochal cyst (Fig 29–1,B and C). The common duct is transfixed at this point with nonabsorbable suture material and transected (Fig 29–1,D). However, the communication between the choledochal cyst and the common duct is frequently so tiny as to be undetectable, the distal end of the choledochal cyst presenting as a blind end. It is interesting that jaundice has not been complete in such patients. In other patients, the distal end of the choledochal cyst can be seen to communicate directly with the pancreatic duct. In such a situation, the choledochal cyst is divided between clamps 1 cm upstream from its junction with the pancreatic duct, after evacuating its contents through the gallbladder catheter. The inner layer of the distal stump is excised or destroyed because it has a high potential for becoming malignant.[8] The remaining tissue is approximated using nonabsorbable transfixing stitches. When the pancreatic duct is inadvertently injured, internal drainage is achieved midway along the Roux-Y loop that is created for a bile conduit.

Dissection of the posterior aspect of the choledochal cyst is extended up-

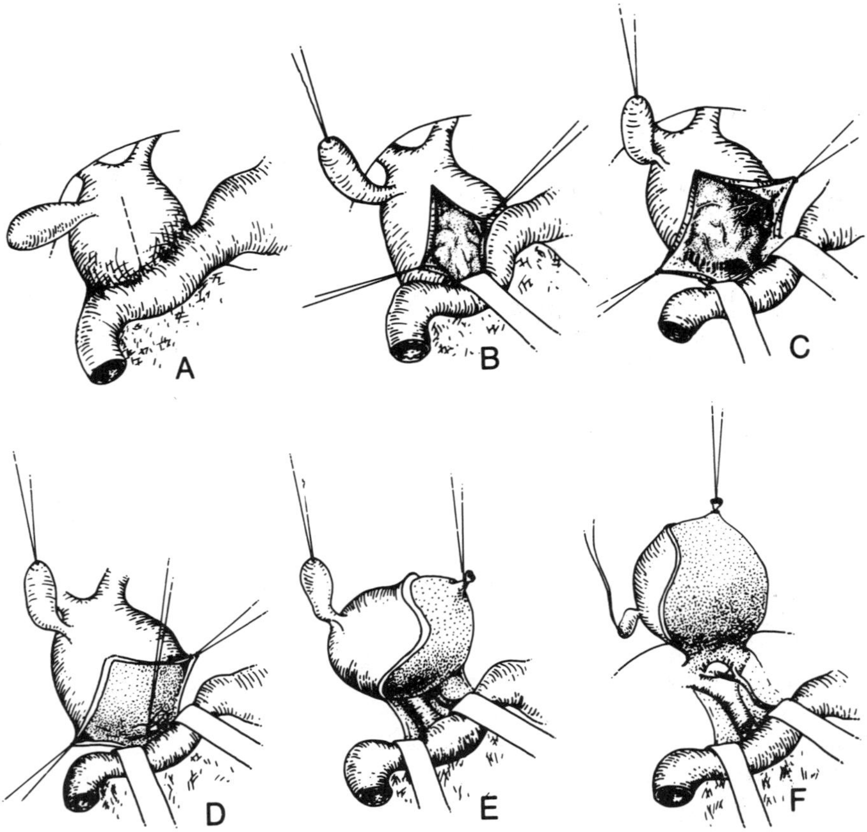

FIG 29–1.
A, serosal incision. **B,** dissection is extended distally with meticulous hemostasis. **C,** the common bile duct communicating with the choledochal cyst is identified and divided **D. E,** the distal end of the choledochal cyst is lifted anteriorly away from the portal vein, under direct vision. **F,** the dissection of the posterior aspect of the choledochal cyst is less difficult.

ward from its divided distal end (Fig 29–1,E and F). A vascular tape or Penrose drain is placed around the hepatoduodenal ligament to protect against inadvertent injury to the portal vein. Dissection of the posterior cyst wall is technically less difficult than that of the anterior wall because the tissue planes are less vascular. The portal vein should be kept under direct vision during this phase of dissection. When the dissection reaches the level of the common hepatic duct, the right hepatic artery is usually observed to cross over the anterior aspect of the cyst. Further dissection toward the hepatic hilus can be facilitated by relocating the entire choledochal cyst anterior to the right hepatic artery.

This is easily done after complete evacuation of the cyst contents. Dissection at the hepatic hilus is complete when both the right and left hepatic ducts have been identified and encircled with tapes. Attention can then be turned to the procedure for constructing the bile conduit.

Reconstruction of the Bile Duct

The proximal jejunum is divided 10 to 15 cm from the ligament of Treitz. Luminal continuity is re-established by an end-to-side anastomosis at 40 cm from the proximal end of the Roux-Y loop. The proximal end of the jejunal loop is brought to the hepatic hilus to meet the hepatic ducts. We prefer an antecolic arrangement of the loop, having experienced an obstruction in the retrocolic jejunal loop in some patients.

When feasible, the common hepatic duct is transected above the dilatation and anastomosed to the jejunal loop in an end-to-end fashion using double suture layers of 4–0 coated Dexon (polyglycolic suture). However, in most patients, dilatation involves both hepatic ducts. In a third of patients, dilatation extends into the intrahepatic bile ducts (Fig 29–2,A). In such patients, the hepatic ducts are transected at a level close to the hepatic hilus and are anastomosed to the jejunal loop in an end-to-side fashion using double-layer sutures of 4–0 coated Dexon. In this anastomosis, the outer layer sutures may have to be placed in the liver capsule. At the completion of bile-conduit reconstruction, a 7-mm, flat Jackson-Pratt drain is placed close to the hepatojejunostomy through a separate stab wound. The laparotomy wound is then closed in layers.

POSTOPERATIVE MANAGEMENT

Immediate Postoperative Management

Patients with a prolonged operation time or with excessive blood loss requiring substantial blood transfusion are admitted to the intensive care unit (ICU) overnight. Blood loss via the drain should be checked frequently, especially in those patients found to have coagulation disorders before surgery. Prophylactic antibiotics (cefazolin 100 mg/kg/day and gentamicin 6 mg/kg/day) are given intravenously until the abdominal drain is removed. Laboratory tests of liver function and serum amylase concentration should be performed on the first postoperative day. The serum bilirubin is usually elevated for the first few days after surgery, and takes about 1 week to return to the normal range. The serum amylase level remains elevated during the period immediately after surgery, gradually returning to normal in several weeks.

Anastomotic leakage is a serious complication after surgery for a choledochal cyst, occuring within a week. The daily discharge through the abdomi-

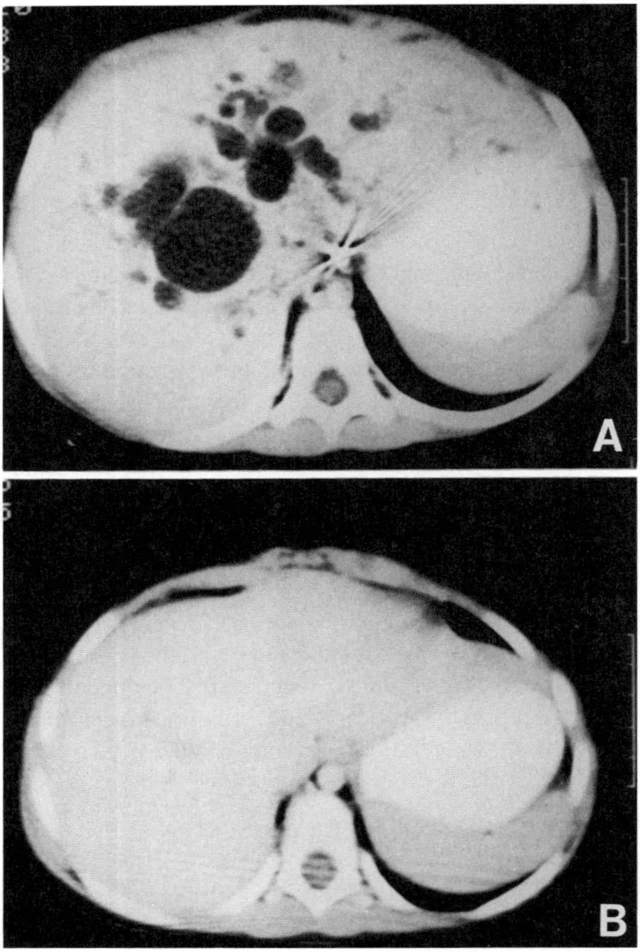

FIG 29–2.
A 4-year-old female patient. **A,** the preoperative CT scan demonstrates remarkable dilatation of the intrahepatic biliary system. **B,** 4 months after surgery, the dilatation has totally disappeared.

nal drain may reach several hundred milliliters and contains bile. Conservative management and continuation of drainage are usually successful in resolving this problem. Exploration is seldom indicated. We routinely leave the abdominal drain in place until oral feedings are tolerated.

Continuous elevation of the serum bilirubin concentration and jaundice suggest obstruction of the bile conduit, usually at the hepatojejunal anastomosis. Percutaneous transhepatic cholangiodrainage is useful for both the diagnosis of this condition and biliary decompression. When repeat cholangiograms via PTCD demonstrate persistent anastomotic obstruction for more than 2 weeks, a revision of the anastomosis should be considered.

Long-Range Follow-up

The patient should be followed every 3 months for the first year after surgery with laboratory tests of liver function and serum amylase concentration. With normal laboratory data, further follow-up should be done on a yearly basis for the next few years. Patients with the preoperatively detected dilatation of the intrahepatic bile ducts should be followed by repeated CT scanning. The dilatation usually disappears within 3 months after surgery (see Fig 29–2).

Cholangitis presenting with jaundice, fever, malaise, abdominal pain, and an elevated leukocyte count may infrequently develop as a late complication after resection of a choledochal cyst. This complication can be successfully managed with intravenous administration of antibiotics for a short period. Pancreatitis is another rare complication and presents with abdominal pain, fever, vomiting, and elevation of the serum amylase level and leukocyte count. The management of this complication is essentially identical to the routine therapy for acute pancreatitis.

REFERENCES

1. Kimura K: Unpublished data, 1990.
2. Babbitt DP: Congenital choledochal cysts: New etiologic concept based on anomalous relationship of the common bile duct and pancreatic bulb. *Ann Radiol* 1969; 7:231–240.
3. Kimura K, Tsugawa C, Ogawa K, et al: Choledochal cyst. Etiological consideration and surgical management of 22 cases. *Arch Surg* 1978; 113:159–163.
4. Todani T, Watanabe Y, Narusue M, et al: Congenital bile duct cysts: Classification, operative procedures, and review of 37 cases including cancer arising from choledochal cyst. *Am J Surg* 1977; 134:263–269.
5. Todani T, Watanabe Y, Fujii T, et al: Anomalous arrangement of the pancreaticobiliary ductal system in patients with a choledochal cyst. *Am J Surg* 1984; 147:672–676.
6. Komi N, Takehara H, Kunitomo K: Choledochal cyst: Anomalous arrangement of the pancreaticobiliary ductal system and biliary malignancy. *J Gastroenterol Hepatol* 1989; 4:63–74.
7. Okada A, Oguchi Y, Kamata S, et al: Common channel syndrome—Diagnosis with endoscopic retrograde cholangiopancreatography and surgical management. *Surgery* 1983; 93:634–642.
8. Okada A, Nakamura T, Okumura K, et al: Surgical treatment of congenital dilata-

tion of bile duct (choledochal cyst) with technical considerations. *Surgery* 1987; 101:238–243.
9. Yamaguchi M: Congenital choledochal cyst. Analysis of 1,433 patients in the Japanese literature. *Am J Surg* 1980; 140:653–657.
10. Miller AJW, Rode H, Buchler J, et al: Whole-gut lavage in children using an iso-osmolar solution containing polyethelene glycol (Golytely). *J Pediatr Surg* 1988; 23:822–824.

30

Cholelithiasis in Children

David E. M. Drucker, M.D.
Arvin I. Philippart, M.D.

A 7-year-old black girl was seen in the hospital emergency room for abdominal pain in the right upper quadrant and fever (38.9° C). She had experienced previous episodes of abdominal pain and had a past history of anemia requiring blood transfusion. She had also recently recovered from a bout of pneumococcal pneumonia. Physical examination showed scleral icterus and right-upper-quadrant tenderness and guarding to palpation at and below the costal margin. Laboratory data demonstrated a hemoglobin of 7.5 g and a serum bilirubin of 8.0 mg/dL with an indirect fraction of 4.5 mg/dL. The white blood cell count was 29,000/mm^3 with a shift to the left on differential smear. Ultrasound of the abdomen showed filling defects within the gallbladder and common bile duct.

The surgical approach to cholelithiasis in children differs little from that in adults: symptomatic gallstones require surgery. While much of pediatric biliary tract disease is idiopathic, children with hemolytic anemias have a high incidence of pigment gallstones. Treatment of the underlying disease in these patients may pose a more significant problem than the surgical management of their gallstones. The presumptive diagnosis in this child is sickle cell anemia (SCA), as evidenced by her manifestation of several of its complications: hemolytic anemia requiring transfusion, previous episodes of abdominal pain, functional asplenia with recent pneumococcal pneumonia, indirect hyperbilirubinemia, gallstones, and now common duct stones with cholangitis. She requires initial confirmatory diagnostic studies and preoperative resuscitation, followed by a cholecystectomy and common bile duct exploration. The timing of the surgery will depend on her response to resuscitation.

In sickle cell anemia, the prevalence of gallstones increases with age, but most remain asymptomatic.[1] The incidence of acute cholecystitis and cholangitis requiring emergency surgery is low at all ages.[2, 3] In the absence of appropriate preparation, the morbidity and mortality from emergency surgery may be high.[4] This has led some centers to perform elective cholecystectomy in patients with SCA and documented cholelithiasis.[4, 5] The rationale is that the complication rate from elective surgery in patients with SCA is much lower than that for emergency surgery. We do not adhere to this policy, because the incidence of surgical emergencies related to the biliary tract in patients with SCA is low. Also, as will be discussed, sickle cell patients can be well and rapidly prepared for urgent surgery if necessary.

DIAGNOSIS

It is unusual for SCA in a child to have remained undiagnosed for 7 years. The severity of the biliary tract disease is also unusual, since most patients do not present with common duct stones and cholangitis. This child will require surgical clearance of her common duct within the next several days. The preoperative preparation will be markedly altered if the diagnosis of sickle cell disease is confirmed. A Wright-stained slide of the patient's peripheral blood should be examined promptly to detect the pathognomonic, sickle-shaped erythrocytes. The hemoglobin solubility test may also be used; it is inexpensive and its results are rapidly available, although not completely accurate. Hemoglobin electrophoresis is definitive. It differentiates homozygous (SS) disease from heterozygous (SC) disease and the sickle thalassemias. In many institutions, however, hemoglobin electrophoresis is not available on short notice. Fortunately this has no practical importance; homozygous sickle cell patients and those with symptomatic sickle variants are prepared for surgery in the same way. Before transfusion therapy is begun (and the patient's blood is diluted with donor cells), a sample should be drawn for hemoglobin electrophoresis so that an exact diagnosis can eventually be made.

Since the introduction of ultrasound, it has been known that the incidence of gallstones in sickle cell patients greatly exceeds the frequency of symptomatic biliary tract disease.[1] In a patient with SCA and right-upper-quadrant pain, tenderness, fever, leukocytosis, and jaundice, the customary differential diagnosis is essentially limited to two possibilities: gallstone disease and abdominal crisis. Acute biliary tract disease is ruled out by a normal ultrasound examination or by a normal hepatoiminodiacetic acid (HIDA) in the presence of ultrasonographically demonstrated gallstones. However, if these studies are abnormal, it does not necessarily mean that the patient has acute cholecystitis.

Asymptomatic patients with SCA often have abnormal ultrasonographic and HIDA studies suggestive of chronic cholecystitis. These include the ultrasonographic finding of a small, shrunken, scarred gallbladder and a HIDA scan demonstrating delayed uptake or release of contrast medium.[6] Therefore, in the symptomatic SCA patient with gallstones demonstrated by ultrasound examination, the diagnosis of acute cholecystitis must usually be made using the clinical evidence present in the history, physical examination, and the response of the patient to treatment.[2]

In SCA, abdominal crises tend to have a prodrome and symptom complex that is characteristic for each patient. Patients presenting with symptoms that do not fit their usual pattern are suspect for surgical disease or some other infection (often pneumonia). Most patients with an abdominal pain crisis are afebrile and have a level of leukocytosis and hyperbilirubinemia that is typical for them. An elevation of temperature, white cell count, or bilirubin beyond the norm for a given patient indicates infection, either surgical or nonsurgical.[2, 7] Finally, given the current management of sickle cell crisis, patients whose pain is not of biliary tract origin will have significant resolution within 12 to 24 hours.[8] In acute cholecystitis, the symptoms will localize to the right upper quadrant by that time.

Occasionally, the diagnosis of acute cholecystitis may be established by the ultrasonographic findings of gallbladder wall edema and pericholecystic fluid, but this is unusual. This girl's case is even more unusual. She presents with both clinical and ultrasound evidence of acute cholangitis with fever, sepsis, jaundice, right-upper quadrant tenderness, and ultrasonographically demonstrated common bile duct stones. This makes an HIDA scan or any further imaging study unnecessary.

In summary, the diagnosis of acute cholecystitis in this patient group is based on the clinical setting and the ultrasonographic findings. We have not found the HIDA scan useful, since abnormal scans are as prevalent in asymptomatic sickle cell patients as in symptomatic ones. This fact renders the HIDA scan unnecessary, and its use, even to confirm the diagnosis, is illogical.

PREOPERATIVE PREPARATION

Proper preoperative preparation can significantly reduce the incidence of complications in sickle cell patients undergoing surgery.[5] Sickling is precipitated by hypoxia, hypovolemia, acidosis, hypothermia, and a high concentration of hemoglobin S. Sickled erythrocytes occlude the microvasculature, resulting in a reduced tissue perfusion that may progress to infarction. Sickle cell patients are also immunocompromised. They are functionally asplenic or hyposplenic and respond to encapsulated bacteria with poor levels of antibody production, opsonization, and phagocytosis. Avoidance of the factors that may cause sickling, and coverage with broad-spectrum antibiotics for any sign of infection, are central to the therapy of acute pain crisis or illness in sickle cell patients.[8]

Oxygen is administered through a warm, humidified mask only if the patient is hypoxic. Intravenous fluids are required. Existing fluid deficits should be corrected promptly. The fluid maintenance requirements are 150% of usual because of the hyposthenuria that is invariably present by this age due to chronic renal medullary infarction. Nasogastric losses are replaced as for any patient, and the electrolyte composition of the administered fluid is adjusted on the basis of frequent determinations of the patient's serum electrolytes and renal function indices. Alkalinization is used only if the patient is acidotic. The patient should be kept warm. Antibiotics are started after blood cultures are obtained. The coverage must be broad enough to include pneumococcus and *Haemophilus influenzae*. In most centers, children with known sickle cell disease are on prophylactic penicillin to reduce the frequency of sepsis from these organisms. When there is a question of cholecystitis, gram-negative coverage must be provided.

Transfusion is used to reduce the concentration of hemoglobin S (Hb S). In vitro studies have demonstrated optimal rheologic characteristics at an Hb S concentration of 30%,[9] but clinical studies demonstrate no additional benefit at 30% vs. 40% to 50% Hgb S.[10] Transfusion also increases the total hemoglobin concentration, from a baseline of 6 to 8 g/dL to 11 to 12 g/dL. This increases the oxygen-carrying capacity of the blood and suppresses further bone-marrow production of sickle erythrocytes.

There are several transfusion techniques. Simple transfusion with no exchange is useful in an emergency, but produces the least decrease in Hgb S concentration per volume of blood transfused. We use a partial exchange technique in which 5 cc of blood per kilogram are withdrawn and replaced by 10 cc per kilogram of washed, packed cells.[10] After one of these cycles the Hb S concentration drops to 60%. After another cycle the Hb S is usually around 45%. A third cycle yields an Hb S of about 30%, with a hemoglobin in the 12 to 13 g/dL range. If the exchange transfusions are performed over a 2- to 3-week period before elective surgery, the benefit of bone-marrow suppression is obtained; the sickle erythrocytes present in the peripheral blood have a much shorter half-life than the transfused cells, and their higher rate of attrition further lowers the Hb S concentration. This may be monitored using the reticulocyte count, which drops when the marrow is suppressed. Hemoglobin electrophoresis can be used preoperatively to confirm the results of therapy.

Cell-separator devices permit rapid exchange transfusion but are rarely used in our institution, except for the treatment of sickle cell patients with cerebral vascular occlusion.[11] Their disadvantages are that large-bore intravenous access is required, they are expensive and not readily available, and they require exposing the patient to multiple donor units of packed red cells in excess of that used for the partial exchange technique (3,000 cc is typical for one exchange). This excess exposure increases the risk to the patient of both transfusion-associated infection and of alloantigen sensitization, which may complicate future red cell crossmatching. Donor erythrocytes may also be subjected to density gradient centrifugation to separate out "neocytes" (young red blood cells) for preferential transfusion.[11] We have not used this technique.

SURGICAL MANAGEMENT

In the more usual case of cholecystitis in a child with SCA, the diagnosis may not be clear until sometime after admission. By then, most patients will have been stabilized on medical therapy and can be discharged following resolution of the acute inflammation. Interval cholecystectomy can be scheduled, preceded by partial exchange transfusions. However, this girl's common bile duct stones require surgical removal during this admission. It is true that pigmented stones may be more likely to pass spontaneously than cholesterol stones, but the risk of recurrent cholangitis in this patient is too significant for delay. If she remains stable or improves during resuscitation, surgery could wait for 2 or 3 days. Transfusion therapy to reduce her Hb S concentration may be used expeditiously either by the preferred exchange method or by simply giving three transfusions of 10 cc/kg of packed cells over 2 to 3 days. Hemoglobin electrophoresis will most likely not be available prior to surgery, but if her hemoglobin is increased to 11 or 12 g/dL, a reasonably low concentration of Hb S is assured.

The surgical plan is straightforward and includes cholecystectomy, cholangiography, common bile duct exploration, T-tube insertion, and completion cholangiography. In the sickle cell patient who is undergoing chronic transfusion therapy, a liver biopsy to assess iron levels can help to determine the need for iron chelation therapy later. Procedures that have been used in adults, such as percutaneous cholangiography and drainage, or endoscopic retrograde cholangiography and sphincterotomy, are temporizing measures only. Furthermore, these require general anesthesia in children, and take longer to perform than definitive surgery. The issue of incidental appendectomy or "inversion appendicoplasty"[12] is objectively unresolved and left to the philosophical determination of the surgeon. However, it is our impression, as well as that of others, that the incidence of acute appendicitis in sickle cell patients is much lower than in the general age-matched population.[2, 3]

POSTOPERATIVE CARE

The postoperative course of the patient with SCA and cholecystitis requires careful attention to hydration, oxygenation, temperature, and acid-base status. Pulmonary complications following right-upper-quadrant operations occur less frequently in children than in adults, but such complications can be significant in sickle cell patients. Any suggestion of right-lower-lobe atelectasis or pneumonia requires vigorous treatment to prevent pulmonary infarction or diffuse sickling.

Prior to discharge, consideration should be given to this child's asplenic state. By her age, all such children should have received pneumococcal and hemophilus vaccines. Administration of these should be scheduled, recognizing that the antibody response may be minimal.[13, 14] Reimmunization may produce a beneficial anamnestic response.[14] Prophylactic penicillin is generally used in age-appropriate doses throughout childhood or beyond. Hematologic consultation for these issues and for chronic care is advisable.

SUMMARY

The frequency of cholelithiasis in patients with SCA increases with age. The indications for cholecystectomy are established by clinical symptoms and radiographic assessment. Appropriate preoperative transfusion therapy reduces complications. Awareness of diminished host defenses is important in postoperative management.

REFERENCES

1. Sarnaik S, Slovis TL, Corbett DP, et al: Incidence of cholelithiasis in sickle cell anemia using the ultrasonic gray-scale technique. *J Pediatr* 1980; 96:1005–1008.
2. Kudsk KA, Tranbaugh RF, Sheldon GF: Acute surgical illness in patients with sickle cell anemia. *Am J Surg* 1981; 142:113–117.
3. McPhillips FL, Bickers JN: Operations on patients with sickle cell anemia at Charity Hospital in New Orleans. *Surg Gynecol Obstetr* 1972; 135:870–872.
4. Stephens CG, Scott RB: Cholelithiasis in sickle cell anemia: surgical or medical management. *Arch Intern Med* 1980; 140:648–651.
5. Bond LR, Hatty SR, Horn MEC, et al: Gall stones in sickle cell disease in the United Kingdom. *Br Med J [Clin Res]* 1987; 295:234–236.
6. Serafini AN, Spoliansky G, Sfakianakis GN, et al: Diagnostic studies in patients with sickle cell anemia and acute abdominal pain. *Arch Intern Med* 1987; 147:1061–1062.
7. Bonadio WA: Clinical features of abdominal painful crisis in sickle cell anemia. *J Pediatr Surg* 1990; 25:301–302.
8. Vichinsky E, Lubin BH: Suggested guidelines for the treatment of children with sickle cell anemia. *Hematol/Oncol Clin North Am* 1987; 1:483–501.
9. Lessin LS, Kurantsin-Mills J, Klug PP, et al: Determination of rheologically optimal mixtures of AA and SS erythrocytes for transfusion. *Prog Clin Biol Res* 1978; 20:123–137.

10. Fullerton MW, Philippart AI, Sarnaik S, et al: Preoperative exchange transfusion in sickle cell anemia. *J Pediatr Surg* 1981; 16:297–300.
11. Greenwalt TJ, Zelenski KR: Transfusion support for the hemoglobinopathies. *Clin Hematol* 1984; 13:151–165.
12. Bishop HC, Filston HC: An inversion-ligation technique for incidental appendectomy. *J Pediatr Surg* 1973; 8:889–892.
13. Ahonkhai VI, Landesman SH, Fikrig SM, et al: Failure of pneumococcal vaccine in children with sickle cell disease. *N Engl J Med* 1979; 301:26–27.
14. Broome CV, Facklam RR, Fraser DW: Pneumococcal disease after pneumococcal vaccination. *N Engl J Med* 1980; 303:549–552.

31

Pancreatic Pseudocysts

H. Biemann Othersen, Jr., M.D.

An 8-year-old boy was injured in a fall from his bicycle. In falling, the child struck his abdomen against the bicycle's handlebar. He had multiple abrasions and a painful right wrist. Three hours after the incident he began to experience mild abdominal discomfort and severe wrist pain. He was taken to the emergency room where an x-ray of his wrist showed a fracture that was reduced under sedation and put in a cast. He was given an analgesic and sent home. That night he vomited and had a fever of 38.5° C. The following morning he was able to tolerate clear liquids but maintained a low-grade temperature elevation. He continued to have a poor appetite and nausea. Two days later he began to vomit bilious material. The boy had upper abdominal pain and fullness and was returned to the emergency room for further evaluation.

A history of a bicycle handlebar injury (Fig 31–1) should immediately arouse suspicion of damage to the pancreas, duodenum, or stomach. Trauma from a point source, such as a bicycle handlebar, concentrates the force of the injury into one small area, such as the cross-sectional area of the handlebar itself. Often the rubber grip on a bicycle handlebar prevents laceration or abrasion of the skin and there is no external evidence of injury. However, the child will indicate the exact location of the impingement. Figure 31–2 shows the mechanism of injury. The handlebar catches the pancreas, duodenum, or both, at the level at which they cross the spine and, since they are retroperitoneal and fixed, a severe injury such as disruption and transection may occur. Moreover, the child usually falls on an outstretched arm and there may be fracture of the forearm or wrist. Radiographs usually show the bony fracture but no abdominal abnormalities. Even disruption of the duodenum may not produce free intraperitoneal air, since the bowel is retroperitoneal and air in that location is difficult to detect. A high index of suspicion of this type of injury is necessary in order to make an early diagnosis of pancreatic or duodenal injury.

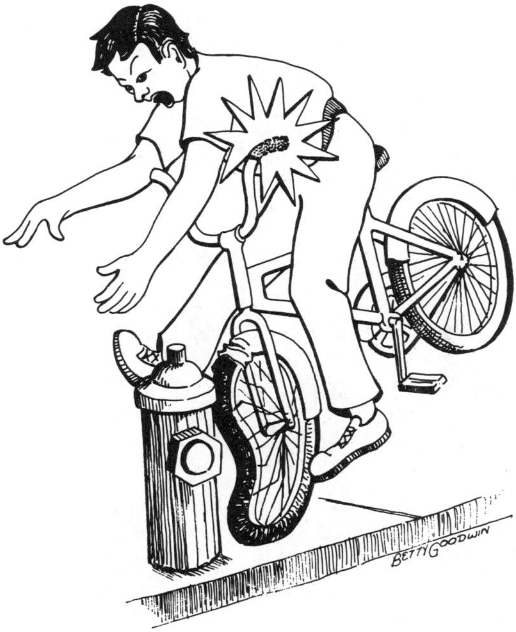

FIG 31–1.
Bicycle handlebar injury.

Physical examination should include careful evaluation of the epigastrium. The skin may look normal, and in the early stages after the injury peritoneal signs may be absent, with no palpable mass. The only finding may be tenderness at the point of injury.

Laboratory aids to the detection of pancreatic injury should include a serum amylase assay and an upper gastrointestinal (GI) series. The contrast study is needed to assess the integrity of the stomach and duodenum. An intramural hematoma of the duodenum or a retroperitoneal leak may be discovered. The pancreas is usually not initially enlarged, and no widening of the C-loop of the duodenum is evident. A computed tomographic (CT) scan or ultrasonography may show only some retroperitoneal edema without fluid collection. Elevation of the serum amylase concentration does not make the exclusive diagnosis of traumatic pancreatitis, since disruption of the intestinal tract may produce the same elevation. If the serum amylase concentration is high and the contrast study of the duodenum shows no leak, the child should be hospitalized for observation and treatment of pancreatic injury. Sometimes, the amylase is elevated initially and then gradually falls, only to rise again as a pseudocyst forms.

If the diagnosis of traumatic pancreatitis is not made on initial evaluation,

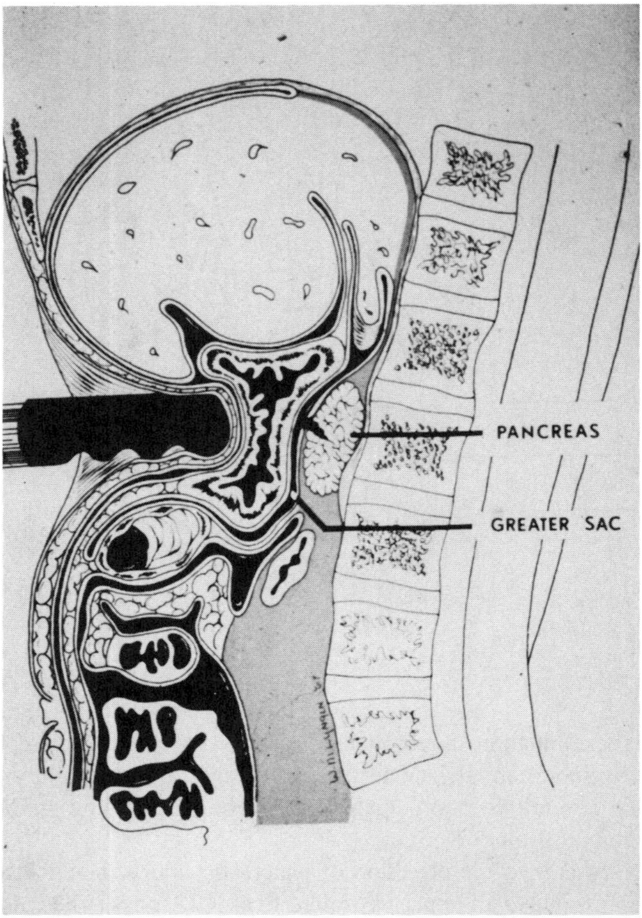

FIG 31–2.
The handlebar or other point source of injury catches the pancreas against the spine and causes parenchymal and ductal injury.

and the child is not admitted until 2 days later, as in this case history, a pancreatic pseudocyst must be sought. If a serum amylase assay has already been done, it should be repeated, since rising levels occur as a pseudocyst develops. A contrast study of the stomach and duodenum, if not performed initially, should be done in order to rule out gastric or duodenal injury. In the case of vomiting, fever, and abdominal pain, ultrasonography or CT scan or both should be done.

The early course of pancreatic injury is difficult to assess. There may be a small retroperitoneal collection of fluid in the lesser sac. All CT examinations of the abdomen should preferably be done with intestinal contrast enhancement, so that air and fluid in the intestines can be differentiated from collections outside the GI tract. In this particular case, the amylase would probably be greatly elevated and ultrasonography and CT scanning would show a pseudocyst of 4 cm or less in diameter. With these findings, the diagnosis of traumatic pseudocyst of the pancreas is made. Figure 31–3 shows the development of a pseudocyst.

Treatment consists of intravenous alimentation and pancreatic rest. Measures for accomplishing this include total parenteral alimentation through a central venous catheter, accompanied by nasogastric suction in order to decrease pancreatic stimulation. The use of systemic antibiotics at this point and without disruption of the GI tract is controversial. However, broad-spectrum coverage, to include enteric organisms, is usually given for 3 to 5 days. Long-term prophylaxis with antibiotics is to be avoided because of the emergence of resistant

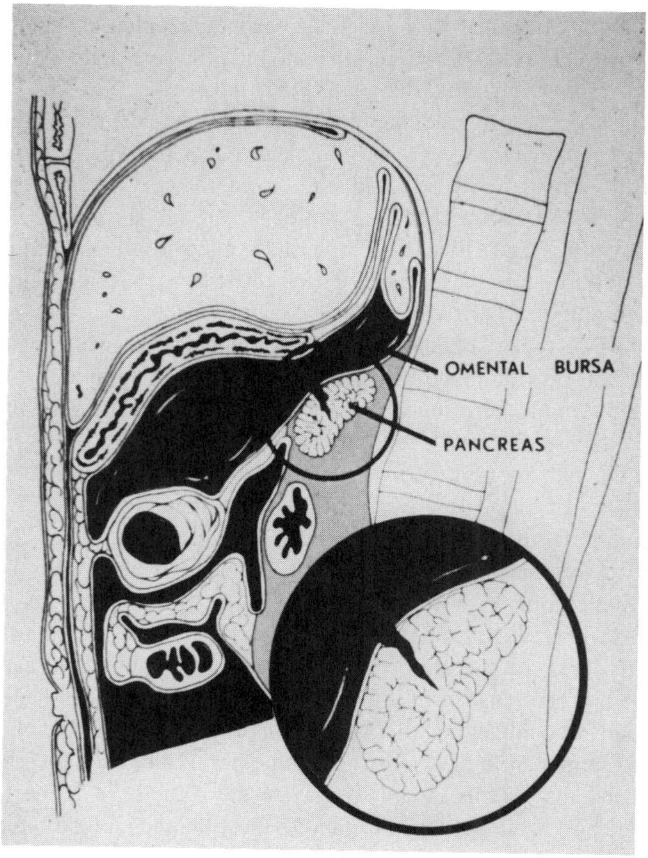

FIG 31–3.
The leaking pancreatic fluid fills the lesser sac.

organisms. Total parenteral nutrition is continued in order to avoid pancreatic stimulation until symptoms and objective findings improve. The parameters for improvement include a decrease in the serum amylase level and reduction of fever and abdominal discomfort. The scanning studies, if abnormal initially, can be repeated and should show a reduction in size of the pseudocyst. Enteral feedings, devoid of fat, are gradually resumed with slow progression to a regular diet. The child may be discharged on parenteral nutrition with orders for the gradual resumption of enteral feedings. Pancreatic injuries are notoriously slow to heal. Exacerbation of injury may occur when pancreatic stimulation produces enzymes that can reactivate a pseudocyst.

If the initial response to pancreatic rest is not gradual improvement, the injury may be severe and a large pseudocyst may develop. With a pseudocyst over 4 cm in diameter, spontaneous resolution is very slow, and complications such as erosion or bleeding may occur. Consideration must then be given to internal or external drainage. It has long been our contention that even with large post-traumatic pseudocysts of the pancreas, internal drainage is rarely indicated in children.[2, 3] Unlike the adult with longstanding pancreatic or biliary problems, the ductal system of the child is usually patent, and gradual healing is to be expected. Only in cases of complete transection of the pancreas with stenosis of the pancreatic duct should some form of direct surgical operation on the pancreas be necessary. External drainage through a catheter, as we described many years ago (Fig 31–4),[2] is sufficient and allows drainage of the pseudocyst. Follow-up studies have shown this therapeutic modality to be effective.[3] Diminution of the cavity can be monitored by injections of contrast medium into the catheter. Our previous recommendations were for simple operative insertion of a drainage catheter. At present, radiographic insertion of a catheter, monitored by ultrasonography or CT scanning, allows the transcutaneous drainage of pseudocysts.[1] This procedure avoids the need for general anesthesia, and the catheter permits external evacuation of the pseudocyst contents. A technical modification involves inserting a catheter through the stomach, with one end in the cyst and the other end in the gastric lumen. Such variations are usually unnecessary. Furthermore, only rarely will internal drainage, such as through a Roux-en-Y cystojejunostomy or cystogastrostomy, be necessary. Both of these procedures are major operations and have attendant morbidity and mortality, and are therefore not considered as early as external drainage. After a tube has been placed into the cyst and external drainage accomplished, it is easy to inject contrast material at intervals and assess the size of the cavity. Repeated CT scans are unnecessary. During external drainage the child can be discharged and the parents taught to irrigate the catheter at home in order to assure its patency. Careful sterile technique must be encouraged, since secondary infection may occur and require cultures and specific antibiotic therapy.

If the pseudocyst persists for longer than 6 months and further reduction in its size does not occur, open drainage must be considered. In this situation,

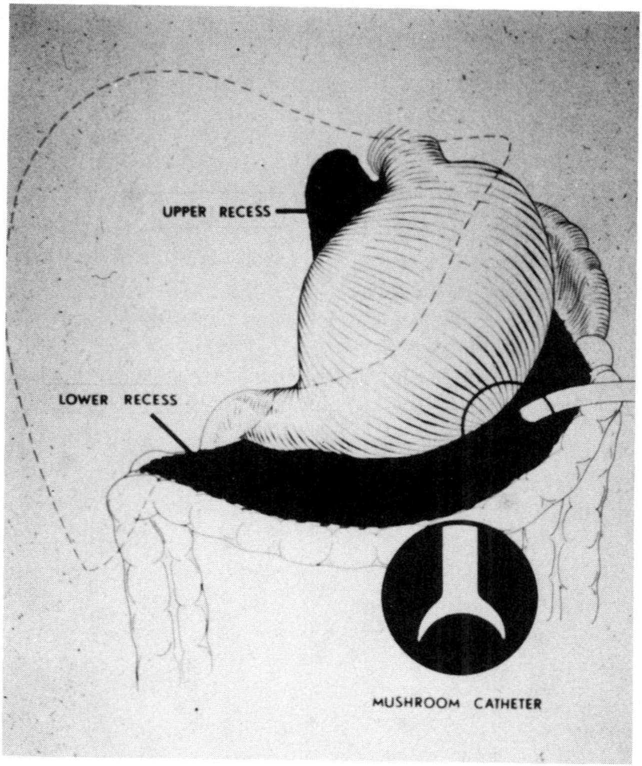

FIG 31–4.
The large pseudocyst was previously drained with a catheter inserted during operation. Now, percutaneous drainage catheters can be inserted with CT guidance.

evaluation of the ductal systems can be accomplished by endoscopic retrograde catheterization of the ampulla of Vater and the injection of contrast medium into the biliary and pancreatic ducts. Surgical procedures for complete ductal disruption with subsequent scarring and obstruction may include internal drainage of the cyst or resection of the distal portion (tail) of the pancreas.

In summary, a conservative and yet aggressive approach to the diagnosis and treatment of a pancreatic pseudocyst means:

1. A high index of suspicion of pancreatic injury in bicycle handlebar accidents, and early diagnosis of the pseudocyst.
2. Monitoring of a pseudocyst by ultrasonography or CT scanning.
3. Treatment by parenteral nutrition and pancreatic rest.
4. If necessary, transcutaneous drainage of the pseudocyst, with guidance by CT or ultrasound.

5. An expectation of slow resolution of the pseudocyst even with good external drainage.
6. Consideration of internal drainage or resection only if the pseudocyst doesn't respond or persists for longer than 6 months.

REFERENCES

1. Jaffe RB, Arata JA Jr, Matlak ME: Percutaneous drainage of traumatic pancreatic pseudocysts in children. *AJR* 1989; 152:591–595.
2. Othersen HB Jr, Moore FT, Boles T: Traumatic pancreatitis and pseudocyst in childhood. *J Trauma* 1968; 8:535–546.
3. Warner RL, Jr, Othersen HB, Jr, Smith CD: Traumatic pancreatitis and pseudocyst in children: Current management. *J Trauma* 1989; 29:597–601.

PART FIVE

Pediatric Trauma

PART FIVE

Pediatric Trauma

32

Resuscitation of the Injured Child

Burton H. Harris, M.D.
Steven Stylianos, M.D.

A 7-year-old boy was riding his bicycle when he veered into the road and was struck by a car. The child was knocked off of the bicycle and landed 6 feet from the automobile on the berm of the road. He was unconscious when the paramedic-supported ambulance arrived. His blood pressure was 70 mm Hg, pulse 130/min, and respiratory rate 26/min and labored. The boy's left leg was slightly foreshortened and externally rotated. There was a hematoma behind the right ear and otorrhea was present.

The quality of treatment in the first 20 minutes after injury is the major determinant of outcome for a multiply-injured child. The physician's responsibilities in this critical period are to preserve life, protect the patient from further injury, begin treatment of the physiologic disorganization that is the invariable consequence of trauma, find all of the child's injuries, and establish treatment priorities.

Errors begin with the unpracticed instinct to rush to the patient's side and attempt several things at once. While each individual procedure for managing trauma is a standard technique, there is a definite sequence in which these tasks are best accomplished.[1] An easy way to keep things in order is to work from a checklist prepared in advance to organize the individual steps for use in the first moments of care. The recommended treatment sequence is given in Table 32-1; this outline of treatment preserves calm and avoids potential omission of important steps.

A multiple-trauma patient entering a medical facility should be treated by

TABLE 31–1.

The Kiwanis Pediatric Trauma Institute Receiving Unit Checklist*

- ❑ Immobilize neck
- ❑ Remove clothing
- ❑ Perform 60-second examination
- ❑ Apply electrocardiographic (ECG) leads
- ❑ Draw blood for complete blood count (CBC), type and crossmatch, analysis, and amylase assay
- ❑ Give nasal oxygen
- ❑ IV
- ❑ Do cutdown
- ❑ Take lateral x-ray of cervical spine
- ❑ Insert Foley catheter and temperature probe
- ❑ Perform endotracheal intubation if necessary
- ❑ Insert nasogastric tube
- ❑ Perform peritoneal lavage
- ❑ Insert arterial line
- ❑ Dress open wounds
- ❑ Complete physical examination
- ❑ Get history
- ❑ Take chest x-ray
- ❑ Check laboratory results
- ❑ Calculate Glasgow coma score and trauma score
- ❑ List positive findings

*Each of these procedures should be considered (but not necessarily performed) for each patient. The trauma team leader makes a do/no-do decision for each step.

an organized team of surgeons, physicians, and nurses. The composition of the team will vary, but the most senior surgeon should be the team leader.

The case presented above is a common pediatric trauma scenario, which always creates several problems in the emergency department to which the injured child is taken. Often there will be little advance notice of the child's arrival and little time to prepare unless a prearranged plan is activated. Usually, those bringing the child to the hospital were not witnesses to the accident. Only a capsule history is available, too sketchy to calculate the application of forces. The parents were not present and the past medical history is unknown.

The first reaction on the part of unprepared medical personnel often seems to be either to talk to the child (to assess consciousness) or to listen to the heart or chest with a stethoscope, but these impulses should be resisted. The first step is prophylaxis against completion of a cervical fracture. If a child arrives without a neck restraint, it is prudent to assume a cervical spine injury until this can be excluded. The "Philadelphia collar," a firm, semiadjustable device, should be applied.

Next, a rapid examination for the ABCs—airway, breathing, and circulation—is conducted. Conceptually, the airway is divided into the upper and lower airway, with the larynx as the dividing line. The frequency of head injury and the large size of a child's tongue relative to the oropharynx make upper airway obstruction far more common. The first maneuver to be attempted in a child with air hunger is the "chin lift," performed by placing the examiner's thumb behind the mandible and forefinger inside the mouth, grasping the mandible, and pulling it forward. In the presence of upper-airway obstruction this maneuver will move the tongue out of the oropharynx and improve breathing almost instantly. If it fails, a quick look should be made inside the child's mouth for foreign objects, and if none are found, lower-airway access should be elected.

Obstruction at or below the larynx requires insertion of an artificial airway. While this can be accomplished by nasotracheal or orotracheal intubation, both are difficult in injured children and may best be left to those with skill and experience. The same is true of tracheotomy, a formidable surgical procedure in a child with an uncontrolled airway in a situation in which instruments, light, and help are not immediately available.

In such instances needle cricothyrotomy can be the safest emergency procedure. The cricothyroid membrane, 1 to 2 cm caudal to the "Adam's apple," is identified. A 12- or 14-gauge angiocatheter is inserted through the cricothyroid membrane, passage through which is noted by a distinct single "pop" as the device enters the lumen of the trachea. The needle is removed, the plastic cannula left in place, the adapter from a size-3 endotracheal tube placed in the Luer lock of the catheter, and an Ambu bag (or the physician's lips) are applied to the adapter and ventilation begun. Needle cricothyrotomy is only a temporary solution. Depending on the age and size of the child, alveolar hypoventilation will eventually occur, but in children of 5 to 7 years of age, satisfactory blood gas values can be maintained for about 10 minutes.[2] This time should be used to summon expert help and assemble the equipment needed to replace the needle cricothyrotomy with another, more durable form of airway access.

If a patient still has breathing difficulty after the airway is established, the etiology is either serious central nervous system damage or direct injury to the lung or pleural space. The former is treated with a respirator. If hypoxemia continues, pneumothorax or tension pneumothorax are the next most likely diagnoses. Even before an x-ray is obtained, a syringe can be connected to a 12-

gauge angiocatheter and the needle inserted into the pleural space in the third or fourth anterior interspaces of both hemithoraces. If a tension pneumothorax is present, the piston of the syringe will be expelled as the tension is relieved.

Severe multisystem trauma is always characterized by hypovolemia. External hemorrhage should be controlled by direct pressure, but most hypovolemia comes from internal bleeding. All multiple-injury patients require large-bore intravenous access. While peripheral venipuncture can suffice, if the first attempt is unsuccessful, a venous cutdown in the saphenous vein, anterior to the medial malleolus, is recommended instead of the inevitable "one more try." A child with signs of hypovolemia should be assumed to have lost in excess of 20% of blood volume. The first step in replacement of this is calculation of the patient's normal blood volume, which is equal to 80 multiplied by the assumed body weight in kilograms (40 × body weight in pounds). Crystalloid solution, preferably lactated Ringer's solution, is then given by hand in increments of 25% of the calculated blood volume, using a syringe with a three-way stopcock. This method allows the most rapid and positive control of infused volume.

The neck having previously been stabilized and immediate threats to life either excluded or treated, the next priority is to ascertain the status of the cervical spine, particularly in a patient with signs or symptoms of central nervous system injury. A single lateral cervical spine film should be taken at this point, with the shoulder girdle pulled caudad while the film is being taken. It is necessary to visualize all seven cervical vertebrae for a satisfactory study. When cervical spine injury is excluded, the neck restraint can be removed, but it is best to leave it in place until the film is reviewed. In an unconscious patient, another presumption is blunt trauma to the brain, with an elevated intracranial pressure (ICP). The best immediate treatment for a rising ICP, presumed or actual, is hyperventilation sufficient to lower the $Paco_2$ to 20 to 25 mm Hg. Hyperventilation with relative hypocapnia is a benign treatment, and unconscious patients should be hyperventilated as a prophylactic measure.

The next decision is how best to evaluate potential injury to the abdominal viscera. While physical examination can suffice in the alert and cooperative child, the interpretation of abdominal findings is unreliable in head-injured children, even those who have regained consciousness. A more positive method of diagnosis is required. In the hemodynamically unstable patient, quantitative peritoneal lavage (600 mL/m^2 body surface area) is a reliable technique when the effluent contains more than 100,000 red blood cells/mm^3. Patients who are hemodynamically stable should have a double-contrast (intraluminal and intravenous) computed tomographic scan (CT), the single best and most anatomic diagnostic test for abdominal injury. A cranial CT scan can be done at the same time, prior to contrast injection. Before taking a child for these examinations, all other receiving-unit maneuvers should be completed, since most patients will go either to the operating room or to the intensive care unit after their CT examination is complete.

Nasogastric suction is an essential although often neglected resuscitative step. Virtually every pediatric trauma patient has gastric dilatation, which holds the potential for additional injury. A large nasogastric tube should be inserted and the stomach contents removed with suction. In a patient such as the one under consideration, the nasogastric tube should be left in.

The purpose of splinting fractures is to stop motion at the fracture site and reduce additional soft-tissue injury and blood loss. The splinting of fractures is an important part of resuscitation. Physical signs of fractures should be sought; shortening and external rotation of the leg almost always indicates a fracture of the shaft of the femur, and a Thomas or Hare splint should be applied before the patient leaves the receiving unit. If extensive soft-tissue injury is present, or the injury is an open fracture, antibiotic treatment and tetanus prophylaxis should be started. The presence of otorrhea and a hematoma of the mastoid area are evidence of a basilar skull fracture through the posterior fossa (Battle's signs), but these should not be treated with prophylactic antibiotics for fear of selecting a resistant organism.

Management of the multiply-injured child is among the most challenging problems in pediatrics and pediatric surgery. For most practitioners, the occasional trauma patient is best treated with a proven, rehearsed, systematic approach. Preparation is mandatory; institutional preparation requires the prepositioning of equipment appropriate to children of varying ages, and individual mental preparedness is a second vital component. Using established techniques, an hour's work can be accomplished in 20 minutes by the additive efforts of trained medical personnel working in a prepared unit. This "20-minute drill," beginning with the ABCs and continuing through the checklist, is the surest way to individualize treatment for each patient while accomplishing the essential steps of diagnosis and treatment.

REFERENCES

1. Harris BH, Latchaw LA, Murphy RE, et al: A protocol for pediatric trauma receiving units. *J Pediatr Surg* 1989; 24:419–422.
2. Bergman KS, Harris BH: Percutaneous transtracheal ventilation, in Harris BH (ed): *Progress In Pediatric Trauma,* ed 2. Boston, Nobb Hill, 1987, p 126.

33

Blunt Abdominal Trauma

L. R. Scherer III, M.D.
J. Alex Haller, Jr., M.D.

An 18-month-old boy is brought to the emergency room by his mother and her boyfriend because of vomiting of 2 days duration. The child is whimpering, listless, and pale. On physical examination a bruise is noted across the upper abdomen. The upper abdomen is tender to palpation and guarding is elicited. Multiple bruises are also noted on both lower extremities and the child's buttocks. The infant's systolic blood pressure is 80 mm Hg and its pulse rate is 148/minute. A chest x-ray is obtained and shows old rib fractures with callus formation. Skull x-rays show an eggshell appearance of old multiple skull fractures. Erect and supine abdominal x-rays show free fluid in the abdomen with an adynamic ileus pattern. The hemoglobin is 8.5 g, the hematocrit is 26%, and the serum amylase is 200 IU. Urinalysis shows no red cells. The urine specific gravity is 1.028 with 2+ ketones. A computed tomographic scan of the abdomen shows a large subcapsular hematoma of the liver. There is a fluid collection in the subhepatic space along the right colonic gutter and in the pelvis.

The presentation of this child represents an unfortunately increasing etiology of abdominal trauma, namely child abuse. The mechanisms of injury are low-velocity blunt forces rather than the high-velocity forces that create multisystem injury from motor vehicle accidents.

INITIAL ASSESSMENT AND MANAGEMENT OF THE PEDIATRIC PATIENT

The early priorities in evaluation and treatment of the pediatric patient with blunt abdominal trauma focus on an adequate airway, ventilation, and an intact cardiovascular system. A child who is unconscious or unable to protect its airway requires immediate endotracheal intubation for management of the airway. Venous access is required for stabilization of the cardiovascular system and the correction of intravascular volume deficits. In the presence of hypotension and tachycardia, an initial intravenous bolus of 20 cc/kg of lactated Ringer's solution should be given. If the patient remains hypotensive, this should be repeated as many as two additional times and should be followed by 10 cc/kg of packed red blood cells. The specific details of the resuscitation of an injured child are further discussed in Chapter 32.

ASSESSMENT OF ABDOMINAL INJURIES

The history is especially important in cases of child abuse, as in the treatment of any trauma victim. The history gives the physician information needed for seeking potential injuries. During the primary and secondary survey the history should include the mechanism and time of injury, the child's clinical status at the scene and during transport to the hospital, the child's level of consciousness, past illnesses, medications, and allergies. In cases of suspected child abuse, the physician should note any discrepancy in the history or alterations in the history as elicited from the custodian of the child. This information needs to be carefully documented in the medical record.

The physical examination is an important tool in the diagnosis of intra-abdominal injuries, although it may not be specific to the injured organ. The examination includes inspection, auscultation, percussion, and palpation. The physician should look for external signs of intra-abdominal injury, such as abdominal wall contusions, abrasions, ecchymosis, or abdominal distention. A lack of bowel sounds may be indicative of intra-abdominal injury. One of the more difficult parts of the abdominal examination is palpation of the abdomen, which requires a cooperative patient and a reassuring observer. The goal is to differentiate between abdominal-wall and intra-abdominal injuries. This requires light palpation of the abdominal wall in an attempt to elicit involuntary guarding. Percussing or shaking of the abdomen may help determine the presence of peritoneal irritation.

An integral part of the evaluation of an intra-abdominal injury includes examination of the pelvis, which begins with palpation of the bony pelvis and visualization of the perineum and rectum. An unstable or tender pelvis often means injury to other pelvic structures. The observer should look for blood at the urethral meatus and for contusions, ecchymoses, and lacerations of the perineum. The rectal examination should include an evaluation of sphincter tone and the position of the prostate gland, an investigation for the presence of blood, and an evaluation of the integrity of the pelvic floor and rectal wall.

Diagnostic studies should begin with the hematologic tests obtained during the primary survey, and should include a blood type and crossmatch test, complete blood count (CBC), platelet count, prothrombin time (PT), partial thromboplastin time (PTT), amylase assay, liver functions tests, and arterial blood gas measurements. During this initial assessment, a urinalysis should be obtained to evaluate for urologic trauma. Every child with a significant mechanism of injury should have upright and lateral chest, abdominal, and pelvic radiography. One should evaluate for fractures of the ribs, spine, and pelvis; air in the retroperitoneum; an abnormal bowel gas pattern; and free intraperitoneal air.

During the past 10 years, abdominal computed tomography (CT) has become the single most useful diagnostic test for evaluating a pediatric patient with intra-abdominal injuries. Ninety percent of major intra-abdominal trauma involves solid-organ injury of the spleen, liver, or kidney.[3] The CT scan is sensitive to lacerations or fractures of the parenchyma, extravasation of blood or urine, and free fluid or blood within the abdominal cavity. The indications for the use of abdominal CT scanning include a Glasgow Coma Scale of less than 10, an unreliable abdominal examination, injuries suggestive of abdominal trauma, or a significant mechanism of injury that may cause intra-abdominal injury.[1] An additional advantage of CT scanning is its noninvasive nature. This allows the physician to continue further reliable physical examination of the child.

Other radiographic techniques that may help in the evaluation of abdominal trauma include abdominal ultrasonography and retrograde urethrocystography. The abdominal ultrasound examination is especially useful in assessing biliary, pancreatic, or duodenal injury. Retrograde urethrocystography and cystography are very useful in the evaluation of patients with pelvic injury that may be associated with urethral injury. Such a study should be done when lower-tract injury is suspected.

Diagnostic peritoneal lavage is generally useful in evaluating intra-abdominal trauma, but is rarely used in children because blood in the peritoneum is no longer an absolute indication for laparotomy. At present, diagnostic peritoneal lavage is indicated in the hemodynamically unstable patient or in the patient undergoing extra-abdominal surgery and who cannot be closely monitored under anesthesia.

There are several pitfalls in the assessment of abdominal injuries. Gastric distention causes a visceral peritoneal stretching and irritation that often mimics intra-abdominal pain. Therefore, in evaluating a child for abdominal injuries, nasogastric decompression is always required. Because bleeding from solid-organ injury in children often produces subtle signs of hypovolemia, children who present with a significant mechanism of injury, tachycardia, and a normal blood pressure should be suspected of having intra-abdominal hemorrhage.

Closed-head injuries are among the most frequent injuries associated with intra-abdominal injury. Hypotension in the presence of a head injury should alert the physician to blood loss that is not in the head. The child who presents with hypovolemic shock is often inadequately resuscitated, since fluid is given to produce a normal blood pressure but the child remains tachycardiac, poorly perfused, and acidotic. Shock may be further aggravated by an inadequate airway, which will cause further tissue hypoxia and cellular injury. Finally, the most unrecognized pitfall is the failure to suspect child abuse.

After the primary survey and stabilization, further therapy depends on the physiologic response and homeostasis of the patient, the mechanism and signs of injury, and the organs that are injured (Fig 33–1). In the presence of documented solid-organ injury and hemodynamic stability requiring less than 50% replacement of the patient's blood volume, nonsurgical management may be considered. The child must be closely monitored after stabilization in a pediatric intensive care unit. Exploration is necessary in children with persistent unstable vital signs despite adequate volume resuscitation, in whom more than 50% of the blood volume has been replaced, or with peritonitis, pneumoperitoneum or positive findings in diagnostic peritoneal lavage.

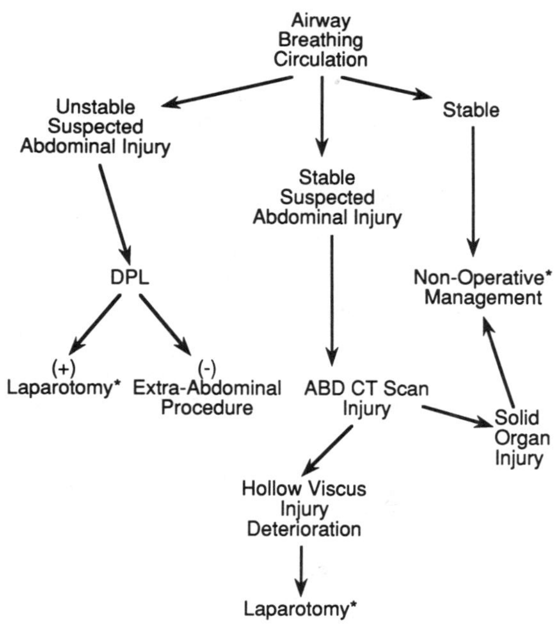

FIG 33–1.

Algorithm for the management of life-threatening blunt abdominal pediatric trauma. ⋆ = see text for specific organ injury.

TREATMENT OF SPECIFIC ORGAN INJURY

The liver and spleen represent the two most commonly injured abdominal organs in children. The pliable thoracic cage offers little protection to compressive and rapid decelerative forces on the chest and abdomen. The child with liver or spleen injuries or both may be asymptomatic, have signs of a chest-wall or abdominal-wall injury, or present with varying signs of blood loss. If the child can be stabilized with replacement of less than 50% of its blood volume, it may be observed in an intensive care unit following serial measurements of the hematocrit and abdominal examinations. Nonsurgical treatment is successful in 80% to 90% of children suffering from hepatic or splenic injuries.[3] Surgical exploration is indicated only if the child requires replacement of more than 50% of its blood volume or is or becomes hemodynamically unstable.

Surgical intervention for splenic injuries begins with control of the splenic hilum and complete mobilization of the spleen into the surgical field. Splenectomy may be required for injuries that traverse the splenic hilum, whereas polar lacerations and large hematomas respond to debridement of devitalized tissue, control of polar vessels with separate ligatures, and mattress suturing of the splenic parenchyma with or without hemostatic pledgets. Hemostatic agents such as thrombin and absorbable gelatin sponge (Gelfoam), collagen fiber, or fibrin glue have been used as adjuvants to obtain capillary hemostasis. Splenectomy is rarely indicated for blunt abdominal trauma in children.

Liver injuries require surgical management only for continued hemorrhage. This may result from extensive parenchymal injury or a significant biliary or vascular injury. Parenchymal injuries can be treated similarly to splenic injuries, with the ligation of larger vessels and bile ducts. Injuries to the retrohepatic veins and inferior vena cava may require the addition of a median sternotomy for control of the vena cava through the use of an intracaval shunt between the right atrium and suprarenal vena cava. Through use of the Pringle maneuver, blood flow to the liver is isolated, allowing time for repair of hepatic vein injuries. Hepatic vein injuries represent unusual and often lethal injuries in children.

The pancreas and duodenum are uncommonly injured, owing to their retroperitoneal position. A more extensive discussion of pancreatic and duodenal injuries is found in Chapter 35. Briefly, these injuries in children are due to compressive forces against the vertebral column from blows to the epigastrium or from striking of the abdomen against such objects as the handlebars of a bicycle. The child often presents with epigastric pain, tenderness, or an upper abdominal mass. The diagnosis is made with an upper gastrointestinal series, ultrasound examination, or CT scan. A duodenal hematoma or traumatic pancreatitis is treated with gastric decompression and total parenteral nutrition for

2 to 3 weeks. Pancreatic duct injury or duodenal perforation is often difficult to diagnose and may require further diagnostic procedures. These injuries require complex surgical intervention involving resection, repair, bypass, and drainage of the affected organ.

Perforation of the small bowel may result from even mild blunt abdominal trauma. Injury may result from lap seat belts or severe blows to the abdomen. The diagnosis of these small bowel injuries requires a high index of suspicion, frequent examination of the abdomen, and the use of radiographic studies including plain films, upper gastrointestinal series, and CT scans.[2] The child may complain of discomfort after seemingly mild trauma, and if a perforation is unrecognized, peritonitis may develop within 24 hours. A crush injury of the jejunum overlying the vertebral column may require 3 to 4 days for perforation and peritonitis to develop. Pneumoperitoneum may occur in perforation of the proximal bowel only. The only radiographic evidence of distal bowel perforation may be fluid within the pelvis and dilated or thickened bowel loops. Peritoneal lavage is helpful in identifying a bowel perforation, since the effluent may contain bacteria, bile, or intestinal debris, or have an elevated amylase concentration.

A small-bowel perforation is best repaired by debriding devitalized tissue and closing the enterotomy in a transverse direction. If necessary a segmental resection and anastomosis may be done to maintain an uncompromised intestinal lumen. In the patient who is unstable or has purulent peritonitis, exteriorization of the injured bowel may be the best decision. Broad-spectrum antibiotics are required in the perioperative period, and if the abdominal cultures are positive, specific antibiotics are added for 7 to 10 days postoperatively.

In blunt abdominal trauma, colon and rectal injuries are extremely uncommon; rectal injuries are, however, encountered in child abuse. These injuries are associated with insertion into the rectum of a blunt object that can cause rectal laceration and perforation. Specific findings in such rectal injuries include a patulous anus and evidence of blood within the rectal vault. If a perforation is present, the child often complains of lower abdominal and pelvic pain. Definitive diagnosis usually requires an examination under anesthesia, including sigmoidoscopy, to fully evaluate the perineum. In the female patient, endoscopic evaluation of the bladder and vagina is also indicated. Mucosal lacerations of the rectum respond to antibiotic therapy and bowel rest. If a perforation is suspected, a laparotomy is often required to evaluate the rectum above the peritoneal reflection. If a perforation is noted, a proximal diverting colostomy, repair of the perforation, and drainage of the injury are usually necessary.

Pelvic injuries are commonly associated with abdominal injuries from motor vehicle accidents and falls. Injuries associated with pelvic fractures include injuries to the bladder, urethra, lumbosacral spine, and proximal femur. The detection of urethral or perineal injury requires a urethrocystogram prior to urethral catheterization. The diagnosis of pelvic fracture is confirmed by plain x-ray films and further defined by CT scan. The primary treatment of pelvic fractures involves the replacement of lost blood with 20 to 40 cc/kg of blood. The remainder of the treatment consists of bedrest and immobilization. With more severe pelvic fractures and massive bleeding, immobilization with a pneumatic antishock garment may help, with subsequent external fixation or angiographic embolization of the internal iliac vessels. Fortunately, even though the injury may be severe, children recuperate from pelvic fractures without long-term sequelae when the injury is recognized early and the appropriate steps in management are followed.

In this case history, the child presents with a 2-day history of abdominal trauma with hemodynamic evidence of a 30% to 35% loss of blood volume. Furthermore, he has evidence of intra-abdominal injury with ileus, vomiting, a tender abdomen, and peritoneal irritation. There is also evidence of previous child abuse. Diagnostic studies show the patient to be anemic and hypovolemic. A serum amylase of 200 IU suggests intra-abdominal injury. Radiographic imaging shows free fluid in the abdomen, with an adynamic ileus pattern. A CT scan of the abdomen shows a contained hematoma within the liver capsule and a fluid collection in the subhepatic space, right colonic gutter, and pelvis.

In the management of this child, crystalloid and blood should be given during the primary survey, as outlined in Chapter 32. The child's mental status may be affected because of shock or associated injuries. If his mental status does not improve after the volume resuscitation, then a neurosurgical evaluation, including CT scan of the head, is indicated.

After resuscitation and stabilization of this patient, further treatment should involve maintaining the intravascular volume, serial measurement of the hematocrit, intensive care monitoring, and repetitive clinical evaluations. If the child becomes unstable or requires more than 50% replacement of his blood volume, a laparotomy is indicated.

The child also had physical findings and diagnostic studies suggestive of other abdominal injuries. The mechanism of his injury, the presence of peritoneal irritation, an elevated amylase concentration, and fluid in the abdominal cavity as demonstrated by a CT scan suggest of pancreatic or small-bowel injury. If the peritoneal irritation continues, the amylase remains elevated, or the ileus persists, then further evaluation of the duodenum, small bowel, and pancreas is indicated as outlined above. Diagnostic peritoneal lavage or laparotomy is indicated if further evaluation is nondiagnostic or a hollow viscus injury is strongly suspected.

Finally, the etiology of this child's injuries must be examined. He has evidence of previous injuries, including the fractures shown in skull films and the multiple bruises on his abdomen, lower extremities, and buttocks. Further evidence should be obtained with radiographs of the long bones. If there is evidence of abuse, the child protection service must be notified of his case.

REFERENCES

1. Beaver BL, Colombani PM, Fal A, et al: The efficacy of computed tomography in evaluating abdominal injuries in children with major head trauma. *J Pediatr Surg* 1987; 22:1117–1122.
2. Cobb LM, Vinocur CD, Wagner CW, et al: Intestinal perforation due to blunt trauma in children in an era of increased non-operative management. *J Trauma* 1986; 26:461–463.
3. Oldham KT, Guice KS, Ryckman F, et al: Blunt liver injury in childhood: Evolution of therapy and current perspective. *Surgery* 1986; 100:542–549.

34

Thoracic Trauma in Children

Martin R. Eichelberger, M.D.

A 4-year-old boy is struck by an automobile while crossing the street. The youngster sustains a basilar skull fracture associated with a right cerebral contusion, fractures of the right sixth through tenth anterior ribs, a right pulmonary contusion, and tension pneumothorax. Additionally, he suffers abdominal injury consisting of a deep laceration of the right lobe of the liver, renal contusion, and a laceration of the tail of the spleen. Also noted is a fracture of the right midshaft of the femur and a right nondisplaced fracture of the tibia and fibula. The youngster manifests multiple abrasions of the right flank and lower extremity. His scalp has a laceration that measures 4 cm in the occipital region of the skull. The child dies 2 days after admission from refractory high intracranial pressure and hypoxia.

Thoracic trauma exists in 4.4% of children admitted for blunt and penetrating trauma.[1] The mean age of these children is 6.2 years, with almost 50% being less than 5 years of age.[2] Injury to the chest is most frequently associated with motor vehicle-related incidents, with the child either an occupant, pedestrian, or bicyclist.

An analysis of children who manifest an injury to the chest reveals that 82% have multisystem trauma and that 58% of such injuries involve the head. Chest injury is usually associated with a lower mean trauma score, a higher mean injury-severity score, a longer mean length of hospitalization, a higher intensive-care-unit (ICU) admission rate, and a higher mortality than non-chest injuries.[2] Trauma injury severity score (TRISS) analysis reveals that the mean probability of survival equals 0.701 (Ps), which reflects the high mortality associated with chest trauma.[3] The severity of the injury differs according to the mechanism of injury; abused children sustain the most severe injuries followed by traffic-related injuries, which are moderate to severe.

The mortality from thoracic injury is exceedingly high.[2] Despite the fact that thoracic injury occurs in only 4.4% of children who sustain blunt or penetrating trauma, the mortality is 26%, which is significantly higher than the overall mortality rate of 2.4% for childhood injury. Unfortunately, 40% of the deaths with associated thoracic injury occur at the scene of the trauma or during transport for definitive care. Late deaths, 72 hours after injury, are rare and occur in less than 4% of cases.

The child under 14 years of age who experiences a thoracic injury commonly sustains intrapleural injury, rib fracture, or pulmonary contusion.[2] Rarely, injury occurs to the heart and great vessels or to the tracheobronchial tree. Occasionally, laryngeal trauma secondary to intubation or esophageal injury from caustic ingestion occurs in young children.

Blunt trauma to the chest wall results in pneumothorax, which frequently progresses to tension pneumothorax. Tension pneumothorax in children produces profound physiologic derangement, manifested by abnormalities in ventilation and perfusion that result from mediastinal displacement. As air enters the thorax, intrapleural pressure increases and the heart shifts to the contralateral side, compressing the opposite lung. The return of blood to the right side of the heart diminishes and affects the ability of the left side of the heart to eject oxygenated blood into the arterial system. Clinical signs of this derangement are hypotension, acute respiratory distress, tracheal deviation, cyanosis, and unilateral diminution of breath sounds. Open pneumothorax or flail chest is rare.

Even though the ribs of a child are relatively elastic, excessive kinetic energy from blunt impact will result in a fracture.[4] Fracture of the ribs in childhood is a marker of severe intrathoracic trauma and is associated with an increased mortality. The degree of physiologic derangement, extent of anatomic injury, and mortality rate worsen as the number of rib fractures increases.

A motor-vehicle collision with a pedestrian is the most common cause of rib fracture. Unfortunately, the second most common etiology of rib fracture is child abuse. The child with rib fracture usually manifests multisystem injury with head trauma; a lethal combination that results in a high probability of death.

Pulmonary contusion with parenchymal hemorrhage and edema commonly occurs in blunt trauma to the chest wall. Frequently, a radiograph manifests a pulmonary infiltrate that is evidence of a pulmonary contusion. A recent analysis revealed that chest x-ray underestimates the severity of pulmonary injury in 38% of children.[5] Computed axial tomography is the technique of choice for evaluating severe thoracic injury. The anatomic derangement that is not evident in plain film radiography is shown clearly by this technique. Frequently, the computed tomographic (CT) scan demonstrates bilateral, basilar atelectasis; parenchymal contusion; or a lung laceration. Pneumothorax, which is occult on a plain film, is also evident in a tomographic scan. The clinical signs that raise the suspicion of an intrapulmonary lesion are a normal plain chest x-ray associated with hypoxia (PO_2 of less than 100 torr; FIO_2 = 1), intrapulmonary shunting, and respiratory failure. These children require CT scanning for proper diagnosis of their injury and for the development of an appropriate management scheme.

Injuries to the heart and great vessels most commonly occur with penetrating trauma to the sternum or left sternal border of the chest.[2, 6] Gunshot or stab wounds to this region require a high index of suspicion for cardiac injury, especially when the child manifests hypotension, cyanosis, and respiratory distress. Adequate volume replacement and pericardiocentesis are essential therapeutic maneuvers. Expedient median sternotomy for evaluation of the heart is imperative, since suture repair of a myocardial injury is lifesaving. The great vessels are infrequently injured, but can be injured by blunt force to the thorax in a child. A flexible mediastinum permits motion of the aorta at the ligamentum arteriosum, reducing the incidence of aortic laceration in childhood. Nevertheless, a wide mediastinum on an anteroposterior (AP) chest film raises the suspicion of aortic laceration and requires evaluation by arteriography.

Another clinical syndrome is traumatic asphyxia, which results from direct, forceful compression in the region of the epigastrium. Children run over by a motor vehicle that traverses their upper abdomen will manifest this syndrome. The cephalad transmission of pressure from the intra-abdominal vena cava causes an increase in the postcapillary pressure. Disruption of the capillary produces petechiae of the face, neck, arms, and upper chest. Also evident are periorbital edema and subconjunctival hemorrhage. Traumatic asphyxia is significant, since pulmonary injury, cardiac contusion, and hepatic trauma commonly accompany it.

Initial management of the child in the clinical case described above requires adequate preoxygenation by bag-mask ventilation before endotracheal intubation. Children who sustain significant thoracic injury benefit from endotracheal intubation and neuromuscular-junction blockade to improve the efficiency of ventilation. The combination of thiamylal sodium (Surital), a short-acting barbiturate, and pancuronium (Pavulon), a nondepolarizing muscle relaxant, provides the best conditions for intubation. This is also optimal treatment for children with increased intracranial pressure. Maintenance of adequate muscle relaxation is usually satisfactory with intermittent administration of pancuronium (0.1 mg/kg). Children with an endotracheal tube in place are at high risk for inadvertent malpositioning of the tube in the esophagus. This results in gastric distention, diaphragmatic impingement, and restricted pulmonary efficiency.

Treatment of the child with thoracic trauma requires evaluation of physical signs associated with chest injury. Routine observation for symmetric chest expansion, auscultation for bilateral equal breath sounds, and an evaluation of mental status reflect the physiologic condition of the injured child. Oxygenation from ventilation is adequate if the skin is pink and the oxygen saturation is greater than 90% by pulse oximeter. Arterial blood-gas evaluation should confirm that the Po_2 is equal to 100 torr and the Pco_2 is less than 35 torr, which are objective measures of proper ventilation and perfusion. Nevertheless, clinical assessment is usually reliable.

Auscultation of the thorax is the most sensitive means for demonstrating abnormal accumulation of air or blood in the hemithorax. When the suspicion of abnormal ventilatory mechanics arises, a needle thoracentesis should be done to exclude pneumothorax or hemothorax. A tube thoracostomy in the midaxillary line of the fourth intercostal space constitutes definitive treatment for most children with an intrapleural injury. Proper siting of the tube thoracostomy prevents the accumulation of air, which will result in tension pneumothorax. In the event of hemothorax, the child will require acute infusion of fluid or blood to re-establish a circulating blood volume. In the rare event of an unstable chest wall (flail chest), endotracheal intubation is helpful for administering positive-pressure ventilation, which improves oxygenation.

Provision of intravenous access by a left saphenous vein cutdown would permit rapid volume resuscitation of the youngster in this case with 20 cc/kg of lactated Ringer's solution. A second infusion is necessary before a clinical assessment of perfusion and oxygenation shows improvement (i.e., a decrease in the capillary refill time and heart rate and an increase in blood pressure). Infusion of 10 cc/kg of universal red blood cells is necessary to improve the oxygen-carrying capacity of the blood, since blood loss is significant. Following infusion of the fluid and blood, the patient's vital signs should become stable.

The abdominal assessment is remarkable for the tenderness it reveals in the right upper quadrant. A chest x-ray will confirm proper placement of the endotracheal tube, expansion of the right lung, and opacification of the right lower lobe of the lung consistent with pulmonary contusion. Examination of all extremities reveals the displacement of the right femur, which requires manual traction and application of a posterior splint to immobilize the femur, tibia, and fibula. The child responds to the fluid infusion, permitting transfer to the radiology suite for a CT evaluation of the head, chest, and abdomen.

The child continues to remain stable despite CT evidence of increased intracranial pressure and a right cerebral contusion. Further tomography of the abdomen reveals a large laceration of the right lobe of the liver, a splenic laceration of the tail of the spleen, and a kidney that demonstrates good perfusion without urine extravasation, although hematuria is noted on urinalysis. Exploratory laparotomy is unnecessary since the patient's bleeding abates. The fractures of the femur, tibia, and fibula are confirmed by plain radiography.

This child requires volume resuscitation despite increased intracranial pressure (30 to 40 torr), which is monitored by an intracranial pressure monitor. Similarly, ventilation is extremely difficult because of the bilateral pulmonary contusion evident on the CT scan. Tube thoracostomy is efficient in evacuating air and blood from the hemithorax and re-expansion of the lung. This reduces the flow of blood from laceration of the injured lung parenchyma. Children who bleed from a thoracostomy tube at a rate of 1 to 2 cc/kg/hr require exploratory thoracotomy for hemostasis. Surgical intervention for thoracic injury is necessary in only 7% of children.[2]

Children in cardiopulmonary arrest from blunt trauma have a 95% mortality. Nevertheless, attention to the mechanics of ventilation is important in resuscitation. The child with blunt trauma requires endotracheal intubation, placement of bilateral thoracostomy tubes, intravenous fluid infusion, and pericardiocentesis if hypotension persists. Children who do not respond to this scheme usually succumb rapidly.

In summary, children infrequently sustain a thoracic injury, but the mortality from such injury is extraordinarily high. The injury to the thorax is usually associated with head trauma and injury to the organs of the upper abdomen; consequently, both of these areas require evaluation. Rib fractures are also a mark of severe injury, and are accompanied by increased mortality. Children who manifest multiple injury with chest trauma require rapid assessment and reconstitution of the mechanics of ventilation to improve the likelihood of their survival.

REFERENCES

1. Peclet MH, Newman KD, Eichelberger MR, et al: Patterns of injury in children. *J Pediatr Surg* 1990; 25:85–91.
2. Peclet MH, Newman KD, Eichelberger MR, et al: Thoracic trauma: An indicator of increased mortality in children. *J Pediatr Surg* 1990; 25:961–966.
3. Eichelberger MR, Mangubat EH, Sacco WS, et al: Outcome analysis of blunt trauma in children. *J Trauma* 1988; 28:1109–1117.
4. Garcia VF, Gotschall CS, Eichelberger MR, et al: Rib fractures in children: A marker of severe trauma. *J Trauma* 1990; 30:695–700.
5. Sivit, CJ, Taylor GA, Eichelberger MR,: Chest injury in children with blunt abdominal trauma: Evaluation with CT. *Radiology* 1989; 171:815–818.
6. Newman KD, Eichelberger MR: The child with thoracic trauma, in Turney S, Rodriguez A (eds): *Management of Cardiothoracic Trauma*. Baltimore, Williams & Wilkins, 1990.

35

Pancreatic and Duodenal Trauma

David E. Wesson, M.D.

A 9-year-old boy fell from a tree limb onto the back of the chair he had used for climbing. He landed on his right upper abdomen and epigastrium. He recovered promptly and resumed his activity. After returning home he developed upper abdominal discomfort characterized by a sensation of fullness and minimal pain. At dinner he developed nausea and vomited bilious material. He attempted to drink water an hour later and vomited again. He was brought to the emergency room. He had minimal right-upper-quadrant pain on physical examination. Plain abdominal x-rays showed a distended stomach and sentinel small-bowel loop in the upper mid-abdomen. A barium swallow showed a compression of the third portion of the duodenum, with a coil-spring appearance.

Pancreatic and duodenal injuries comprise approximately 5% of blunt abdominal injuries requiring hospitalization. They are often difficult to diagnose and can be very difficult to treat. Recently, computed tomography (CT) and ultrasonography have made accurate diagnosis much easier and have allowed us to adopt a conservative, nonsurgical approach in the vast majority of cases of such injury.

Pancreatic and duodenal injuries fall into two large groups according to the way in which they present. Most are isolated, low-energy injuries caused by a direct blow to the upper abdomen by a bicycle handlebar, hockey stick, or other object. These injuries may present from several hours to several days after they are sustained. A full recovery is the rule. The case presented above would fall into this group.

The second group consists of high-energy injuries, often caused by motor-vehicle accidents. Such cases usually have multiple injuries that are reflected in high injury severity scores. Patients in this group usually present early. However, the diagnosis of pancreatic or duodenal injury may be delayed. The prognosis in high-energy trauma is much worse than in low-energy trauma.

CLINICAL FEATURES

In most cases of pancreatic and duodenal trauma, there is a history of a direct blow to the epigastrium, often with a blunt object such as the back of the chair in the case under discussion. Victims of motor-vehicle accidents and other high-energy injuries seldom give a clear history pointing to pancreatic or duodenal injury.

The onset of symptoms may be delayed from several hours to several days after the injury. Epigastric pain, sometimes radiating into the back, occurs even with mild duodenal or pancreatic trauma. Nausea and bilious vomiting are also common, particularly in cases of duodenal hematoma with obstruction.

In most cases, the vital signs are normal because neither bleeding nor frank peritonitis is common. However, in the small minority of cases with duodenal perforation or pancreatic transection, secondary peritonitis develops with fever and tachycardia.

Inspection of the abdomen may reveal a lap-belt bruise which, if present, suggests a bowel, pancreatic or spinal injury. Abdominal tenderness in the mid-epigastrium or right upper quadrant is to be expected with all pancreatic and duodenal injuries, but frank peritonitis is rare. Occasionally, a mass can be felt in the presence of a large duodenal hematoma.

Routine laboratory investigations should include microscopic urinalysis and a serum amylase assay, which almost always gives an elevated result. In the case outlined above, the history suggests a direct blow to the duodenum by the chair. Frank perforation did not occur, but a hematoma developed over several hours, leading to obstruction of the duodenum.

PATHOLOGY AND PATHOPHYSIOLOGY

The pancreas and duodenum are well protected in the retroperitoneum. However, when a blunt object is forced into the epigastrium, the duodenum and pancreas can be damaged by compression between the intruding object and the spine. This may happen more frequently in children because the costal margin is relatively higher and more flared, and offers less protection to the pancreas and duodenum than in adults.

The most common injury to the duodenum is an intramural hematoma. This is the most likely diagnosis in the case under discussion. Rarely, free perforation of the duodenum occurs. This may be difficult to diagnose because, at least for a time, the spillage of duodenal contents is confined to the retroperitoneum. We have recently recognized a new injury called obstructive pancreatitis in association with duodenal hematoma.[1] In this condition, ultrasonography shows some thickening of the pancreas and frank dilatation of the pancreatic duct, presumably because of obstruction at the duodenum.

The most common pancreatic injuries are contusion, laceration with or without major duct injury, and transection. Laceration and transection may be complicated by the development of a pancreatic pseudocyst. Major combined pancreaticoduodenal injuries with tissue loss or devascularization, and penetrating injuries, are rare in children.

DIAGNOSIS

In most cases of abdominal trauma, including the present one, a preliminary diagnosis of pancreatic or duodenal injury can be made on clinical grounds. The key diagnostic step is to rule out perforation of the duodenum, major pancreatic duct injury, or complete transection of the pancreas. For this reason, further investigation is always indicated. Although not very sensitive, plain films may reveal retroperitoneal air, a pneumoperitoneum, or both, indicating perforation of the duodenum. Plain films may also show a double bubble sign in children with obstruction of the duodenum by a duodenal hematoma. The plain films in this case suggest duodenal obstruction and possibly also direct pancreatic trauma because of the sentinel loop of bowel.

Ultrasonography has revolutionized the treatment of pancreatic and duodenal injuries, and in the fully conscious patient with no clinical features of peritonitis, ultrasonography alone, without a gastrointestinal (GI) constrast study or CT scan, is sufficient to guide treatment. Ultrasonography can provide a definitive diagnosis of duodenal hematoma.[2] The typical feature is a sonolucent mass anterior to the right kidney. In pancreatic injuries, the ultrasound examination may show enlargement of the gland, a peripancreatic fluid collection, or duct dilatation. It can also reveal the earliest signs of pseudocyst development, often within a few days of the injury. In such cases, serial ultrasound examinations are invaluable.

A barium contrast study of the upper gastrointestinal tract, as performed in this case, is a very satisfactory alternative to ultrasound examination. It has the added advantage of ruling out a perforation in equivocal cases. The typical coiled-spring obstruction confirms the diagnosis of duodenal hematoma.

When clinical examination is unreliable or suggestive of a possible perforation of the duodenum or major pancreatic injury, we perform a CT scan with intravenous and enteric contrast enhancement, mainly to rule out perforation of the duodenum.

Endoscopic retrograde cholangiopancreatography (ERCP) is almost never indicated in the acute situation, but is useful in cases of chronic or recurrent pancreatitis following blunt abdominal trauma, to rule out a stricture of the pancreatic duct.

Hyperamylasemia is almost always present in pancreatic injuries. When the serum amylase is elevated, serial determinations are indicated until it returns to normal. A rising amylase level may be an early indication of a pseudocyst.

Diagnostic peritoneal lavage is rarely helpful in diagnosing pancreatic or duodenal injuries. We occasionally use this method in equivocal cases, to rule out peritonitis from intestinal perforation when a CT scan is not diagnostic.

TREATMENT

All patients with pancreatic or duodenal trauma require nasogastric drainage and intravenous fluids, at least in the beginning of their treatment. In most cases of duodenal hematoma, obstructive pancreatitis, or pancreatic contusion, the treatment is nonsurgical. Spontaneous recovery occurs in almost all such cases. Total parenteral nutrition (TPN) via a peripheral vein may be used, but gut function usually resumes promptly, allowing normal enteric feeding within a week. Patients treated nonsurgically are followed in the hospital with serial ultrasound examinations and amylase determinations. Enteric feeding is resumed when the results of these procedures return to normal and when nasogastric drainage decreases, indicating that the duodenal obstruction has resolved.

When duodenal peforation or major pancreatic injury are suspected, immediate laparotomy is indicated. In these cases, or when such injuries are found at laparotomy for other reasons, treatment is tailored to the surgical findings. In simple duodenal perforation, primary repair and drainage are sufficient. For major pancreatic duct disruption or transection to the left of the superior mesenteric vessels, distal pancreatectomy with preservation of the spleen and drainage of the proximal pancreatic stump is indicated. Pancreatic contusions discovered at laparotomy should be drained, but duodenal hematomas should be left alone. In cases of major duodenal disruption, particularly with tissue loss or extensive laceration of the head of the pancreas, primary repair supplemented by wide drainage, and pyloric exclusion with gastrojejunostomy should be considered. Pancreaticoduodenectomy is rarely if ever indicated.

When a pseudocyst develops, the patient should be kept on TPN to suppress pancreatic exocrine secretion and to allow spontaneous resolution of the pseudocyst. If the pseudocyst persists for more than 2 weeks, drainage is indicated to prevent bleeding, sepsis, perforation, and obstruction of the bowel. Percutaneous drainage under sedation, using a pigtail catheter and ultrasonographic guidance, is almost always successful. It is no longer necessary to wait 4 to 6 weeks in order to allow "maturation" of the pseudocyst so that internal drainage to either the stomach or small bowel can be performed. In our experience, neither recurrence nor external fistula formation has been a problem following percutaneous drainage of post-traumatic pancreatic pseudocyts.

Once the cyst has been drained percutaneously, the patient may resume a normal diet. The drainage usually stops in a few days, at which time the catheter can be removed and the patient discharged.

PROGNOSIS

Most duodenal hematomas, such as the one described here, resolve in 5 to 7 days. In cases of simple laceration of the duodenum, primary healing with prompt recovery is to be expected within a similar period. Rapid recovery is also the rule after distal pancreatectomy.

When major devascularizing injuries to the duodenum or head of the pancreas occur, external duodenal fistulae are common. They may require a long

TABLE 35–1.
Current Treatment Protocol for Pancreatic and Duodenal Trauma

- Immediate operation for
  - Pancreatic transection on CT scan
    - Distal pancreatectomy
  - Duodenal disruption on upper gastrointestinal series or CT scan
    - Repair, duodenal decompression, drainage, and bowel rest
  - Other injuries requiring laparotomy
    - Intraoperative evaluation of the pancreas and duodenum, with treatment as necessary
- Nonsurgical management for all others
  - In-hospital observation, bowel rest, and TPN
  - Serial abdominal ultrasound and serum amylase determinations
  - Resumption of enteric feeding when spontaneous resolution is complete (amylase normal, pancreatic ultrasound examination normal)
- Complications
  - Pseudocyst
    - Percutaneous drainage if symptomatic or persistent (>2 weeks)
  - Chronic or recurrent pancreatitis
    - ERCP and distal pancreatectomy if ductal stricture present
  - Pancreatic abscess
    - Surgical debridement and drainage
  - Duodenal fistula
    - Adequate drainage, skin protection, fluid and electrolyte replacement, and TPN

period of TPN. However, provided that adequate external drainage is maintained, parenteral feeding is given, and the skin is protected properly, spontaneous healing usually results.

SUMMARY

Most pancreatic and duodenal injuries in children are isolated, low-energy injuries from a direct blow to the epigastrium. Most such injuries, including duodenal hematomas, as described in this case, heal spontaneously with gut rest and TPN. Perforation of the duodenum and complete transection of the pancreas or one of its major ducts are uncommon. The most notable complication is a pancreatic pseudocyst, which may be treated by external drainage if it does not resolve spontaneously.

Our approach to the treatment of pancreatic and duodenal injuries is summarized in Table 35–1.

REFERENCES

1. Gorenstein A, O'Halpin D, Wesson DE, et al: Blunt injury to the pancreas in children: selective management based on ultrasound. *J Pediatr Surg* 1987; 22:1110–1116.
2. Winthrop A, Wesson DE, Filler RM: Trauma duodenal hematoma in the pediatric patient. *J Pediatr Surg* 1986; 21:757–760.

PART SIX

Head and Neck Lesions

36

Congenital Cysts and Sinuses of the Neck

Charles H. Stolar, M.D.

An 18-month-old girl presents with a small compressible mass in the upper left neck (anterior triangle), medial to the sternocleidomastoid muscle. A small sinus tract is also observed in the lower third of the neck, medial to the sternocleidomastoid muscle. Stringy mucus is noted at the sinus-tract site. No other abnormalities are noted. A contrast sinogram performed with a 24-gauge Silastic catheter demonstrates passage of contrast material superiorly into the cystic mass in the upper neck, near the angle of the jaw.

The child in this case history presents with a congenital anomaly of the branchial apparatus. Each groove, cleft, pouch, and arch of the branchial apparatus has its own unique embryologic destination, deviation from which produces characteristic anomalies. The branchial apparatus is apparent during the fifth week of gestation, and is marked externally by four ectodermal clefts and internally by four endodermal pharyngeal pouches. Within this "sandwich" is a mesodermal branchial arch that generates a skeletal element as well as a blood vessel connecting the dorsal and ventral aortae. In the fully developed human infant, the first cleft becomes the external auditory canal, the first pouch becomes the eustachian tube, and the mesoderm becomes the tympanic membrane. The second, third, and fourth clefts become obliterated by fusion with the underlying arches. The second pouch becomes the tonsillar fossa and the third pouch becomes the pyriform recess, while the other pouches are unrepresented.

Anomalies of the first branchial cleft are uncommon, but are manifested as agenesis, atresia, stenosis, or duplication of the external auditory canal. They are often heralded by a deformed pinna and may be associated with recurrent infections and drainage behind the pinna. Hearing deficits are the rule. Surgical excision is needed through a parotidectomy incision, taking care to avoid injury to the facial nerve. Anomalies of the second branchial cleft are the most common abnormalities of the branchial apparatus, and such an anomaly is the likely diagnosis in the case presented above. These remnants can present as a cyst, sinus, or fistula, and can be referred to synonomously as branchial cleft cyst, sinus, or fistula. The branchial cleft cyst results from persistence of a squamous epithelium-lined space as the cleft is obliterated. The cyst is located below the angle of the jaw and deep to the anterior border of the sternomastoid muscle. The diagnosis is usually obvious, although it is possible for such a cystic lesion to be confused with a parotid tumor. Such lesions can appear at any age from infancy to adulthood, and are treated by surgical excision. During the excision, care must be taken to avoid injury to the facial and greater auricular nerves. On occasion there is a tract that extends from the posterior aspect of the cyst, through the carotid bifurcation, and to the tonsillar fossa, where it ends and should be ligated and divided. During dissection within the carotid bifurcation, care must be taken to avoid injury to the hypoglossal and glossopharyngeal nerves.

On other occasions a sinus will present itself somewhere along the anterior border of the sternomastoid muscle. As in the above case, it will often drain a mucoid/saliva-like secretion and communicate with the cyst itself. Injection of the opening with radiopaque contrast medium can confirm the diagnosis if it is not clear on physical examination. If a sinus is present, an incision at the level of the sinus will need to be complemented by a counterincision at the level of the carotid bifurcation for en bloc removal of the entire complex with the best cosmetic result. The dissection may be facilitated by filling the entire complex with a vital dye such as methylene blue. Supervening infection, usually polymicrobial, will have to be treated with antibiotics, and occasionally with incision and drainage, before excision of the cyst complex. Anomalies of the third branchial cleft are unusual, but present as a sinus opening low on the neck at the anterior border of the sternomastoid muscle. They communicate with the pyriform fossa by a tract that passes from the neck superiorly and medially to loop over the hypoglossal nerve, run inferiorly medial to the carotid artery, and enter the pyriform sinus after piercing the thyrohyoid membrane. Anomalies of this type are treated with the same surgical principles described above.

First- and second-branchial-pouch remnants are rare and of little clinical importance. Third- and fourth-pouch abnormalities are also unusual but, because these structures are involved in the development of the thymus and parathyroid glands, they are important. Absence of the third and fourth pouches results in the DiGeorge syndrome, which features agenesis of the parathyroid and thymus glands. This results in disordered calcium homeostasis and impaired cellular immunity. Rarely, the third pouch persists as a cul-de-sac from the pyriform sinus that can become infected and present as an anterior neck mass. It may fistulize to the overlying skin. Also rarely, ectopic thymus rests can become cystic and present as masses anywhere from the anterior sternomastoid muscle to the mediastinum. There are anecdotal reports of malignancy in these thymic cysts, and all of them should be removed surgically.

Although the thyroid gland is not a derivative of the branchial arches, its role in the development of the thyroglossal-duct cyst is important. The gland arises from the midline floor of the pharynx at what becomes the foramen caecum. It then descends into the neck to its final position, by the eighth week of gestation. A communication with the foramen caecum may persist, although the usual remnant is represented by a pyramidal thyroid lobe. During the thyroid descent, the hyoid bone is formed from the second branchial arch. As a result of the intimate relationship between the hyoid bone and the thyroglossal duct, the duct can become surrounded by or displaced anteriorly or posteriorly to the hyoid bone. It is also possible for the duct to end at the hyoid bone. Persistence of the thyroglossal duct in any form will present as a thyroglossal-duct cyst. At presentation the cyst may be an asymptomatic midline mass directly overlying the hyoid bone or an infected mass. If there is communication with the skin, a clear mucoid material may be draining. Supervening infection is treated by appropriate antibiotics and drainage if needed. The operation for a thyroglossal-duct cyst is characterized by an incision over the mass, with careful dissection of the mass to the hyoid bone. The thyrohyoid and sternohyoid muscles are released from the central portion of the bone, which is then divided on either side of the midline. Not to remove the central portion of the hyoid bone is to do an incomplete operation. Remaining duct is sought behind the hyoid bone, where it is dissected to the base of the tongue, ligated, and divided. Because the hyoid bone cannot be reapproximated after the removal of its central portion, the remaining space is obliterated as best as possible and a small drain is left in place to be removed after 48 hours. Recurrent thyroglossal-duct cyst is usually a consequence of an incomplete initial operation.

SUMMARY

The 18-month-old girl in this case, with a neck mass, has had a radiographic demonstration of its communication with the pharynx. The diagnosis can be nothing other than a branchial cleft cyst and sinus arising from the second branchial cleft. The only management is surgical excision. For completeness we have also reviewed the embryology, clinical spectrum, and surgical treatment of abnormalities of the branchial apparatus.

37

Cystic Hygroma

Dennis W. Shermeta, M.D.

A 3.5-kg, full-term infant boy presents with a large, soft, compressible lesion that fills the right side of the neck, and has intermittent episodes of labored breathing. The mass extends across the midline to the left. The lesion extends superiorly to the angle of the jaw, inferiorly beneath the clavicle, and laterally into the posterior neck triangle. The mass transilluminates and has a few areas of hemorrhage. X-rays of the neck reveal tracheal narrowing at the level of the sternal notch. Ultrasound examination is consistent with a large, multiloculated cystic structure that extends into the upper mediastinum.

Cystic hygroma presents as a soft, cystic, discrete mass at the time of birth. Its equal sex distribution favors a random accidental failure of the normal development of the lymphatic system. A lack of lymphatic-to-venous drainage results in the proliferation and infiltration of sequestered lymphatic structures, usually characterized by endothelium-lined cystic structures actively producing lymph, with varying amounts of fibrous stroma. Seventy-five percent of cystic hygromas occur in the cervical area, most commonly on the left side. Their size at birth may occasionally be great, with extension beyond the midline and below the clavicle into the superior mediastinum. The larger hygromas will most likely be infiltrative in distribution making en bloc resection both impractical and technically impossible without sacrificing important cranial nerves.

Hemorrhage into cystic cavities may occur secondarily to birth trauma, with subsequent expansion of the cystic spaces causing compression of adjacent structures. When such compression involves the upper airway, rapid therapeutic measures may be lifesaving. Ultrasonography frequently provides antenatal diagnosis of a cervical mass of cystic nature with the possibility of airway compression. Rapid and skilled endotracheal intubation immediately after birth may be lifesaving. Significant deviation of the trachea, as well as massive enlargement of the tongue, may make intubation extremely difficult, and emergency tracheotomy may be the only means of affording ventilation upon delivery. If ultrasonography indicates a mass of extreme size, both the personnel and equipment for emergency tracheostomy must be available. A cesarean-section delivery may be the best way of ensuring optimal neonatal airway management.

As described, this neonate had involvement of the right neck extending from the angle of the mandible into the superior mediastinum. The management scheme may be divided into three anatomic areas. While the initial surgical therapy will probably involve all three areas, the unique problems associated with each are best discussed individually.

The first and most critical problem is the involvement of the trachea described above, with definite respiratory compromise. Since the compromise is intermittent, one must assume that it either occurs on a postural basis or is related to the level of agitation of the child (i.e., occurring only when the infant is crying). If the respiratory difficulties are pronounced and constant at the time of delivery, immediate endotracheal intubation is obviously the first step. It is then essential to determine the level of airway obstruction. If the obstruction is due to a hygroma compressing the trachea at the level of the thoracic inlet, surgical decompression at this narrow space may be curative. The hygroma will usually occupy the scalene fat pad and extend into the thoracic inlet in the groove between the trachea and esophagus. Identification and preservation of the phrenic nerve is crucial, and is usually readily accomplished by spreading of the curved hemostat in a vertical direction until the scalene muscle is identified. Simple spreading of the hygroma over the nerve then allows it to be completely and safely exposed. Similar blunt dissection in the groove between the trachea and esophagus, as well as in the retroesophagus, facilitates safe identification of the right vagal trunk. Removal of all other soft tissue, excepting muscle, will usually result in complete removal of the hygroma with decompression of the trachea, and will prevent recurrent difficulties.

The most common respiratory obstruction caused by a hygroma results from involvement of the base of the tongue and hypopharynx. Since these structures cannot be sacrificed, this level of respiratory obstruction must be managed with a tracheostomy. Following creation of an unobstructed airway, evaluation of the extent of pharyngeal and hypopharyngeal involvement including subglottic and esophageal extension, may be done endoscopically. Involvement of the epiglottis often precludes oral alimentation, necessitating the insertion of a gastrostomy tube. If the hypopharynx is free of hygroma, the surgical treatment will be greatly simplified.

The second compartment, the anterolateral and occasionally the posterior compartment at the neck, usually contains the bulk of the hygroma mass. Total excision without compromise of cranial nerves, blood vessels, or the thyroid gland is rarely accomplished and usually not necessary. This dissection should be done slowly, with meticulous attention to preserving neurovascular structures. Although the first resection is usually the easiest, as it becomes increasingly difficult to differentiate postoperative scar tissue from cystic hygroma, multiple resections are usually the reality. The mandibular branch of the facial nerve and the hypoglossal nerve are the easiest to damage, and should be identified in order to allay fears of surgical misadventure. Injury to the hypoglossal nerve in a patient who has extensive involvement of the floor of the mouth and tongue may occur at several sites. The first site is in the neck, where the nerve crosses in front of the external carotid artery. Since it is coursing perpendicularly to the main neurovascular channels, it may be cut if not identified. It is also in jeopardy when the hygroma is being excised through the floor of the mouth and base of the tongue. The hypoglossal nerve enters the tongue in the midline and then branches laterally. Wedge resection of the lateral portion of the tongue, in an attempt at debulking, can also injure branches of the lingual nerve if the extent of the resection is too great.

The use of sclerosing agents has had variable success. The floor of the mouth, base of the tongue, and hypopharyngeal structures would be best suited to such treatment if it were successful. Among the agents that have been used are ethanolamine oleate, bleomycin, and most recently OK-432, a lyophilized extract of a mixture of human, low-virulence Su strain of type III group A streptococcus pyrogens with potassium penicillin G. While previous agents had significant side effects, OK-432 was associated only with transient fever and an inflammatory reaction at the injection site. If the fibrosis that follows the injection of OK-432 into the epiglottis, subglottic trachea, and base of the tongue does not significantly impair function, this agent may be a significant adjunct to surgical therapy for hygroma.

The final and most difficult area of involvement by a cystic hygroma is the intraoral hypopharyngeal area with bilateral involvement of the tongue, epiglottis, and larynx. Since successful resection can occur only if critical function is preserved, hygroma in this area usually defies resection. Multiple debulking procedures are usually successful in maintaining a patent entry into both the trachea and esophagus, with laser resection of tracheal involvement having produced acceptable results.

Long-term surgical problems in the treatment of cystic hygroma usually center around postoperative neurovascular deficiencies. Most commonly, injuries to branches of the facial or hypoglossal nerves result in corresponding muscular atrophy. Wound healing has not been a significant problem, although excessive scar formation has been the rule rather than the exception.

Perhaps the most challenging sequela to a large cystic hygroma such as described in this case has been the tremendous enlargement of the size of the mandible, which in some cases has approached twice the size of the maxilla (Fig 37–1). Thinning of the bone, with exposure of the roots of developing

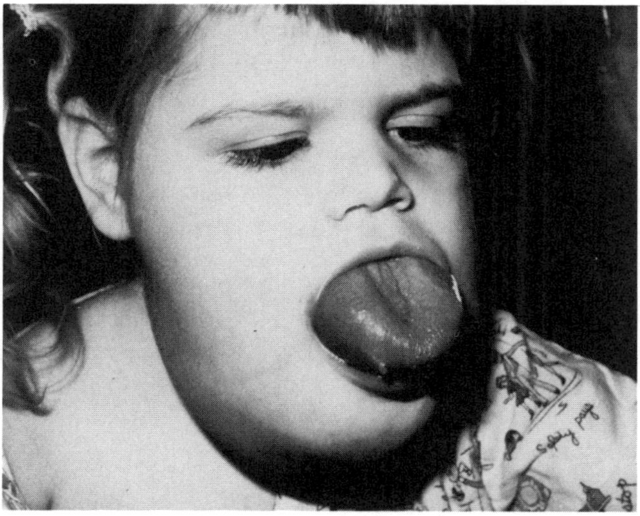

FIG 37–1.
A 2-year-old girl after resection of all of a cystic hygroma.

teeth, has made proper dental occlusion impossible. Early mandibular osteotomies have not been practical, since fixation for postoperative stabilization has not allowed the aggressive oral hygiene necessary in extensive hypopharyngeal hygromas. The appropriate timing of facial reconstruction is the single most difficult challenge to be solved in the future management of large cystic hygromas.

38

Management of Cervical Lymphadenopathy

R. Peter Altman, M.D.

A 5-year-old girl presents with a mass in the right preauricular area of 8 weeks' duration. The mass was erythematous and was treated with ampicillin for 10 days by her referring physician, with no therapeutic effect. There was no history of travel to any unusual geographic locations. The family history was negative for tuberculosis and other contagious disorders. The family acquired a kitten 3 months prior to the development of the mass. On physical examination the preauricular mass is fixed and tender to palpation. Enlarged lymph nodes are also palpable in the anterior triangle of the neck. The lesion is solid on ultrasound examination of the neck.

Chronic cervical lymphadenopathy, defined as adenopathy persisting for more than 3 weeks, raises the question of an inflammatory vs. a neoplastic etiology. Often the issue can be resolved only by surgical excision and microscopic examination of the involved tissues. Malignant adenopathy is beyond the scope of this discussion, which will be confined to a consideration of adenopathy of infectious etiology.

The case history rarely provides insight into the etiology of the adenopathy. Viral infections of the upper respiratory tract are probably the most common causes of cervical lymphadenopathy. These usually resolve within a week or so and require only symptomatic therapy. Among the other agents causing cervical adenitis are *Staphylococcus aureus* and group A *Streptococcus*. Regional infection with gram-positive cocci results in rapid nodal enlargement and systemic signs and symptoms including fever, tenderness, and erythema. There is usually a history of antecedent respiratory infection. On physical examination these nodes are exquisitely tender and there are obvious signs and symptoms of regional inflammation. The process runs a more fulminant course. The lymph nodes may suppurate, in which circumstance the patient presents with a fluctuant mass that may drain spontaneously or require surgical drainage. Surgical drainage and appropriate antibiotic therapy is curative, although induration may persist for many weeks.

The more indolent chronic adenopathy is less commonly associated with systemic illness. The patient usually feels quite well or has only a low-grade fever and mild respiratory symptoms. The adenopathy most often affects the anterior cervical or submandibular nodes, but multiple sites may be involved. The history may be helpful but is sometimes misleading. When one confirms the presence of a pet cat in the house, a causative relationship is suspected. Cat-scratch disease is caused by the cat-scratch bacillus. The syndrome is characterized by regional adenopathy, fever, and malaise. If the cat-scratch antigen is available, the diagnosis can be established by skin testing. These children are usually acutely ill, in contrast to those with atypical *Mycobacterium* infection, and their lymphadenopathy may take many weeks to resolve. The diagnosis can be confirmed by histologic examination of the lymph nodes (Warthin-Starry stain).

Among the most common causes of chronic cervical lymphadenopathy in children is infection with atypical mycobacteria. In the immunocompetent host these infections are rarely systemic and are almost invariably confined to regional nodes (occasionally involving other than cervical lymph nodes). The findings are usually unilateral and anterior or submandibular, but bilateral cervical node involvement is present in 10% of cases. The nodes are rarely tender, often agglutinated, and relatively fixed. The surrounding tissues are slightly indurated. If the condition has persisted for many weeks, the nodes may suppurate and form draining sinuses to the skin, a reliable sign of atypical (or occasionally tuberculous) *Mycobacterium* infection. Tuberculous adenitis (caused by *Mycobacterium tuberculosis*) is re-emerging as patients migrate to urban centers from underdeveloped regions. Occasionally one can elicit a history of exposure to an adult carrier of tuberculosis. Adenopathy caused by *Mycobacterium tuberculosis* is often associated with pulmonary findings, including hilar adenopathy. Tuberculous adenitis is responsive to pharmacotherapy.

The definitive diagnosis of adenopathy related to atypical *Mycobacterium* infection cannot always be established preoperatively. Skin-test results are variable. Most patients will exhibit a mildly positive purified-protein-derivative (PPD) reaction. Specific atypical tuberculosis skin-test antigens are not readily available, but the skin reaction to these antigens is usually positive.

Cervical adenitis due to atypical mycobacterial infection is caused by one of several strains of the bacillus. It is more commonly encountered in North America than is infection with *Mycobacterium tuberculosis*. It is important to differentiate between the two, since the treatment for tuberculosis is medical. In fact, one of the features that specifically characterizes atypical mycobacteria is their failure to respond to antituberculous drug therapy (isoniazid, streptomycin, para-aminosalicylic acid, or rifampin).

SURGICAL TREATMENT

The surgical treatment of atypical mycobacterial adenopathy is accomplished by making an elliptical incision over the mass, which, whenever feasible, should be placed under the jaw for cosmetic advantage. When the skin is particularly erythematous or indurated, it should be excised. Any pre-existing cutaneous fistulae must be included with the resected specimen. When submandibular lymph nodes are involved, the mandibular branch of the facial nerve is often closely related to the mass, and distortion of the normal anatomy demands special care in isolating and protecting this branch of the nerve during dissection of the lymph nodes. The corner of the mouth is exposed in the operative field so that nerve function can be ascertained intraoperatively, with a nerve stimulator. An extensive en bloc lymph-node dissection is unnecessary. Surgical treatment involves removing the obvious and largest of the involved nodes. The wound is closed without drainage, and good healing can be anticipated after resection and primary closure if the abnormal overlying skin and any draining sinuses have been removed. The strains of atypical mycobacteria vary in their culture characteristics. A definitive diagnosis is based on the growth of these organisms in culture. Recurrence is unusual and surgical excision is generally curative.

39

Vascular Access

Howard C. Filston, M.D.

A 19-month-old boy presents with bilateral orbital ecchymosis. A large abdominal mass is palpated in the left flank. The child has lost 2 lb in the past month and appears pale. Abdominal roentgenograms demonstrate calcifications in the mass. A ^{99m}Tc-pertechnetate bone scan shows multiple lesions consistent with metastases. The child was anergic to multiple skin-test antigens. Pertinent laboratory data show an elevated urinary vanillylmandelic acid excretion and anemia. Bone-marrow biopsy shows rosettes of tumor cells consistent with the diagnosis of neuroblastoma. Multiple venipunctures to obtain blood samples for laboratory tests, and infiltration of peripheral intravenous infusion sites make venous access extremely difficult.

This is a child over the age of 1 year with apparent stage IV neuroblastoma. Although there is no clear evidence that adjuvant therapy makes a difference in survival in the neuroblastoma population above a year of age, treatment will require prolonged vascular access for chemotherapy. In addition, the child's anemia and weight loss will create additional demands for access to his vascular system for the replacement of blood products and the provision of nutrition, especially during periods of chemotherapy, when he may have vomiting and anorexia as side effects.

Central vascular access would provide a point of dependable entry into his vascular system for drawing blood, administering blood products and chemotherapeutic agents, and providing intermittent parenteral nutritional supplementation.

In contradistinction to these positive effects of central vascular access, negative concerns include the risks of gaining central access, the long-term complications of an indwelling catheter, and the increased risk of catheter-related infection in a child who is already anergic from his tumor and who will probably have current and future periods of immune deficiency due to his tumor and to the suppressive effects of the chemotherapeutic agents used for treating neuroblastoma. Nonetheless, it has been shown that central-access catheters can be used successfully to facilitate the treatment of childhood tumors with an acceptable and controllable rate of infection.

PREOPERATIVE EVALUATION

Before the placement of a central access catheter is undertaken, the child's general condition should be assessed, with particular attention to his pulmonary function, any cardiac abnormalities, and his electrolyte balance, since in most small children general anesthesia will be required for placement of a central catheter. The child's platelet count and clotting factor levels should be carefully assessed. The inability to correct his platelet count and clotting factor levels toward near normal is a contraindication to placement of a central access catheter.

It is the surgeon's responsibility to be certain that the parents have had a fair discussion of the access device, including its advantages and disadvantages. Too often, the medical people involved paint a glowing picture of the ease of access and emotional benefits for the patient, and fail to give the parents a clearly defined discussion of the risks and complications of central access devices. Although serious and life-threatening events are unusual complications of these devices, they do occur, even when the most careful protocols for catheter placement and care are followed.

SITES OF VASCULAR ACCESS

Successful access to the superior vena cava can best be obtained by either percutaneous entry into the subclavian veins or by incisional access to the external or internal jugular veins.

The advantages of the subclavian access route include the need for minimal incision and dissection. Subclavicular access to the subclavian vessels provides convenience and stability; furthermore, advancement into the superior vena cava and right atrium is easy from the subclavian vessels, and the subclavian vessels usually remain patent and available for frequent recannulation.

The disadvantages of subclavian access are the greater skill and experience required for consistently successful access and the increased risk associated with the "blind nature" of the access. Injury to the pleura may produce a pneumothorax, and entry into the subclavian artery can, if done in an inappropriate fashion, produce severe hemorrhage requiring major surgical exposure for control. The small percentage failure rate associated with the subclavian approach is minimized by increased experience.

In the hands of an experienced surgeon, neck-vein access has the advantage of direct exposure of the vessels by incision and dissection, with minimal risk of injury to surrounding structures. However, vital structures course through the neck and can be injured if such exposure is attempted by one who is not familiar with the anatomy.

The disadvantage of neck-vein access is that there is often an undependable central course to the external jugular vein, with the result that threading of the catheter into the central system may be difficult. In addition, the incisional exposure and necessary ligation of the vessels to control hemorrhage in the dissected tissues means that each such exposure eliminates a vessel for subsequent cannulation.

TECHNIQUE

Jugular Venous Insertion

Incisional access to the neck veins is the more commonly used approach to insertion of a central venous catheter, especially in small infants and particularly in neonates and premature infants. The first choice should be any obvious external jugular vein. An incision of less than 1 cm can be used to expose the vessel, which is then elevated into the wound. Absorbable sutures are passed around the vessel proximally and distally, with the more proximal location being ligated. An incision is then made in the vessel and a guidewire is passed centrally under fluoroscopic guidance. A previously tunneled catheter is laid out over the image of the guidewire, from the point of entry to the estimated point of junction of the superior vena cava and right atrium. The catheter is cut to this length and the guidewire is then removed. The catheter is inserted into the superior vena cava to the point of juncture with the right atrium. A distal ligature is then tied snugly but not occlusively around the catheter and the incision is closed with appropriate subcuticular sutures and dressed.

If successful entry into the external jugular system is not possible, the deep jugular vessel itself can be exposed and a fine purse-string suture placed in its anterior surface, with entry then being made by incision within the circle of the purse-string. Further entry of the catheter is achieved in a fashion similar to that described for external jugular access, except that only the purse-string is tied around the catheter, with no proximal ligation of the internal jugular vein. Alternatively, the facial vein can be identified as a proximal branch of the deep jugular vein and utilized as an entry point. This obviates the need to either incise or partially ligate the deep jugular vein itself.

Subclavian Access

I prefer the "percutaneous" subclavian approach over incisional access to the neck veins.[1] The catheter passes more easily and in a more gentle curve into the superior vena cava from the left subclavian vein. The right side can be successfully cannulated if necessary, and this approach is sometimes chosen if, for instance, a ventriculoperitoneal shunt has been placed on the left side. However, I have found that the right-sided approach more frequently leads to the catheter passing up into the jugular system in a retrograde fashion, or crossing over into the left subclavian vein.

SURGICAL TECHNIQUE

The patient is anesthetized and restrained on the operating table to keep him from slipping off head first when put in the Trendelenburg position. The head is extended and taped in place with the face forward, and a sizable roll of padding is placed between the child's scalpulas to bring his chest forward and shoulders back. The neck and chest are then prepped with antiseptic solution and draped in an appropriate fashion, leaving both areas exposed in the field. An incision is made just beneath the clavicle at the midpoint between the sternal notch and the deltopectoral groove. The groove between the first rib and the clavicle can be palpated deep beneath the clavicle.

The child is then placed in an extreme Trendelenburg position to allow good filling of the upper trunk vessels, and an 18-gauge, 30-cm Intramedicut catheter-introducer system is used for initial access (Fig 39–1). This consists of a short introducer cannula with a needle stylet and outer plastic sheath, attached to a syringe that is inserted through the small infraclavicular incision and passed into the tissues to a depth that will place it at the deep surface of the clavicle. The introducer is then lined up parallel to the deltopectoral groove and the syringe flattened against the chest to force the needle stylet and cannula tightly beneath the clavicle. This introducer is then advanced into the subclavian vessel.

Aspiration of blood confirms entry. The blood is then reinjected forcefully from the syringe, which should "balloon up" the vein, allowing the needle to be passed further in, thus allowing the plastic cannula, which ends approximately 1 mm proximal to the bevel of the needle, to enter the vein. The needle stylet is then removed from the plastic cannula, and if free flow of blood is not evident, the plastic cannula is slowly backed out of the tract until free flow of blood is established. During all manipulations in which the needle stylet is used, the child is kept apneic by the anesthesiologist.

The plastic catheter is then introduced through the plastic cannula introducer, and under fluoroscopic guidance it is passed into the superior vena cava and well into the right atrium to demonstrate that it has followed a normal course. If any doubt arises, the catheter is injected with a small amount of radiographic contrast material. The cannula is advanced fully and the catheter removed and replaced by a flexible guidewire. The cannula is then removed and

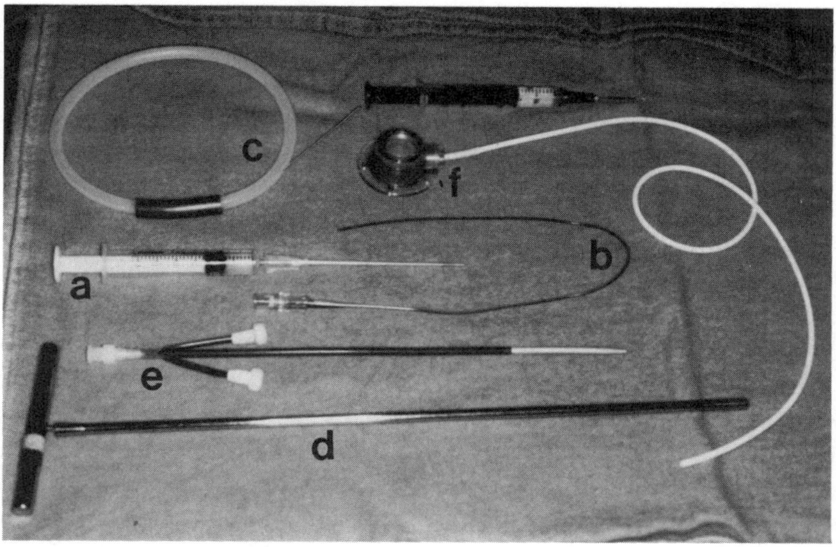

FIG 39–1.
Equipment for percutaneous subclavian insertion of the Infuse-a-port device (Shiley Infusaid Inc., Norwood, MA 02062.) Intramedicut cannula *(a)*. Intramedicut catheter *(b)* (Argyle Intramedicut Catheter Kit, Sherwood Medical, St. Louis, MO 63103). Guidewire *(c)*. Tunneling device *(d)*. Tearaway sheath introducer and sheath *(e)* (Peel-away Introducer Set, Cook, Bloomington, IN 47402). Infuse-a-port with catheter *(f)*.

the guidewire is left in the right atrium. Care must be taken to ensure that the guidewire is not causing any arrhythmias from abutting against any elements of the conduction system of the heart.

Depending on whether a Broviac catheter or implanted port is chosen, the next step is to fashion either an insertion site for the catheter in the paraxiphoid area or a pocket for the port through an incision on the lower chest, on the same side on which entry was made into the subclavian vessel. When a port is chosen it is sutured into the pocket with heavy absorbable suture material, and a tunnel is then fashioned between the pocket incision and the subclavicular incision. The catheter is threaded through this tunnel and brought out through the subclavicular incision.

If a Broviac catheter is chosen,[2] the cuff on the catheter is advanced until it is 1 to 2 cm distal to the site of entry of the catheter in the paraxiphoid area. In either case, the catheter emerging from the infraclavicular incision is then laid out on the chest over the guidewire image, and, under fluoroscopic control, is cut to such a length that its tip will lie at the junction of the superior vena cava and right atrium. There is approximately a 1-cm tolerance proximally and distally to this ideal point. A tearaway sheath-introducer system is then passed over the guidewire and inserted into the central system, again under fluoroscopic control. The introducer is then removed and the catheter passed into the tearaway sheath. When the catheter is fully inserted, the tearaway sheath is removed, leaving the permanent catheter in place. The wounds are closed and dressed appropriately.

A chest radiograph is then obtained to assure proper location of the tip of the catheter and to search for any sign of pneumothorax or hemothorax as a result of the insertion procedure.

EXTERNAL CATHETER (BROVIAC/HICKMAN) VS. TOTAL IMPLANTATION OF THE ACCESS DEVICE

Generally, there are two types of access device. The first is some variation of the Broviac or Hickman Silastic catheter that provides an external cannulation site, with a catheter that enters at some distance from the actual point of entry to the vascular system and is tunneled through the subcutaneous tissue to the point of vascular entry. These catheters usually have a cuff just distal to the coupling site that allows for the ingrowth of fibroblasts to seal the tract and hold the catheter firmly in place.

The implanted port is totally buried beneath the skin, with no external component whatsoever. Access to the port is gained by inserting a percutaneous needle into the central, self-sealing diaphragm of the port. Special (Huber) needles must be used because standard injection needles may core out a piece of the self-sealing diaphragm of the port.

The external catheter is more easily placed and is more easily removed than the implanted port. Only a small incision and local anesthesia are required. It is also more easily flushed in cases of occlusion by clot or precipitates from infused fluids. It is ideal in circumstances in which continuous vascular access is planned, such as in long-term nutritional support.

The disadvantage of the external catheter is the external part of the device itself, which can be damaged or worn thin. However, repair kits are available for dealing with such events. There is a greater likelihood of contamination with the external catheter, since there is an open wound with a foreign body running into it, and it is more susceptible to dislodgement despite the cuff with the bond of fibrous-tissue attachments. The external catheter requires dressing changes and some type of totally sealed dressing for such activities as swimming.

The implanted device, with its lack of any external equipment, allows for normal activities, although for some contact sports it might be wise to fashion some sort of protective device for the lower chest. In addition, the presence of the implanted device is less obvious than is that of the external catheter.

The main disadvantage of the port is that a second course of general anesthesia is usually required for its removal. Also, local extravasation of medications from misplaced access needles may cause sloughing of tissue or begin the process of infection. The implanted device is also more costly and more difficult to declot and clear of any obstructing materials.

COMPLICATIONS OF LONG-TERM CENTRAL VASCULAR ACCESS

Immediate complications of central venous access, at the time of entry, include failure to achieve successful access, pleural entry with laceration and pneumothorax, arterial entry with potential laceration and severe hemorrhage leading to hemothorax and possible shock, and extravascular placement of the catheter with subsequent infusion into extravascular structures, which may lead to necrosis, infection, airway compression, and pericardial tamponade. Careful fluoroscopic evaluation and assurance of free blood return make undetected extravascular positioning unlikely. In experienced hands, pneumothorax occurs once or twice in a hundred insertions and responds to tube thoracostomy.

Although entry into the subclavian artery rather than the subclavian vein occurs with some frequency, hemorrhage from the former vessel generally stops with 4 or 5 minutes of compression. We have not seen a major arterial injury in 17 years of routinely using the subclavian vessels for access in infants ranging from 24-week, 400-g prematures to adult-sized children. With rigorous adherence to the rule of never changing direction once the needle point passes beneath the clavicle, serious injury during insertion is highly unlikely.

The most common long-term complication of central catheterization is infection, either a bacteremia as a result of contamination from the catheter, or locally along the catheter tract or in the Infusaport pocket. The latter type of infection is far less common than the former. The second most common complication, occlusion of the catheter, is due to backup of blood, with clotting, or to precipitates of injected materials, such as when calcium and phosphorus are being given along with parenteral nutrition fluids and lipids.

A less common long-term complication is gradual erosion of the catheter through the wall of the vessel, with extravasation of infused materials, such as chemotherapeutic agents or parenteral nutrition fluids, into the extravascular space. With a properly placed catheter whose tip originally was at the junction of the superior vena cava and right atrium, this would usually result in either a mediastinitis or a pericardial effusion with potential pericardial tamponade. The best guard against this complication is to make the parents aware that any chest symptom should be thoroughly investigated by assuring free withdrawal of blood through the catheter and by radiographic confirmation of continued proper catheter positioning.

The catheter can act as a nidus for the deposition and propagation of thrombus, which can lead to occlusion of the subclavian or jugular vessels or of the superior vena cava itself. As with any thrombus, embolism from the thrombus is an ever-present risk.

Occlusion of the catheter by thrombus can be treated by flushing it with increasingly concentrated solutions of heparin; when heparin flushing fails, an appropriate amount of urokinase can be inserted into the catheter and left until the clot dissolves.

The risk of any of these thrombotic complications can be reduced by the routine use of heparin in the system, with 1 unit of heparin used for each milliliter of solution infused through the catheter. A somewhat more concentrated solution of 5 units of heparin per milliliter should be used whenever the catheter is to be flushed and capped without a continuous infusion.

Catheter breakage occurs both within the vascular system, where a catheter may break off and embolize to the heart, and at the external site. External breakages can usually be repaired with an appropriate-size replacement device from a repair kit. However, there is eventually too little external catheter to allow attachment of a new repair extension, and the entire catheter must be replaced. Catheter emboli can usually be retrieved by a competent vascular radiologist.

Children with malignant tumors have a depressed immune mechanism and are frequently malnourished, and the chemotherapeutic agents used in their treatment directly suppress their immune response and bone marrow. Nevertheless, the infection rate is acceptable and the infections treatable, and the benefit of central access devices can therefore be offered to these children with a relatively high degree of safety.

Infection is best prevented by developing careful protocols for the handling of central catheters and for gaining access to them. They should never be accessed by inexperienced personnel, and great care should always be taken to assure aseptic entry into the catheter. Parents often do a better job of avoiding catheter contamination than do hospital personnel. Continuous education of all personnel involved with catheterized children is essential to minimizing the rate of contamination and subsequent infection.

Minor infections at the site of entry of an external catheter can often be treated with antibiotics given both locally and systemically. A well-sealed cuff will usually prevent extension of a tract infection into the vascular system itself. Infection of the pocket containing the implanted port is more problematic and less likely to respond to antibiotics, especially if the infection results from extravasation of fluid or hemorrhage around the device, with subsequent infection of the hematoma or extravasated fluid. Most frequently, such infections require removal of the device, clearing of the infection, and reinsertion of a new device at an alternate site.

Bacteremia and septicemia can usually be cleared by treating the patient with appropriate antibiotics through the catheter itself.[2, 3] Only recurrent infections of the catheter line caused by the same organism require removal of the device to allow clearing of the infection. Repeated infections with different organisms can be treated with appropriate antibiotics, with the access system being left in place if the infection clears.[4] Should the patient remain toxic after 24 hours of therapy, or should subsequent blood cultures continue to show the presence of the organism, the device must be removed.

A not infrequent source of catheter infection is the fungus *Candida albicans*. Once it is established, this organism can rarely be cleared from a catheter device by antifungal agents alone, and the identification of a fungal septicemia generally requires removal of the device.

REFERENCES

1. Filston, HC, Grant, JP: A safer system for percutaneous subclavian venous catheterization in newborn infants. *J Pediatr Surg* 1979; 14:564–570.
2. Gauderer, MWL, Stellato, TA: Subclavian Broviac catheters in children—Technical considerations in 146 consecutive placements. *J Pediatr Surg* 1985; 20:402–405.
3. Wallace, J, Zeltzer, PM: Benefits, complications and care of implantable infusion devices in 31 children with cancer. *J Pediatr Surg* 1987; 22:833–838.
4. Olson, TA, Fischer, GW, Lupo, MC, et al: Antimicrobial therapy of Broviac catheter infections in pediatric hematology oncology patients. *J Pediatr Surg* 1987; 22:839–842.

40

Parenteral Nutrition

Arnold G. Coran, M.D.

At 34 weeks' gestation, a 2.2 kg infant boy is born with evisceration of the intestine through a gastroschisis defect. Careful inspection of the viscera documents the presence of an associated bowel atresia. After fluid resuscitation, the patient is taken to the operating room. The viscera are reduced and primary abdominal-wall closure and formation of an end-intestinal stoma are performed. During the postoperative course, the infant has a prolonged adynamic ileus and cannot tolerate enteral feedings. The serum albumin is 2.9 gm/dL, the transferrin level is 70 mg/dL. The infant's weight at 2 weeks of age is the same as his birth weight.

The intestine of infants born with gastroschisis is usually severely inflamed and edematous at birth. In addition, there is often a fibrinous peel over the intestinal serosa. These three abnormalities result in a significant adynamic ileus in these neonates, which may last for as long as 4 to 5 weeks following surgery. Also, these abnormalities make it very difficult for the surgeon to determine whether or not a true congenital bowel atresia is present or whether the areas of narrowing noted in the small intestine are merely secondary to the inflammation and edema. As a result, some pediatric surgeons prefer not to do anything about a possible intestinal atresia noted at the time of abdominal-wall closure, while others prefer to resect the atresia and create a jejunostomy or ileostomy in the abdominal wall. If a primary closure of the abdominal wall cannot be performed, and a Silastic chimney must be placed, most pediatric surgeons will not create an abdominal stoma because of the significant risk of infecting the Silastic pouch. Under these circumstances, the entire intestine is returned to the abdominal cavity, and if at 3 to 4 weeks postoperatively there is evidence of intestinal obstruction, the re-exportation is performed and the intestinal stenosis or atresia is resected.

The abnormal bowel in the infant with gastroschisis creates two major postoperative problems, one in the immediate postoperative period and the second later on. The inflamed, edematous intestine sequesters a large amount of extracellular fluid (ECF) during the early postnatal and postoperative period, which results in a significant decrease in circulating plasma volume. This phenomenon of "third-spacing" leads to decreased renal perfusion during the first 48 to 72 hours after surgery, which causes very low urine output during this period. We have recently studied this phenomenon in postoperative neonates, using nonradioactive tracers to measure ECF volume and total body water. Sodium bromide was used to measure the ECF volume and deuterium oxide was used to measure total body water.[1] These studies show that infants with gastroschisis have a marked decrease in their ECF volume during the postoperative period, in contrast to other infants who undergo surgery for major congenital anomalies (Figs 40–1 and 40–2). As a result of our clinical observations and the data from our study, we feel that all infants born with gastroschisis need more fluid in the postoperative period than infants who have surgery for other congenital anomalies such as intestinal or esophageal atresia. The second problem arising from the inflamed edematous intestine is the prolonged ileus, which, as mentioned above, can last for as long as 4 to 5 weeks. This adynamic ileus obviously precludes enteral feeding of the infant during this period. Therefore, parenteral nutrition should be started in the immediate postoperative period, once the early additional fluid requirements of the infant have been met.

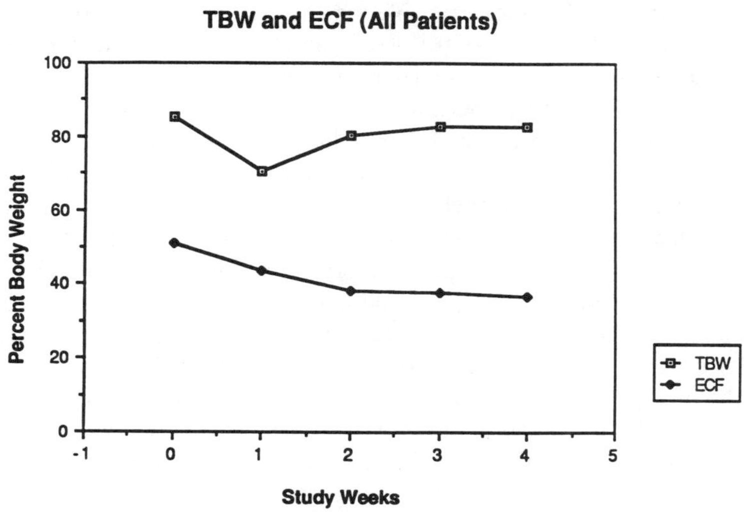

FIG 40–1.
Total body water and extracellular fluid changes in postoperative neonates. Note that the total body water value of 80% does not change during the study period; however, the extracellular fluid volume decreases from 56% to 40% during this period.

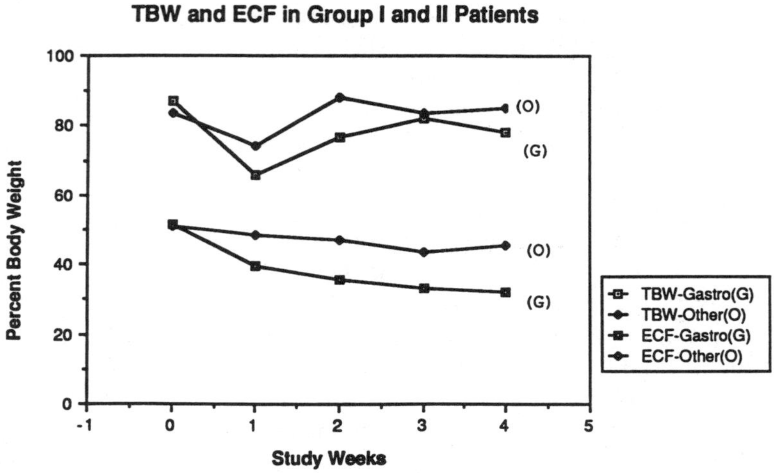

FIG 40–2.
Total body water and extracellular fluid changes in postoperative neonates. Infants with gastroschisis have a significant decrease in their extracellular fluid volume compared with the other postoperative neonates.

There are essentially three approaches to intravenous nutrition in infants: (1) central infusion of hypertonic glucose–amino acid solutions, (2) peripheral infusion of moderately hypertonic solutions of glucose and amino acids along with a fat emulsion, and (3) peripheral infusion of moderately hypertonic glucose–amino acid solutions in large volumes, without fat. Each of these techniques produces nitrogen retention and weight gain. In a difficult case, all three techniques may be required over a long period of time. Our initial approach to the newborn requiring total parenteral nutrition (TPN) is to use the peripheral infusion of moderately hypertonic solutions of glucose and amino acids together with a fat emulsion. The peripheral infusion technique involves the insertion of a 21- or 23-gauge needle into a peripheral vein, usually in the scalp. The intravenous tubing from the bottle containing the glucose–amino acid solution is connected to the needle, and the tubing from the fat emulsion bottle is then inserted piggyback into the rubber nipple at the end of the tubing from the first bottle. A calibrated buret is placed in each intravenous line and the contents of both bottles are infused over 24 hours, using two separate constant-infusion pumps. Since a fat emulsion will not pass through a Millipore filter, the filter is inserted into the line containing the amino acid solution, proximal to the point of entry of the fat solution. The injection site usually must be changed every 2 to 3 days because of infiltration, which is usually bland and nonphlebitic. Warm compresses on the site hasten resolution of the infiltration, and the same vein can usually be used again within 48 hours. The basic peripheral parenteral nutrition solution is made up of equal volumes of 5% amino acids and 25% glucose and water. This solution contains a final concentration of 2.5% amino acids and 12.5% glucose, which yields 0.53 cal/ml. Electrolytes are added to the solution to provide the recommended daily requirements, plus additional needs based on the patient's clinical condition (Table 40–1). A trace-element solution is routinely added to the infusate. Hep-

TABLE 40–1.

Peripheral Parenteral Nutrition With Fat in Infants*

CONSTITUENT	AMOUNTS PER KG PER 24 HR
Glucose	15–20 g
Protein	2.0–4.0 g
Sodium	2–4 mEq
Potassium	2–4 mEq
Chloride	3–6 mEq
Magnesium	0.5–1.0 mEq
Calcium	0.5–3.0 mEq
Phosphate	0.5–1.0 mM
Trace elements†	0.5 mL
Multivitamin infusion (MVI)‡	1.0 mL/day
Vitamin K_1	0.5 mg/day
Vitamin B_{12}	5 μg/day
Folic Acid	50 μg/day
Heparin	1.0 IU/mL
Glucose-protein volume	80–160 mL
Fat	4 g
10% fat emulsion volume	40 mL
Total volume	120–200 mL
Total calories	80–125

*Each 1,000 mL of standard solution is prepared by mixing 500 mL of 25% dextrose and water with 500 mL of 5% amino acids to give a final concentration of dextrose of 12.5% and of amino acids of 2.5%. The appropriate amounts of electrolytes, vitamins, and trace elements are added according to the patient's weight.

†Each 0.5 ml of trace element solution (University of Michigan Pharmacy) contains: zinc, 100 μg; copper, 20 μg; manganese, 10 μg; chromium, 0.2 μg.

‡Each milliliter of MVI (USV Pharmaceutical Corporation) contains: vitamin A, 2000 IU; vitamin D, 200 IU; ascorbic acid, 100 IU; thiamine (vitamin B_1), 10 mg; riboflavin (vitamin B_2), 2 mg; niacinamide, 20 mg; pyridoxine, 3 mg; dexpanthenol, 5 mg; vitamin E, 1 IU.

arin, 1 U/mL, is added to the infusate to help prevent phlebitis. Unless contraindicated, it is advantageous to use an intravenous fat emulsion as a major calorie source in the peripheral feeding program. Up to 4 g of fat per kilogram of body weight per 24 hours may be administered to infants. In addition to providing a major source of calories, the fat-emulsion administration also meets all the essential fatty acid requirements of the infant. The entire peripheral infusate with the fat emulsion provides between 80 and 125 kcal/kg of body weight per 24 hours.

If the infant requires TPN for longer than 3 weeks, then the central intravenous route is utilized at that time. This change is made at this time because venous sites become difficult to find after 3 weeks of peripheral TPN. The high osmolality of the central parenteral nutrition solution requires that it be delivered into an area of very rapid mixing via a central venous catheter. We prefer to use the Broviac silastic catheter (infant size) for central parenteral nutrition in infants. The catheter is inserted in the operating room under general anesthesia with strict aseptic technique. Generally, the catheter is inserted through a cutdown on the external jugular vein, or occasionally on the internal jugular vein; more recently, however, we have successfully inserted these catheters percutaneously into the subclavian vein in neonates and infants. The catheter is tunneled into the infant's chest wall medial to the nipple. The catheter exit site on the chest wall is about 5 cm away from the venous entrance site. This is done to minimize the likelihood of catheter contamination from dressing changes. When the external or internal jugular vein or the subclavian vein are unavailable, the central venous catheter can be inserted into the common iliac vein through a cutdown on the saphenous vein in the groin. This is a less desirable site of insertion because of the greater risk of contamination in the groin. Every 48 hours, the dressing is changed aseptically, the skin cleansed with an antiseptic, and povidone/iodine (Betadine) ointment is applied to the catheter–skin junction to protect against bacteria and fungi. A Millipore filter (0.22 μ) is placed in-line to remove particulate matter such as calcium salts and microorganisms that may have contaminated the solution. A calibrated buret is necessary for accurate monitoring of the volume delivered, and is used even when the solution is infused by a volumetric pump. Injection tubing may also be added to the circuit so that intravenous drugs can be giving aseptically above the filter. To minimize the risk of infection and mechanical failure of the central line, an alternate line should be used whenever possible, for infusing drugs, measuring central venous pressure, and transfusing blood products. All intravenous tubings are changed each day, when the new bottle of infusate is hung. Since the high sugar content of these infusates supports the growth of yeast, the external surfaces of all intravenous tubing should be washed with povidone/iodine (Betadine) once a day to remove traces of nutrient solution that may have dripped from the bottle onto the tubing. Povidone/iodine (Betadine) is also applied to all the joints in the circuit to prevent entry of microorganisms at these points. The infusate is delivered at a uniform rate over a 24-hour period using a volumetric constant-infusion pump.

The composition of the central parenteral nutrition solution is outlined in Table 40–2. The solution contains 25% glucose and 3.5% amino acids. Electrolytes, trace elements, and vitamins are added in appropriate amounts based on the infant's weight. Heparin is included to help prevent platelet thrombi

TABLE 40–2.

Central Parenteral Nutrition in Infants*

CONSTITUENT	AMOUNT PER KG PER 24 HR
Glucose	15–30 g
Protein	2.0–4.0 g
Sodium	2.4 mEq
Potassium	2.4 mEq
Chloride	3–6 mEq
Magnesium	0.5–1.0 mEq
Calcium	0.5–3.0 mEq
Phosphate	0.5–1.0 mM
Trace elements†	0.5 mL
Multivitamin infusion (MVI)‡	1.0 mL/day
Vitamin K_1	0.5 mg/day
Vitamin B_{12}	5 μg/day
Folic acid	50 μg/day
Heparin	1.0 IU/mL
Glucose-protein volume	60–114 mL
Fat	1–4 g
10% fat emulsion volume	10–40 mL
Total volume	70–154 mL
Total calories	70–154

*Each 1000 mL of a standard solution is prepared by mixing 500 mL of 50% dextrose and water with 500 mL of 7% amino acids to give a final concentration of dextrose 25%–amino acid 3.5%. The appropriate amounts of electrolytes, vitamins, and trace elements are added according to the patient's weight.

†Each 0.5 ml of trace element solution (University of Michigan Pharmacy) contains: zinc, 100 μg; copper, 20 μg; manganese, 10 μg; chromium, 0.2 μg.

‡Each milliliter of MVI (USV Pharmaceutical Corporation) contains: vitamin A, 2000 IU; vitamin D, 200 IU; ascorbic acid, 100 IU; thiamine (vitamin B_1), 10 mg; riboflavin (vitamin B_2), 2 mg; niacinamide, 20 mg; pyridoxine, 3 mg; dexpanthenol, 5 mg; vitamin E, 1 IU.

and blood clots from forming at the catheter tip. The final solution contains 1 cal/mL. The infusion of 100 to 120 mL/kg body weight/day of this solution provides an appropriate mixture of glucose, amino acids, and other nutrients to meet the normal infant's need for tissue growth and repair. On the first day, the solution is given at half strength, diluted with equal volumes of 5% dextrose and water, to allow the patient to adapt to the osmotic load, thus preventing osmotic diuresis and hypertonic dehydration. Three-quarter strength solution is infused on the next day. When the patient's tolerance develops, as indicated by appropriate blood glucose levels and diminishing glucosuria, full-strength solution is used. Exogenous insulin is generally not required for nondiabetic children. Iron requirements are met by the daily addition of 2 mL of iron dextran (Imferon) to the solution, starting at 5 weeks of age. Trace elements are added to the basic mixture routinely. Linoleic acid, the essential fatty acid, is provided by the weekly infusion of a commercial fat emulsion in amounts totaling 2% to 4% of the patient's caloric requirements. The fat emulsion can also be used to provide additional nonprotein calories to the infant.

METABOLIC OBSERVATIONS

Infants on parenteral nutrition must be carefully monitored. Essential clinical measurements include daily body weight, weekly body length and head circumference, and accurate intake and output volumes. The urine sugar and acetone content are monitored, initially with each voiding and then, after the patient is stable, once each nursing shift. Judicious and sparing use of blood tests is important in infants, with their small total blood volume. Table 40–3 lists the recommended tests and frequency of monitoring for infants receiving TPN. More frequent monitoring of some parameters may be necessary in patients with spe-

TABLE 40–3.
Blood Values Monitored Routinely During Total Parenteral Nutrition

FREQUENCY OF MONITORING		
AT START OF THERAPY AND WEEKLY	AT START OF THERAPY AND EVERY 2 WK	AS INDICATED
Na, K, Cl	SGOT, LDH, alkaline phosphatase	Copper
Urea	Bilirubin, direct/total	Zinc
Glucose	Creatinine	Iron
Magnesium		Ammonia
Calcium, phosphorus		Osmolarity
Albumin		pH
Hb, Hct, WBC, platelets		

cific abnormalities, such as kidney or liver disease. Weight changes during intravenous nutrition vary with the patient's overall clinical status. During the first 2 weeks of therapy, significant weight gain is not commonly seen in infants who are severely depleted at the start of treatment. Weight gains comparable to those of normal infants may be expected in patients who are not severely malnourished or septic. Increased metabolic demands, such as from sepsis, result in a flatter growth curve. The average weight gain in the neonate on TPN is 15 to 25 g/day.

Positive nitrogen balance has been observed in almost all infants studied while receiving parenteral nutrition. Loss of amino acids from the urine is negligible, except in the very premature infant in whom the parenteral nutrition solution may produce an osmotic diuresis. The large amount of intravenous glucose is well tolerated by most infants, without the need for exogenous insulin. Blood sugar levels generally remain in the high normal range, with urinary glucose levels between 0 and 2+. If hyperglycemia and glycosuria occur, slowing the infusion rate or lowering the concentration of glucose usually solves the problem temporarily unless the patient is septic. Although TPN usually results in a greater excretion of solutes in the urine than is observed during oral feeding, this increased load does not exceed the concentrating ability of the normal kidney. As a result, water balance is usually well maintained.

COMPLICATIONS

The complications seen with parenteral nutrition are either technical or metabolic. All of the technical complications are related to the central venous catheter. The use of nonreactive silicone catheters in place of polyvinyl catheters has reduced the incidence of foreign-body reactions, vein perforation, and subclavian or vena cava thrombosis. The incidence of cardiac arrhythmias due to catheter irritation has been greatly reduced by placing the catheter at the tip of the superior vena cava and right atrium rather than in the heart. Likewise, radiologic control of catheter placement has removed the risk of hepatic necrosis from direct infusion of hypertonic solutions into the hepatic veins. Suturing the catheter to the skin and checking at each dressing change to be sure that the catheter is secured have reduced the frequency of catheter dislodgment. Thrombosis of the superior vena cava is usually well tolerated, but the superior vena cava syndrome does occasionally occur. Although pulmonary embolism is seen at autopsy in infants who have had a central venous catheter placed for TPN, the clinical manifestations of this complication are rare. Almost all of the technical complications inherent in central parenteral nutrition can be avoided by the use of peripheral parenteral nutrition, in which phlebitis and superficial skin sloughing are the most common complications. The incidence of phlebitis is reduced in these patients by the simultaneous infusion of intravenous fat. The infusion of fat reduced the osmolality of the glucose–amino acid solution and increases the pH of the solution, both of which appear to reduce the incidence of phlebitis. In addition, the fat emulsion itself, in some unknown way, appears to protect the vein from phlebitis.

Almost every conceivable metabolic abnormality has been reported during TPN. Table 40–4 lists the more commonly encountered abnormalities. Most of the metabolic complications are a result of administering too much or too little of a particular nutrient. Although serious consequences may ensue if these complications go undetected for any length of time, careful clinical monitoring and appropriate adjustment of the parenteral nutrition solution allow most patients to tolerate TPN quite well. A few of these complications will be discussed in the following sections.

TABLE 40–4.
Potential Metabolic Complications of Total Parenteral Nutrition

- Electrolyte imbalance
  - Hyper- or hyponatremia
  - Hyper- or hypokalemia
  - Hyper- or hypochloremia
  - Hyper- or hypocalcemia
  - Hyper- or hypomagnesemia
  - Hyper- or hypophosphatemia
- Carbohydrate administration
  - Hyper- or hypoglycemia
  - Hyperosmolarity and associated osmotic diuresis with dehydration, leading to nonketotic coma
- Protein administration
  - Cholestatic jaundice
  - Azotemia
  - Hyperchloremic metabolic acidosis (with protein hydrolysate)
- Lipid administration
  - Hyperlipidemia
  - Alteration of pulmonary function
  - Displacement of albumin-bonded bilirubin by plasma free fatty acid
  - "Overloading syndrome" characterized by hyperlipemia, fever, lethargy, liver damage, and coagulation disorders. This has been reported in adults but has been recognized rarely in children.
- Trace-element deficiencies
  - Zinc deficiency
  - Copper deficiency
  - Chromium deficiency
- Essential fatty acid deficiency
  - If lipids not used; manifested by skin rash

Hyperglycemia

Hyperglycemia is most common in the low-birth-weight or premature infant during the first 24 hours postoperatively, or in the presence of systemic sepsis. Once sepsis has been ruled out or effectively treated, hyperglycemia usually responds to diluting the parenteral nutrition solution and gradually increasing its concentration to full strength over a 24- to 48-hour period. If the hyperglycemia cannot be controlled by this manipulation, insulin may be added to the infusate. Nondiabetic infants rarely require added insulin.

Hypoglycemia

Although hypoglycemia has been reported when parenteral nutrition is abruptly terminated, we have never observed this complication, despite many accidental interruptions of infusions.

Hypocalcemia

Premature infants require relatively more calcium than full-term infants, and this must be taken into account when administering TPN to these infants.

Zinc Deficiency

Zinc deficiency is most commonly manifested by a seborrheic type of dermatitis, alopecia, and diarrhea. We have not observed this deficiency in any of our infants since we began to routinely add a trace-element solution to the infusate.

Fatty Acid Deficiency

Chemical signs of essential fatty acid deficiency may occur after as little as 2 to 3 weeks of fat-free parenteral nutrition, and consist of an increased serum level of 5,8,11-eicosatrienoic acid, low levels of linoleic and arachidonic acid, and an eicosatrienoic:arachidonic (triene-tetraene) ratio greater than 0.4. Clinical signs usually of the deficiency do not appear until after 2 to 3 months of fat-free therapy. Typically, a flaking, erythematous, papular skin rash develops, limited to the legs, chest, and face. This deficiency can be corrected by administering 2% to 4% of the patient's daily caloric requirements in the form of linoleic acid. Intralipid (Cutter; Berkeley, Calif.) contains 50% linoleic acid, and Liposyn (Abbott; North Chicago, Ill.) contains 77% linoleic acid. Most patients receiving a fat emulsion have normal serum triglyceride and cholesterol levels; a few who receive parenteral nutrition for longer than 1 month have serum triglyceride levels in the range of 300 to 350 mg/dL (normal: 50 to 100 mg/dL) and serum cholesterol values of 150 to 250 mg/dL (normal: 100 to 150 mg/dL). These mild elevations correct themselves once the fat emulsion is discontinued.

Cholestatic Jaundice

Abnormalities of liver function, such as elevations in serum glutamic oxaloacetic transaminase, (SGOT), lactate dehydrogenase (LDH), serum glutamic pyruvic transaminase (SGPT), and bilirubin have been reported within 2 to 14 days after beginning TPN, but histologic examination of the liver does not reveal any consistent pathologic change in most patients with these elevations. The elevations are variable and intermittent, and the SGOT, LDH, SGPT, and bilirubin levels return to normal once the parenteral nutrition therapy has been stopped. These elevations are seen in patients receiving parenteral nutrition with or without fat. In patients receiving intravenous fat, a fat pigment is usually seen in the Kuppffer cells of the liver after 1 month of therapy. The significance of this pigment is unknown. Severe cholestatic jaundice during TPN is seen only in the newborn, especially the premature newborn. The etiology of this abnormality is unknown, but may be related to the immaturity of the biliary excretory system in the infant. Cholestatic jaundice usually begins after 3 to 4 weeks of TPN and may progress to marked elevations in bilirubin of as high as 35 to 40 mg/dL, with the eventual development of severe cirrhosis. The only successful treatment for this condition is the cessation of parenteral nutrition and the institution of enteral feedings. The success of this treatment in reversing the cholestatic jaundice suggests that biliary stasis may be a significant contributory factor in this condition. Some investigators feel that the elevation of serum bile acids secondary to the bile stasis may contribute to the liver damage. Unfortunately, many of the infants who develop severe cholestatic jaundice cannot be weaned from their parenteral nutrition and placed on enteral nutrition, because their intestinal tract is not functioning. The infant with gastroschisis is a classic example of this dilemma; often, at 3 to 4 weeks postoperatively, the adynamic ileus in the infant has not cleared, and enteral feedings cannot be started. It is usually at this point that the bilirubin is beginning to climb rapidly as a result of the cholestatic jaundice, which rapidly progresses to fibrosis and cirrhosis. We have found that a small amount of enteral feeding at this point, added to the continuing TPN, will often reverse the progressive jaundice. In a recent study at our institution, we have shown that after 6 weeks of TPN in neonates, 45% have developed cholestasis, and by 12 weeks, 100% have cholestatic jaundice (Figs 40–3 and 40–4).[2]

Osmotic Diuresis

Osmotic diuresis occasionally occurs with a 25% glucose infusate, and is secondary to significant glucosuria. The premature infant, with underdeveloped re-

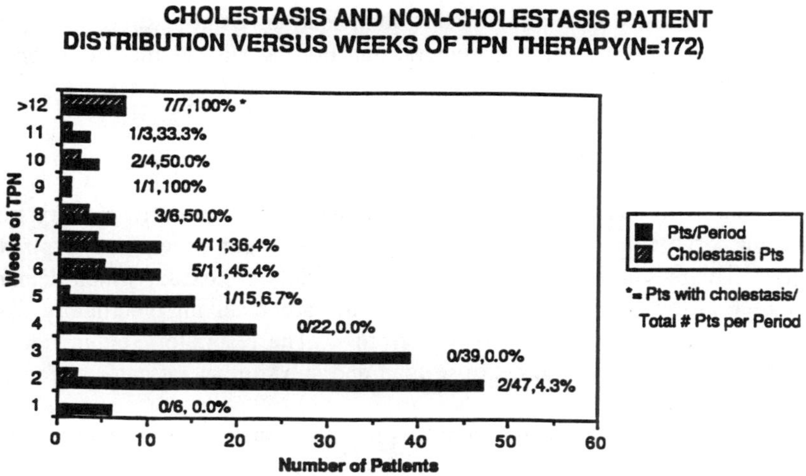

FIG 40–3.
This graph shows the incidence of cholestatic jaundice in relation to the duration in weeks of total parenteral nutrition. Note that by 6 weeks of therapy, 45% of the infants have developed cholestatic jaundice, and that by 12 weeks of therapy, 100% have developed cholestatic jaundice.

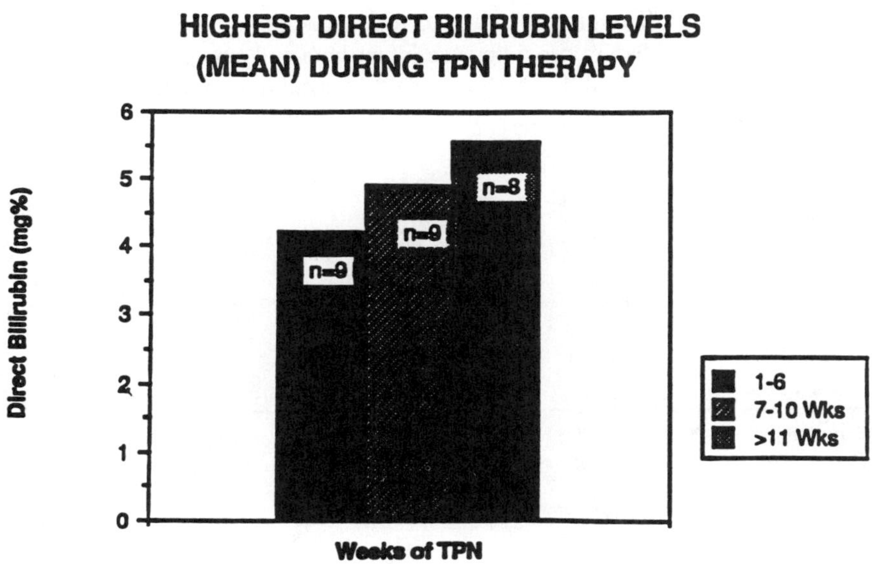

FIG 40–4.
This graph shows the highest direct bilirubin levels achieved by infants suffering from cholestatic jaundice during total parenteral nutrition.

nal tubules, is most susceptible to this complication. Osmotic diuresis is generally not seen with peripheral parenteral nutrition because of the lower tonicity of the infusate.

Respiratory Failure

In patients with obstructive airway disease and compromised respiratory function, the large dextrose load in parenteral nutrition can precipitate respiratory failure. This is due to the high production of carbon dioxide, which demands increased respiratory work. If these patients are receiving ventilatory assistance, they may be difficult to wean from it. The respiratory failure may be resolved by decreasing the dextrose load and substituting fat calories for dextrose calories.

Once the intestines of the infant with gastroschisis begin to work, enteral feedings can be started. Premature infants may have more difficulty with oral feedings than full-term infants because they have not yet fully developed the complex physiology of sucking and swallowing. Under these circumstances, gavage tube feedings can be started and used until the infant is able to feed orally. Oral or tube feedings should be started with small volumes of sugar water, with the volume gradually increased over the next 12 to 24 hours. Infants tolerate increases in volume much better than increases in concentration of the formula, and it is therefore preferable to reach the appropriate volume of formula for the infant before providing the infant with full-strength formula. It is important to keep in mind that high-osmolality formulas are poorly tolerated by infants; this intolerance is usually manifested by diarrhea and vomiting (Table 40–5).

TABLE 40–5.
Composition of Infant Formulas

	KCAL							
FORMULA	(PER OZ)	(PER ML)	NA (MEQ/L)	K (MEQ/L)	CA (MG/L)	P (MG/L)	FE (MG/L)	OSMOLARITY (MOSM/L)
Breast milk	20	0.67	7	14	340	162	1.5	100
Cow's milk	20	0.67	25	35	1240	950	1	270
Enfamil	20	0.67	11	19	546	462	Trace	285
Nutramigen	20	0.67	14	17	630	473	13	460
Portagen	20	0.67	14	21	630	473	13	210
Pregestimil	20	0.67	14	17	630	473	13	311
ProSobee	20	0.67	18	19	788	525	13	250
Similac 20	20	0.67	11	19	580	430	Trace	285
SMA	20	0.67	7	15	400	200	12	250

If the infant has an inadequate amount of small intestine, as can occur in an infant with gastroschisis and intestinal atresia such as the propositus in the case described at the beginning of this chapter, then one is dealing with the short-gut syndrome. A full-term infant is born with approximately 200 cm of small intestine. Although there is no clearly defined lower limit of intestinal length compatible with life, most pediatric surgeons believe that less than 25 to 30 cm of small intestine, with an intact ileocecal valve, is incompatible with survival on oral alimentation. Without an ileocecal valve, approximately 50 cm of small bowel is necessary to sustain life. Once short-gut syndrome is diagnosed, the program for management of the infant is complex and not well defined. In general, the care of these patients requires a combination of parenteral nutrition, elemental diets, and predigested formulas. Gradually, regular feedings are achieved over a period of several weeks to several months. Requirements for growth and development should be kept in mind at all times, and these patients should be maintained on parenteral nutrition with all the necessary carbohydrate, fat, and protein calories while various diets are manipulated. Thereafter, the intravenous nutrition is gradually tapered and the gastrointestinal tract adapts to oral feedings. Since infants with a short bowel have very little tolerance for even moderately hypertonic diets, predigested formulas such as Pregestamil should be administered in very dilute form. The volume is increased gradually over several days to weeks, and only after sufficient volume is tolerated is the concentration slowly increased. If these diets are not well tolerated in any concentration, an elemental diet such as Vivonex can be tried in very dilute form. As the infant grows, its nourishment supplemented by intravenous calories, the intestine begins to adapt through lengthening, dilatation, and villous hypertrophy, and oral diets become more readily tolerated. It is not unusual for these infants to be hospitalized for periods ranging from several months to a year or more. During this time, the infant may have several setbacks that may discourage the parents and the medical staff. This discouragement may lead to decreased attention to the critical details involved in the management of these complex cases. This decreased attention to detail can be countered by maintaining a high morale among the physicians, nutritionists, and nurses caring for these infants.

REFERENCES

1. Coran AG, Drongowski RA: Body fluid compartment changes following neonatal surgery. *J Pediatr Surg* 1989; 24:829–832.
2. Drongowski RA, Coran AG: An analysis of factors contributing to the development of TPN-induced cholestasis. *J Parenter Enter Nutr* 1989; 13:586–589.

41

Airway Management

Keith W. Ashcraft, M.D.

A 3.0-kg neonate aspirated meconium during vaginal delivery and required tracheal suctioning, endotracheal intubation, and ventilator support. After a prolonged course of ventilator support (more than 1 month's duration) the infant improved. Attempts were made to wean the infant from the ventilator. This was successful and a $Paco_2$ of 42 torr and Pao_2 of 75 torr with an Fio_2 of 0.3 was noted on a simple continuous positive-airway pressure (CPAP)-blow-by humidified system attached to the endotracheal tube. Following attempted extubation, however, the infant developed tachypnea and stridor associated with both sternal and intercostal retractions. Repeat blood gas analysis showed a $Paco_2$ of 58 torr and a Pao_2 of 50 torr, with a pH of 7.28.

Prolonged intubation for the ventilatory management of meconium aspiration syndrome is most likely to produce subglottic edema, resulting in the situation described above. An endotracheal tube that is tight enough to prevent leakage under the conditions of high-pressure ventilation needed for the treatment of meconium aspiration will fit the airway most snugly at the level of the cricoid cartilage, just below the glottis. As the patient recovers from meconium aspiration and begins to breathe on his own, the endotracheal tube serves as a means by which the airway is kept open. Although satisfactory ventilation is demonstrated, removal of the tube results in the classic signs of airway obstruction: tachypnea, stridor, retraction, CO_2 retention, and respiratory acidosis. The dilemma facing the surgeon in the neonatal intensive care unit (ICU) at this time is to first determine whether the patient can be safely maintained without reintubation, and second to quickly run through the differential diagnostic list of other possible causes for the child's upper airway obstruction.

Intubation from the first minutes of life is most likely to be the etiology of the subsequent airway obstruction in the infant described above, but by the same token, intubation in the first few minutes of life may have masked a congenital lesion that now only becomes apparent on decannulation of the infant. Table 41–1 includes four lesions that may have been congenital and yet undiscovered in this clinical situation, all exceedingly unusual, and except for tracheomalacia, unlikely to occur as acute obstructive phenomena under the circumstances described in this patient's clinical history. Subglottic hemangioma is often associated with cutaneous hemangioma, and produces its airway obstruction when the patient is crying or otherwise exerting himself, at which time increased venous pressure produces engorgement of the hemangioma and obstruction of the airway. Vascular ring malformations, unless a very tight double aortic arch or a vascular sling malformation in which the left pulmonary artery crosses between the trachea and esophagus, are unlikely to produce airway obstruction as their primary lesion. Most often, the patient with a double aortic arch presents with difficulty in swallowing and breathing at the same time. The malformations most commonly associated with the vascular sling are complete cartilaginous rings in a very small trachea, extending down to and sometimes beyond the carina, an obstructive situation that is usually not relieved by endotracheal intubation. A bronchogenic or esophageal cyst compressing the trachea may produce acute obstruction upon removal of the endotracheal tube. These lesions are so uncommon as to not be in serious consideration in this clinical picture. Tracheomalacia is usually associated with esophageal atresia, which produces compression of the tracheal cartilages as they develop. It is unlikely to be an isolated lesion.

Pulmonary interstitial edema (PIE) or bronchopulmonary dysplasia (BPD) are other possible causes for the patient's clinical picture, and may be a result of the barotrauma from the treatment of meconium aspiration syndrome. The physiologic disorders occurring as a result of PIE or BPD, however, should produce hypoxia and hypocarbia, even when the patient was intubated but not being ventilated.

TABLE 41–1.

Lesions Producing Airway Obstruction or Hypoventilation in the Newborn

Lesions Producing Airway Obstruction or Hypoventilation in the Newborn
Subglottic hemangioma
Vascular ring
Bronchogenic/esophageal cyst
Tracheomalacia
Pulmonary interstitial emphysema (PIE) or bronchopulmonary dysplasia (BPD)
Vocal cord ulceration
Vocal cord paralysis
Subglottic edema
Subglottic stenosis

The most likely causes for the patient's clinical picture are subglottic edema, as was mentioned earlier, ulceration of the vocal cords, or subglottic stenosis obstructing the patient's airway. Edema is the most likely acute situation. Cord ulceration is uncommon in our experience. Congenital paralysis of the vocal cords may produce the clinical picture described. We have seen two patients with this lesion, both of whom had esophageal atresia. Subglottic stenosis, as a result of prolonged intubation, is a very real possibility, but would be a diagnosis that could only be established upon endoscopy.

The etiology of both subglottic edema and its sequela, subglottic stenosis, is the pressure of the endotracheal tube on the narrowest portion of the airway. The airway mucosa is very subject to edema formation, as is evident by the response of the airway to any sort of viral illness or bacterial invasion. We have long entertained the belief that a nasotracheal tube moves less in the pharynx, and that less motion therefore occurs in the subglottic region than occurs with an orotracheal airway, which is subject to the action of the mandible and tongue. Although I know of no evidence to prove that subglottic edema and stenosis occur less commonly in nasotracheally intubated infants, we have always preferred that route of intubation. The neonatologists in our institution, however, prefer the orotracheal tube, especially in those infants who might have to be put on extracorporeal membrane oxygenation (ECMO) and require anticoagulation, thinking that it produces less risk of bleeding from the turbinates. Lateral pressure from the tube on the subglottic area, and friction from motion, will rapidly result in edema formation. Should the subglottic area have been compressed to the point of erosion or necrosis of the mucosa, scar formation will occur around the tube. Upon removal of the tube, airway obstruction becomes apparent.

This postulate fits with the clinical situation of the patient described above, who breathes satisfactorily with the endotracheal tube in place but quickly develops hypercarbia and acidosis once the tube is removed.

The definitive diagnosis of subglottic edema or stenosis can often be made indirectly. Our plan of attack would be to attempt to avoid further acidosis while trying to avoid reintubation. Dexamethasone (Decadron), administered in a dose of approximately 1 mg/kg, will sometimes relieve acute subglottic edema to the point at which the patient can breathe comfortably and maintain satisfactory respiration until the acute edema has further cleared and the patient's airway is once again as patent as it can be. If given our choice, we would administer the dexamethasone perhaps an hour before extubation, simply to avoid, if possible, the situation in which the steroid must exert its effect while the patient is in respiratory distress. If, however, the patient has been extubated, is laboring to breathe, and is becoming acidotic, we would very carefully monitor the respiratory effort and the blood gases while giving dexamethasone and hoping for the best. The action of the dexamethasone and the relief of the respiratory effort should occur within 30 minutes if it is going to be effective. If the patient is becoming more acidotic or has flaring of the nostrils and is obviously exerting increasing effort to breathe, then reintubation is certainly necessary, with perhaps a half-millimeter smaller tube than was previously placed. Mechanical ventilation may be needed for a period of time in order to allow the child to rest while the blood gases are normalized. Our approach would be to leave the patient intubated overnight and to administer another dose of dexamethasone about 1 hour before the next decannulation.

If the obstruction-acidosis situation again occurs, reintubation is done and plans are made for further diagnostic study. At the time of reintubation, some assessment of vocal-cord motion is made. We would then plan a rigid bronchoscopy to inspect the airway from above the glottis to the carina and beyond. This would be done under general anesthesia in the operating room. Subglottic edema can be differentiated bronchoscopically from a firm subglottic stenosis, which is the likely etiology of this extended scenario. Supraglottic cysts or webs, granulomas, or other obstructive lesions may certainly be visualized and, if the patient is only lightly anesthetized, tracheomalacia or other obstructive lesions of the trachea will likewise be apparent. The diagnostic accuracy of rigid bronchoscopy under anesthesia is immeasurably superior to flexible bronchoscopy in the conscious patient at our institution.

Following establishment of the diagnosis of subglottic stenosis, we would once again attempt extubation. If subglottic stenosis is to be successfully managed without tracheostomy, the child should be able to breathe and maintain "satisfactory" blood gas tensions, although some CO_2 retention is commonly seen for a while. The definitive test of whether satisfactory ventilation is possible is to observe whether the patient can breathe, eat, and gain weight. Growth may well be the only fully satisfactory treatment for subglottic stenosis. As the patient grows, the stridor, retraction, and hypercarbia will resolve. If the patient is unable to gain weight under these conditions, then the establishment of a tracheostomy is in order.

Once the tracheostomy has been placed, a surgical approach to the subglottic stenosis may be selected. We have successfully used dilatations in many instances of subglottic stenosis, sometimes in association with intralesional steroid injections, but we have found the steroid injections to be of very little benefit in the management of rigid fibrous subglottic stenosis. We have had no experience with laser resection of subglottic stenosis and will therefore not comment further on it. Should resolution of the stenosis not be apparent after several dilatations, then surgery is indicated. We have tried many different surgical approaches to subglottic stenosis, but by far the best is the procedure described by Gerwat and Bryce,[1] which is an anterior wedge resection of the cricoid cartilage (Fig 41–1). In our experience, this works quite well and is far preferable to either the Cotton operation, which turns a block of thyroid carti-

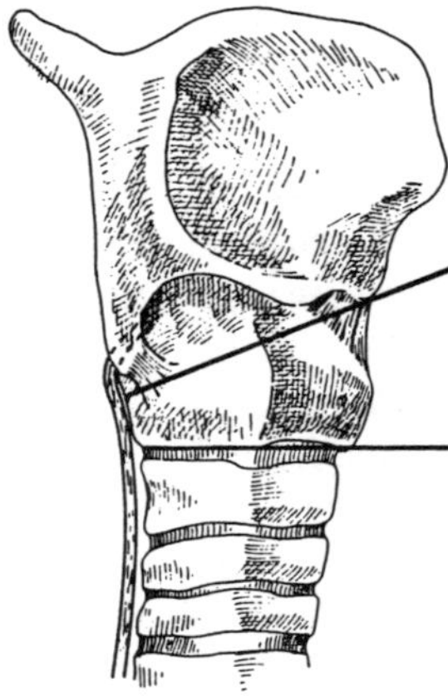

FIG 41–1.
Subtotal cricoid resection for subglottic stenosis after the method of Gerwat and Bryce.[1] The cricoid is wedged out, removing essentially all of the narrowed area, anteriorly and on each side, preserving the articulation of the cricoid cartilage with the thyroid cartilages posteriorly, and thereby protecting the recurrent laryngeal nerves. The first tracheal ring is then sutured to the cricothyroid membrane, which remains. Stents are not used, but a tracheostomy is required. (From Gerwat J, Bryce DP: *Laryngoscope* 1974; 84:940–957. Used with permission.)

lage down to insert into the anteriorly opened cricoid cartilage, or the Evans procedure, which is an extensive procedure used to enlarge the cricoid ring. The anterior cricoid wedge resection requires no stenting of the airway, and allows immediate relief with quite satisfactory preservation of cord function because the recurrent nerves are not at risk. The cords are not subjected to long-term stenting, which has reduced the success rate for the other procedures.

REFERENCES

1. Gerwat J, Bryce DP: The management of subglottic laryngeal stenosis by resection and direct anastomosis. *Laryngoscope* 1974; 84:940.

42

Bleeding and Clotting Disorders

Amy Shapiro, M.D.

A 2-month-old boy entered the ambulatory surgical suite for outpatient repair of an inguinal hernia. The child was a full-term infant who had had an uneventful spontaneous vaginal delivery. Physical examination showed a well-nourished and -developed infant boy with a large right inguinoscrotal bulge. The 4.0-kg infant had not been circumcised. His preoperative hemoglobin was 12.0 g and his hematocrit was 39%. Herniorrhaphy was performed under general anesthesia. The procedure was complicated by continual oozing from the subcutaneous and deep tissues. Use of an electrocoagulator appeared to resolve the problem. Pressure was kept on the subcuticular closure for 5 minutes to stop oozing from the skin edges. The patient was brought to the recovery area. Approximately 15 minutes later, the wound was checked by the nurse, who noted that the dressings were soaked with blood. A repeat hemoglobin was 8.0 g with a hematocrit of 26%. The partial thromboplastin time was approximately twice the upper limit of normal.

This case illustrates a child with abnormal bleeding in association with a surgical procedure. The hemorrhage has been significant, with a subsequent decrease in the hemoglobin. Disorders leading to abnormalities of hemostasis need to be considered. The initial laboratory workup should include a basic hemostatic screen to evaluate for the more common disorders of coagulation. A basic hemostatic screen includes a prothrombin time (PT), partial thromboplastin time (PTT), fibrinogen, thrombin time (TT), fibrin split products (FSP), and bleeding time (BT), as well as a complete blood count with platelet count. The initial laboratory evaluation in this child revealed a PTT of approximately twice normal.

Evaluation should proceed rapidly in a bleeding child, to determine the cause of the prolongation of the PTT. A study should be performed to determine if the prolongation of the PTT is secondary to a coagulation factor deficiency or to the presence of an inhibitor. This is accomplished by repeating the PTT after mixing test plasma with normal plasma. Complete correction of the PTT is characteristic of a coagulation-factor deficiency; lack of complete correction indicates the presence of an inhibitor. This child had complete correction of the PTT.

Further evaluation includes specific coagulation factor analysis. Abnormalities of the procoagulants XII, XI, IX, VIII, as well as the contact factors, which include high-molecular-weight kininogen (HMWK) and prekallikrein (PK), lead to prolongation of the PTT with a normal PT. A deficiency of factor XI, factor IX, and factor VIII may lead to a bleeding diathesis, whereas a deficiency of the remaining procoagulants, XII, HMWK, PK, is not associated with a hemorrhagic tendency. It is vital that the specific coagulation factor deficiency be established in order for optimal therapy to be instituted.

BACKGROUND

The most common factor deficiencies leading to a hemorrhagic tendency are often referred to as the hemophilias. The hemophilias are in inheritable group of bleeding disorders characterized by absent or decreased quantities of functional procoagulants. The most common of these disorders are hemophilia A (factor VIII deficiency), hemophilia B (factor IX deficiency), hemophilia C (factor XI deficiency), and von Willebrand's disease.

Factor VIII and factor IX deficiencies are inherited as sex-linked recessive traits. Males are affected and females are carriers. Factor XI deficiency is seen most commonly in persons of Ashkenazi Jewish descent, and is inherited as an autosomal recessive trait, with males and females equally affected. Von Willebrand's disease is most commonly inherited in an autosomal dominant fashion, with males and females equally affected. A rarer form of von Willebrand's disease (type III) is severe and inherited in an autosomal recessive pattern. Individuals with type III von Willebrand's disease may have bleeding patterns similar to those with severe hemophilia. Individuals with hemophilia A or B may not have a family history of other affected individuals. Lack of a family history of hemophilia may occur in sporadic cases secondary to new mutations, or may be due to the deficiency having been previously carried silently within the family.

Hemophilia A and B are divided into three groups based on the level of procoagulant. Severely deficient individuals have levels below 1%, moderately deficient individuals have levels between 1% and 5%, and mildly affected individuals have levels greater than or equal to 5% and usually below 30%. These categories are associated with differing patterns of bleeding episodes. Patients with a severe deficiency may experience spontaneous bleeding episodes, often starting when they become mobile in childhood. Bleeding episodes in severely deficient patients may occur as frequently as two to four times per month, and often involve, but are not limited to, the joints, muscles, and skin. Moderately deficient patients have less frequent bleeding episodes. Often a history of injury may be elicited. Mildly affected individuals bleed infrequently, and usually only in association with injury, trauma, or surgery.

Individuals with von Willebrand's disease most commonly have bruising and bleeding from their mucous membranes. Hemorrhage after dental work, surgery, or laceration; spontaneous epistaxis; bruising; menorrhagia; postpartum hemorrhage; and gastrointestinal-tract bleeding constitute the most common bleeding episodes in individuals with von Willebrand's disease. Von Willebrand's disease is divided into subtypes based on the plasma and platelet multimeric structure of the von Willebrand factor. The disease may be associated with abnormalities in factor VIII coagulant activity, in the von Willebrand factor antigen, in the ristocetin cofactor activity of the von Willebrand factor, in the bleeding time, and in the in vitro platelet response to ristocetin.

TREATMENT

In a bleeding child with a suspected disorder of coagulation, it is imperative to maintain intravenous access. Frequent monitoring of vital signs should be done and an ongoing estimate of blood loss should be obtained. As the diagnostic work-up is rapidly pursued, a type and crossmatch analysis for packed red blood cells should be performed. Fresh-frozen plasma (minimum: 10 to 20 cc/kg) should be set aside for use if the bleeding is uncontrollable with local measures and a specific diagnosis is not yet available. Fresh-frozen plasma contains the full complement of coagulation factors, but its use may result in difficulty restoring the deficient procoagulant to a hemostatic level (approximately 20%) in individuals with severely deficient hemophilia. The rate of transfusion of the fresh-frozen plasma should be based on the status of the child's blood volume. Packed red blood cells and fresh-frozen plasma are more efficient than fresh whole blood for replacing lost red blood cell mass and providing deficient procoagulants.

Once a definitive diagnosis is established, specific replacement of the coagulation factor will rapidly correct the bleeding diathesis.

FACTOR VIII DEFICIENCY

In children with hemophilia A who are experiencing active bleeding in association with a surgical procedure, the factor VIII level should be corrected to approximately 80% to 100% activity. One unit of factor VIII equals the activity of factor VIII in 1 cc of normal plasma. The number of units needed to achieve a desired level is based on the patient's weight in kilograms and the volume of distribution of factor VIII, which is approximately 0.5. Therefore, in a 4-kg child:

$$\text{Number of units} = \text{level desired} \times \text{weight (kg)} \times 0.5$$

$$\text{Number of units} = 100\% \times 4 \times 0.5$$

$$\text{Number of units} = 200$$

Vials of factor concentrate are tested for activity and labeled with the number of units contained. The assay of each vial is the number of units it contains. The closest assay vial in relation to the number of calculated units needed should be used. All of the units contained within the vial should be infused into the patient rather than discarded, since they represent a costly product. Factor VIII concentrate may be given by an intravenous bolus over the relatively short period of approximately 5 minutes. Each package of factor VIII concentrate comes with the supplies needed for reconstitution of the lyophilized coagulation factor, as well as directions for its reconstitution and administration.

Much progress has been made in developing new factor VIII concentrates through advanced technologies. Close attention should be given to the factor concentrate chosen for children who have never been exposed to blood products, including factor concentrates. Products are available that are pure and safe from transmitting blood-borne viral infections such as hepatitis B, hepatitis non-A/non-B, and the human immune deficiency virus (HIV), which causes AIDS. A national network of comprehensive hemophilia centers exists throughout the United States and Canada, and has available the most up-to-date information about product availability.

FACTOR IX DEFICIENCY

In children with hemophilia B who are experiencing active bleeding in association with a surgical procedure, the factor IX activity should be corrected to approximately 80% to 100% of its normal activity. One unit of factor IX equals the amount of factor IX activity in 1 cc of normal plasma. The number of units needed to achieve a desired activity level is based on the patient's weight in kilograms and the volume of distribution of factor IX, which is approximately 1.0. Therefore in a 4-kg child:

$$\text{Number of units} = \text{level desired} \times \text{weight (kg)} \times 1.0$$

$$\text{Number of units} = 100\% \times 4 \times 1.0$$

$$\text{Number of units} = 400$$

As detailed in the discussion of factor VIII deficiency, the vial with the closest assayed content of factor IX concentrate to that which is needed should be chosen, and the entire contents infused. Factor IX concentrate should be infused over approximately 10 to 20 minutes, with adjustments for side effects associated with these products, such as activation of the coagulation, complement, and bradykinin systems.

Unfortunately, advances in technology that have greatly improved the available factor VIII concentrates have lagged behind in the development of pure factor IX concentrates that do not transmit blood-borne viral infections. Consultation with a comprehensive hemophilia center is imperative when determining the best product available for use in a previously untransfused, factor IX-deficient hemophila patient. Until factor IX concentrates shown in clinical studies not to transmit blood-borne viral infections are readily available, one should assume that hepatitis may be transmitted in currently available products, and appropriate measures should be taken to minimize exposure to it. Comprehensive hemophilia centers may have access to promising new products that are available through clinical trials. In emergent situations requiring the infusion of a factor IX concentrate that is not free of the risk of transmitting hepatitis, hepatitis immune globulin should be administered concomitantly. All hemophilia patients must receive the hepatitis B immunization series, which should be instituted as soon as the diagnosis of hemophilia has been established.

OTHER DEFICIENCIES

Deficiency of procoagulants other than factor VIII or factor IX may lead to a bleeding diathesis. Treatment of the rarer procoagulant factor deficiencies is best done in collaboration with a comprehensive hemophilia treatment center.

Optimal therapy for patients with von Willebrand's disease is determined by the subtype of the disease. In emergent situations, therapy consists of replacement with exogenous, normal von Willebrand factor. Von Willebrand factor is contained in cryoprecipitate. Calculation of the necessary dosage for patients with von Willebrand's disease is the same as that in factor VIII deficiency. It is assumed that each unit of cryoprecipitate contains approximately 100 units of factor VIII. The usual factor concentrates used to treat factor VIII-deficient hemophilia patients will not achieve hemostasis in an individual with von Willebrand's disease, since they do not contain intact von Willebrand factor. However, there exist factor VIII concentrates that are pasteurized and also contain von Willebrand factor. These products and how to obtain them are best discussed with the regional comprehensive hemophilia center.

FURTHER MANAGEMENT

The treatment discussed thus far deals with the immediate management of a bleeding child with an inherited deficiency of coagulation. Once the diagnosis has been established and acute management has been instituted, with the establishment of hemostasis and stable hemodynamics, a plan should be formulated for deciding the duration and frequency of replacement therapy. This plan is based on the half-life of the deficient factor and the period required for healing. Surgical procedures such as uncomplicated herniorrhaphies require replacement therapy for at least 10 days.

The half-life of factor VIII is approximately 12 hours, while that of factor IX is closer to 18 to 20 hours. Therefore, once the patient has received a bolus infusion of factor VIII concentrate, one expects the factor VIII level to be approximately half of the infused dose in 12 hours. Continuous infusion of factor VIII concentrate is possible, and allows the maintenance of a steady level of factor VIII activity. Continuous infusion of factor IX concentrate is not possible, and intermittent bolus infusions are necessary to maintain hemostasis. Thrombotic episodes have been reported as complications of either large doses or in association with prolonged use of factor IX concentrate. Daily monitoring of the activity level of the deficient factor, PT, PTT, fibrinogen, FSP, TT, and complete blood count with platelet count is important in the postoperative management of the hemophilia patient.

SUMMARY

The case described at the beginning of this chapter involves a child with abnormal bleeding after a surgical procedure secondary to an inherited disorder of coagulation. Rapid evaluation and prompt intervention are required in order to achieve hemostasis. A hematologist with knowledge and experience in the management of individuals with inherited disorders of coagulation should be involved at the earliest possible time, so that appropriate planning and optimal management will be achieved. A network of regionalized comprehensive hemophilia centers exists throughout the United States to provide up-to-date information and assistance in the treatment of individuals with hemophilia.

Index

A

Abdomen
  mass in, in preoperative evaluation of choledochal cyst patient, 207–208
  pain in, in immunosuppressed patient, 108–111 (*see also* Typhlitis in immunosuppressed patient)
  trauma to, blunt, 236–243
    assessment of, 237–239
      initial, 236–327
    management of, initial, 236–237
    treatment of specific organ injury in, 240–243
  viscera of, evaluation of, in resuscitation of injured child, 234–235
Abused child, blunt abdominal trauma in, 236–243
Achalasia of esophagus, 162–167
  clinical presentation of, 162–163
  diagnostic evaluation of, 163
  differential diagnosis of, 163–165
  therapeutic options and outcomes for, 165–167
Age, risk of pelvic inflammatory disease and, 93–94
Airway
  examination of, in resuscitation of injured child, 233
  management of, 290–294
    dexamethasone in, 292–293
    tracheostomy in, 293–294
  obstruction of, postextubation, differential diagnosis of, 290–292
Anemia, sickle cell, cholelithiasis and, 215–220
Anesthesia for hernia in premature neonate, 7–8
Aortic injury from thoracic trauma, 246
Apnea after hernia in premature neonate, 7
Appendices, gonadal, torsion of, 64
Appendicitis, acute, 71–76
  diagnostic tests for, 73
  differential diagnosis of, 75
  history of, 71–72
  pathogenesis of, 71–72
  physical examination in, 72
  treatment of, 75–76
Asphyxia, traumatic, from thoracic trauma, 246
Atresia
  biliary, 197–204 (*see also* Biliary atresia)
  esophageal, 141–153 (*see also* Esophageal atresia)
Autotransplantation of abdominal testes into scrotum for bilateral undescended testes, 56

B

Bacteremia complicating long-term central vascular access, 275
Barium swallow in gastroesophageal reflux diagnosis, 170
Bethanechol in gastroesophageal reflux management, 173
Bile duct reconstruction after choledochal cyst resection, 211
Biliary atresia, 197–204
  diagnostic evaluation of, 197–198
  pathology of, 198–199
  postoperative complications in, 201–203
  prognosis in, 204
  surgical management of, 200–201
Bleeding disorders, 295–300 (*see also* Clotting disorders)
Bowel
  disease of, inflammatory, 113–118 (*see also* Crohn's disease (CD))
  incarceration of, complicating inguinal hernia in premature neonate, 3–4
  perforation of, complicating intussusception, 80–81
  small, blunt trauma to, treatment of, 241
Branchial cleft cyst, 257–258
Breathing
  examination of, in resuscitation of injured child, 233–234
  periodic, after hernia in premature neonate, 7
Bronchogenic cyst, airway obstruction from, 291
Bronchopulmonary dysplasia (BPD)
  airway obstruction from, 291
  complicating hernia in premature neonate, 6
Broviac/Hickman catheter vs. total implantation of vascular access device, 272–273

C

Catheter(s)
  breakage of, complicating long-term central vascular access, 274
  external, vs. total implantation of vascular access device, 272–273
Caustic stricture of esophagus, 175–183
  conservative management of, 176
  emergency room management of, 175–176
  esophageal perforation complicating, 179–180
  intraluminal esophageal stent for, 176–177
    discussion of, 181–183
    results of, 180–181
Cervical lymphadenopathy, management of, 264–266
Cervical spine
  examination of, in resuscitation of injured child, 234
  stabilization of, in resuscitation of injured child, 233
Child abuse, blunt abdominal trauma from, 236–243
Cholangitis complicating surgery for biliary atresia, 201–203
Choledochal cyst, 206–213
  postoperative management of, 211–213
  preoperative evaluation of, 207–208
  resection of, 209–211
  surgery for
    preparation for, 208
    procedure for, 208–211
Cholelithiasis, 215–220
  postoperative care in, 219–220
  in sickle cell anemia patient
    diagnosis of, 216–217
    preoperative preparation in, 217–219
  surgical management of, 219
Cholestatic jaundice complicating parenteral nutrition, 286, 287
Chronic ulcerative colitis (CUC), 113, 114, 115
Cimetidine in gastroesophageal reflux management, 173
Circulation, examination of, in resuscitation of injured child, 234
Cisapride in gastroesophageal reflux management, 173

Clotting disorders, 295–300
background of, 296–297
from factor IX deficiency, 298–299
from factor VIII deficiency, 297–298
management of, 300
treatment of, 297
in von Willebrand's disease, 299–300
Colitis, ulcerative, chronic, 113, 114, 115
Colon for esophageal replacement, 155
left, retrohilar route for, 157–158
right, retrosternal route for, 157
Computed tomography (CT) scanning
abdominal, for blunt abdominal trauma evaluation, 238
in typhlitis, 110
Congenital cysts and sinuses of neck, 257–259
Constipation, acute appendicitis differentiated from, 74
Contraceptives, risk of pelvic inflammatory disease and, 94
Crohn's disease, 113–118
clinical presentation of, 114
endoscopy in, 114–115
roentgenographic studies in, 115
therapy of, 116–118
Cryptorchidism, 51–58
bilateral, 55–58
impalpable, 58
in premature neonate, inguinal hernia and, 3
unilateral, 51–54
orchiopexy for, 52–54
Cyst(s)
bronchogenic, airway obstruction from, 291
choledochal, 206–213 (*see also* Choledochal cyst)
congenital, of neck, 257–259
esophageal, airway obstruction from, 291
Cystic hygroma, 260–263
management of
anterolateral and posterior compartment in, 261–262
intraoral hypopharyngeal area in, 262
trachea in, 261
sequela of, 262–263

D

Deafness, congenital, Hirschsprung's disease and, 125
Dexamethasone for subglottic edema/stenosis, 292–293
DiGeorge syndrome, 258
Diuresis, osmotic, complicating parenteral nutrition, 286, 288
Diverticulectomy, prophylactic, in Meckel's diverticulum, 130–131
Diverticulum, Meckel's, 127–131
Down's syndrome, Hirschsprung's disease and, 125
Duodenum, trauma to, 249–254
blunt to, treatment of, 240–241
clinical features of, 250
diagnosis of, 251–252
high-energy, 249–250
low-energy, 249
pathology of, 250–251
pathophysiology of, 250–251
prognosis for, 253–254
treatment of, 252–253

E

Edema
bronchopulmonary, airway obstruction from, 291
subglottic, airway obstruction from, 292
Endoscopy
in Crohn's disease, 114–115
in gastroesophageal reflux diagnosis, 171–172
Enterocolitis
necrotizing, 132–138 (*see also* Necrotizing enterocolitis)
superimposed on Hirschsprung's disease, 119–126 (*see also* Hirschsprung's disease with superimposed enterocolitis)
Epididymo-orchitis, testicular torsion differentiated from, 64–65
Erosion of catheter through vessel/wall complicating long-term central vascular access, 273
Esophageal atresia (EA), 141–153
with tracheoesophageal fistula, 141–147
assessment of, 142–145
esophageal, 143–144

Esophageal atresia (EA) *(cont.)*
evaluation in, 144–145
other anomalies in, 144
pulmonary status in, 144
postoperative management of, 146
presentation of, 141–142
results in, 146–147
surgical management of, 145–147
type A, 148–153
esophagoesophagostomy in, 152–153
gastrostomy in, 149
stretching of upper esophageal segment in, 150–152
Esophagoesophagostomy in type A esophageal atresia, 152–153
Esophagomyotomy, Heller, modified, for achalasia of esophagus, 166
Esophagoscopy in gastroesophageal reflux diagnosis, 171–172
Esophagus
achalasia of, 162–167 (*see also* Achalasia of esophagus)
atresia of, 141–153 (*see also* Esophageal atresia)
caustic stricture of, 175–183 (*see also* Caustic stricture of esophagus)
cyst of, airway obstruction from, 291
replacement procedures for, 154–160
colon in, 155
operative procedures for, 157–158
complications of, 160
gastric tube in, 155–156
operative procedures for, 158–159
jejunum in, 156
operative procedures for, 159–160
operative procedures for, 156–160
postoperative care in, 160
stomach in, 156
operative procedures for, 159
spasm of, diffuse, achalasia of esophagus differentiated from, 165
External catheter vs. total implantation of vascular access device, 272–273

F

Factor VIII deficiency, 297–298
Factor IX deficiency, 298–299
Factor XI deficiency, 296
Fat malabsorption complicating surgery for biliary atresia, 203
Fatty acid deficiency complicating parenteral nutrition, 285–286
Feeding, thickened, in gastroesophageal reflux management, 173
Fistula, tracheoesophageal, esophageal atresia with, 141–147 (*see also* Esophageal atresia (EA) with tracheoesophageal fistula)
Fracture(s)
of rib from thoracic trauma, 245
splinting of, in resuscitation of injured child, 235
Fundoplication, Nissen, for gastroesophageal reflux, 173–174

G

Gallstones, 215–220 (*see also* Cholelithiasis)
Gastric scintiscan in gastroesophageal reflux diagnosis, 170–171
Gastric tube for esophageal replacement, 155–156
simultaneous esophagectomy without thoracotomy with, 158–159
Gastroenteritis, acute appendicitis differentiated from, 74
Gastroesophageal disorders, 139–194
Gastroesophageal reflux (GER), 169–174
achalasia of esophagus differentiated from, 163–164
diagnostic studies in, 170–172
discussion of, 169–170
medical management of, 172–174
surgery for, 173–174
Gastroschisis
management of, 276
parenteral nutrition in, 278–289 (*see also* Parenteral nutrition in gastroschisis)
postoperative problems in, 276–277
Gastrostomy in type A esophageal atresia, 149

Genitourinary symptoms, risk of pelvic inflammatory disease and, 94
Gonadal appendices, torsion of, 64

H

Heart injury from thoracic trauma, 246
Heller esophagomyotomy, modified, for achalasia of esophagus, 166
Hemangioma, subglottic, airway obstruction from, 291
Hemophilia A and B, 296–297
Hepatic portoenterostomy for biliary atresia, 200–204
Hepatobiliary disorders, 197–220
Hernia
  inguinal, 3–35 (*see also* Inguinal hernia)
  umbilical, 36–48 (*see also* Umbilical hernia)
Hirschsprung's disease with superimposed enterocolitis, 119–126
  colostomy for, 121–122
    closure of, 125
  conditions associated with, 125
  definitive operation for, 122–124
  diagnosis of, 121
  postoperative complications in, 125–126
  results in, 126
Hydrometrocolpos, 104–107
Hygroma, cystic, 260–263
Hyperglycemia complicating parenteral nutrition, 285
Hypertension, portal, complicating surgery for biliary atresia, 203
Hypertrophic pyloric stenosis (HPS), 184–188
  diagnosis of, 184–185
  postoperative course in, 187–188
  preparation for surgery on, 185–186
  surgical correction of, 186–187
Hypocalcemia complicating parenteral nutrition, 285
Hypoglycemia complicating parenteral nutrition, 285

I

Ileus, prolonged, in gastroschisis, 277
Immunosuppressed patient, abdominal pain in, 108–111 (*see also* Typhlitis in immunosuppressed patient)
Incarcerated hernia in infant, 9–15
  clinical presentation of, 10–13
  complications of, 14–15
  embryology of, 9–10
  management of, 13–14
  reduction of, 13
Incarceration of bowel complicating inguinal hernia in premature neonate, 3–4
Infant(s), incarcerated hernia in, 9–15 (*see also* Incarcerated hernia in infant)
Infarction, testicular, complicating incarcerated hernia, 14
Infection(s)
  complicating long-term central vascular access, 273, 274–275
  upper respiratory, acute appendicitis differentiated from, 74
  urinary tract, acute appendicitis differentiated from, 74
Inflammatory bowel disease, 113–118 (*see also* Crohn's disease)
Inguinal hernia, 3–35
  incarcerated
    in infant, 9–15 (*see also* Incarcerated hernia in infant)
    testicular torsion differentiated from, 65
  in premature neonate, 3–8
    complications of, 3–4
    emergency surgery for, 5
      anesthesia for, 7–8
      care during, 5–7
      complications of, 4, 6
      postoperative care for, 7
    reduction of, 4
  recurrent, 29–35
    after repair in infant, 15
    prevention of, 30
    technique of preperitoneal repair of, 31–35
    treatment of, 30–31
  ventriculoperitoneal shunt patient, 17–27
  in ventriculoperitoneal shunt patient
    incidence of, 21–23
    intra-abdominal pressure increase and, 24–25
    precipitating factors for, 23–25

Inguinal hernia *(cont.)*
processus vaginalis patency rate and, 23–24
repair of
clinical experience with, 19–23
complications of, 25–26
discussion of, 23–26
postoperative complications from, 20–21
recommendations for, 26–27
shunt infection prevention in, 25–26
Intersex, bilaterally impalpable testes with, 58
Intravaginal testicular torsion, 62–63
Intussusception, 77–83
clinical presentation of, 77
complications of, 80
diagnosis of, 79–81
idiopathic, 77–78
physical examination in, 78–79
treatment of, 79–83

J

Jaundice
cholestatic, complicating parenteral nutrition, 286, 287
in preoperative evaluation of choledochal cyst patient, 207
Jejunum for esophageal replacement, 156
operative procedure for, 159–160
Jugular venous route of vascular access, 268–269

L

Ladd procedure for malrotation with midgut volvulus, 88–89
Laparotomy in surgery for choledochal cyst, 208
Liver, blunt trauma to, treatment of, 240
Lung(s), contusion of, from thoracic trauma, 245–246
Lymphadenopathy, cervical, management of, 264–266

M

Malrotation
classification of, 85–86
embryology of, 85
with midgut volvulus, 84–90
clinical presentation of, 86–88
diagnosis of, 86–88
outcome of, 90
treatment of, 88–90
Mandible, enlarged, in cystic hygroma, 262–263
Manometry, esophageal, in diagnosis of achalasia of esophagus, 163
Mayer-Rokitansky syndrome, 106–107
Meckel's diverticulum, 127–131
description of, 127–128
diagnosis of, 128–129
prophylactic diverticulectomy for, 130–131
treatment of, 129–130
Medication in gastroesophageal reflux management, 173
Menstruation, risk of pelvic inflammatory disease and, 94
Metoclopramide in gastroesophageal reflux management, 173
Midgut volvulus, malrotation with, 84–90

N

Nasogastric suction in resuscitation of injured child, 235
Neck, congenital cysts and sinuses of, 257–259
Neck-vein route of vascular access, 268–269
Necrotizing enterocolitis, 132–138
clinical presentation of, 134
diagnosis of, 134–135
low-birth-weight and, 132–134
treatment of, 135–138
Neonate, premature, inguinal hernia in, 3–8
Neurologic syndromes, Hirschsprung's disease and, 125
Night-time stooling after surgery for Hirschsprung's disease, 125–126
Nissen fundoplication for gastroesophageal reflux, 173–174
Nutrition, parenteral, 276–289 (*see also* Parenteral nutrition)

O

Orchiopexy
for bilateral undescended testes, Fowler-Stephens technique of, 56
late, in prune-belly syndrome, 57–58
for unilateral cryptorchid testicle, 52–54
Osmotic diuresis complicating parenteral nutrition, 286, 288
Ovary, torsion of, 100–103

P

Pain, abdominal, in immunosuppressed patient, 108–111 (*see also* Typhlitis in immunosuppressed patient)
Pancreas, trauma to, 249–254
blunt, treatment of, 240–241
clinical features of, 250
diagnosis of, 251–252
high-energy, 249–250
low-energy, 249
pathology of, 250–251
pathophysiology of, 250–251
prognosis for, 253–254
treatment of, 252–253
Pancreatic pseudocysts, 222–228
diagnosis of, 223–225
treatment of, 225–227
Pancreatitis in preoperative evaluation of choledochal cyst patient, 207
Parenteral nutrition, 276–289
in gastroschisis
approaches to, 278
central, 280–282
complications of, 283–289
cholestatic jaundice as, 286, 287
fatty acid deficiency as, 285–286
hyperglycemia as, 285
hypocalcemia as, 285
hypoglycemia as, 285
osmotic diuresis as, 286, 288
respiratory failure as, 288–289
zinc deficiency as, 285
metabolic observations during, 282–283
peripheral, 278–280
total, for pancreatic and duodenal trauma, 252–253
Pelvic inflammatory disease (PID), 92–99
diagnosis of, criteria for, 93
laboratory assessment of, 95
management of, 96–98
past history of, risk of pelvic inflammatory disease and, 94–95
risk factors for, 93–95
surgical assessment of, 95–96
treatment of, 96–98
ultrasonographic diagnosis of, 96
Pelvis, blunt trauma to, treatment of, 241–242
Peptic ulcer, acute, 190–194
medical treatment of, 191
surgical management of, 191–193
types of, 190–191
Periodic breathing after hernia in premature neonate, 7
Pneumatic dilatation for achalasia of esophagus, 165–166
Pneumothorax from thoracic trauma, 245
Portal hypertension complicating surgery for biliary atresia, 203
Portoenterostomy, hepatic, for biliary atresia, 200–204
Positioning in gastroesophageal reflux management, 172
Premature neonate, inguinal hernia in, 3–8
Prune-belly syndrome, bilateral undescended testes in, 55–58
Pseudocysts, pancreatic, 222–228
Pulmonary interstitial edema (PIE), airway obstruction from, 291
Pyloric stenosis, hypertrophic, 184–188 (*see also* Hypertrophic pyloric stenosis (HPS))
Pyloromyotomy for hypertrophic pyloric stenosis, 186–187
postoperative course after, 187–188

R

Ranitidine in gastroesophageal reflux management, 173
Rectum, blunt trauma to, treatment of, 241

Reflux, gastroesophageal, 169–174 (*see also* Gastroesophageal reflux (GER))
Respiratory complications of emergency surgery for inguinal hernia in premature neonate, 6
Respiratory distress syndrome complicating hernia in premature neonate, 6
Respiratory failure complicating parenteral nutrition, 288–289
Respiratory tract, upper, infection of, acute appendicitis differentiated from, 74
Resuscitation of injured child, 231–235
  treatment sequence for, 231–235
Rib fracture from thoracic trauma, 245
Roentgenographic studies in Crohn's disease, 115

S

Scintiscan, gastric, in gastroesophageal reflux diagnosis, 170–171
Scleroderma, achalasia of esophagus differentiated from, 164–165
Scrotal edema, idiopathic, testicular torsion differentiated from, 65
Septicemia complicating long-term central vascular access, 275
Sexual activity, risk of pelvic inflammatory disease and, 94
Sexually transmitted disease (STD), past history of, risk of pelvic inflammatory disease and, 94–95
Shunts, ventriculoperitoneal, inguinal hernia repair with, 17–27 (*see also* Inguinal hernia in ventriculoperitoneal shunt patient)
Sickle cell anemia, cholelithiasis and, 215–220
Sinuses, congenital, of neck, 257–259
Spasm, esophageal, diffuse, achalasia of esophagus differentiated from, 165
Spine, cervical
  examination of, in resuscitation of injured child, 234
  stabilization of, in resuscitation of injured child, 233
Spleen, blunt trauma to, treatment of, 240
Splinting of fractures in resuscitation of injured child, 235
Stent, esophageal, intraluminal, for caustic esophageal stricture, 176–179
  discussion of, 181–183
  results of, 180–181
Stomach for esophageal replacement, 156
  transposition procedures with, 159
Stricture of esophagus, caustic, 175–183 (*see also* Caustic stricture of esophagus)
Subclavian route of vascular access, 268
  technique for, 269–270
Subglottic edema/stenosis, airway obstruction from, 292
Subglottic hemangioma, airway obstruction from, 291
Supravaginal testicular torsion, 61–62

T

^{99m}Tc-pertechnetate scan in Meckel's diverticulum diagnosis, 129
Technetium-99m iminodiacetic acid (IDA) in biliary atresia diagnosis, 197–198
Testicle(s)
  cryptorchid, 51–58 (*see also* Cryptorchidism)
  infarction of, complicating incarcerated hernia, 14
  torsion of, 60–67 (*see also* Torsion of testicles)
Testis(es), undescended, 51–58 (*see also* Cryptorchidism)
"Third spacing" in gastroschisis, 277
Thorax, trauma to, 244–248
  aortic injury from, 246
  cardiac injury from, 246
  initial management of, 246
  pneumothorax from, 245
  pulmonary contusion from, 245–246
  rib fracture from, 245
  traumatic asphyxia from, 246
  treatment of, 246–248

Thrombus formation complicating long-term central vascular access, 274
Thyroglossal-duct cyst, 259
Torsion
of gonadal appendices, 64
of ovary, 100–103
of testicles, 60–67
diagnosis of, 65–66
differential diagnosis of, 64–65
intravaginal, 62–63
supravaginal, 61–62
treatment of, 66–67
types of, 61
Total parenteral nutrition (TPN) for pancreatic and duodenal trauma diagnosis, 252–253
Tracheoesophageal fistula, esophageal atresia with, 141–147 (*see also* Esophageal atresia (EA) with tracheoesophageal fistula)
Tracheomalacia, airway obstruction from, 291
Tracheostomy in airway management, 293–294
Trauma, 229–254
abdominal, blunt, 236–243
duodenal, 249–254 (*see also* Duodenum, trauma to)
pancreatic, 249–254 (*see also* Pancreas, trauma to)
resuscitation following, 231–235
thoracic, 244–248
Traumatic asphyxia from thoracic trauma, 246
Typhlitis in immunosuppressed patient, 108–111
case report on, 108–109
clinical presentation of, 110
imaging of, 110
outcome of, 111
pathogenesis of, 109
pathology of, 109–110
treatment of, 110–111

U

Ulcer, peptic, acute, 190–194 (*see* Peptic ulcer, acute)
Ulcerative colitis, chronic, 113, 114, 115
Ultrasonography
abdominal, in acute appendicitis diagnosis, 73
in hydrometrocolpos, 104, 105
in pancreatic and duodenal trauma diagnosis, 251
in pelvic inflammatory disease diagnosis, 96
in typhlitis, 110
Umbilical hernia, 336–48
anatomy of, 37–38
clinical manifestations of, 40–41
complications of, 43, 48
embryology of, 36–37
incidence of, 38–40
natural history of, 40
operative technique for, 42–43, 44–48
treatment of, 41–42
Undescended testis, 51–58 (*see also* Cryptorchidism)
Urinalysis in acute appendicitis diagnosis, 73
Urinary tract infection, acute appendicitis differentiated from, 74

V

Vaginal anomalies, hydrometrocolpos and, 105–107
Varicocele, testicular torsion differentiated from, 65
Vascular access, 267–275
external catheter vs. total implantation of access device for, 272–273
jugular venous insertion technique for, 269
long-term, complications of, 273–275
neck-vein route of, 268–269
preoperative evaluation for, 268
sites of, 268–269
subclavian route of, 268
technique for, 269–270
surgical technique for, 270–272
technique of, 269
Vascular ring malformations, airway obstruction from, 291
Ventriculoperitoneal shunts, inguinal hernia repair with, 17–27
Volvulus, midgut, malrotation with, 84–90

von Willebrand's disease, bleeding disorders in, 296, 297, 299–300

W

Waardenburg's syndrome, Hirschsprung's disease and, 125

White blood cell (WBC) count in acute appendicitis diagnosis, 73

Z

Zinc deficiency complicating parenteral nutrition, 285